Blockchain Technology in Healthcare Applications

T0332910

Advances in Smart Healthcare Technologies

Series Editors
Chinmay Chakraborty and Joel J. P. C. Rodrigues

Blockchain Technology in Healthcare Applications: Social, Economic, and Technological Implications
Bharat Bhushan, Nitin Rakesh, Yousef Farhaoui,
Parma Nand Astya and Bhuvan Unhelkar

Digital Health Transformation with Blockchain and Artificial Intelligence
Chinmay Chakraborty

Blockchain Technology in Healthcare Applications

Social, Economic, and Technological Implications

Edited by
Bharat Bhushan
Nitin Rakesh
Yousef Farhaoui
Parma Nand Astya
Bhuvan Unhelkar

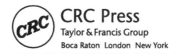

CRC Press
Taylor & Francis Group
Boca Raton London New York

CRC Press is an imprint of the
Taylor & Francis Group, an **informa** business

First edition published 2022
by CRC Press
6000 Broken Sound Parkway NW, Suite 300, Boca Raton, FL 33487-2742

and by CRC Press
2 Park Square, Milton Park, Abingdon, Oxon, OX14 4RN

ISBN: 9781032123196 (hbk)
ISBN: 9781032123226 (pbk)
ISBN: 9781003224075 (ebk)

DOI: 10.1201/9781003224075

Typeset in Times
by codeMantra

Contents

Preface

Nowadays, healthcare organizations are transforming themselves into more user-centered, coordinated and efficient systems employing various multimedia techniques. However, data management within such systems demands huge human efforts and faces the threat of security breaches. Integration of Internet of Things (IoT) and healthcare mitigates such threats, reduces overall cost and improves the standard of patient care. However, these IoT devices are susceptible to a huge range of attacks. As healthcare data contains sensitive and personal information, it might be of interest to various cybercriminals. Blockchain is regarded as the most disruptive and revolutionary technology, which will provide protection and secrecy of control systems in real-time environment. Blockchain technology is capable of tracking, organizing and bearing out communications by storing the data received from numerous devices and forming parties without the need of a federal cloud. Furthermore, blockchain facilitates patient data accessibility and captures patient record and intermediate activity information. However, research in the field of blockchain is still in a nascent stage. This is evident from the fact that there exist numerous open challenges that restrict the widespread adoption of blockchain in healthcare applications. This book focuses on techniques, experiences and lessons learned with respect to state-of-the-art security, privacy, interoperability solutions for DLT, secure multimedia processing and blockchain technology. The core of the book is focused on explaining how such technologies are disruptive, and, further, it explores the concrete consequences of these disruptions in terms of technological, economic and social consequences. This book provides theoretical concepts, empirical studies and a detailed overview of various aspects related to the development of healthcare applications from a reliable, trusted and secure data transmission perspective. Further, it also intends to induce further research about the ethical impact of the new "distributed trust" paradigm resulting from the surge of such a disruptive technology.

Editors

Dr. Bharat Bhushan is an Assistant Professor in the Department of Computer Science and Engineering (CSE) at School of Engineering and Technology, Sharda University, Greater Noida, India. He received his undergraduate degree (BTech in Computer Science and Engineering) with distinction in 2012, postgraduate degree (MTech in Information Security) with distinction in 2015 and doctorate degree (PhD Computer Science and Engineering) in 2021 from Birla Institute of Technology, Mesra, India. He earned numerous international certifications such as CCNA, MCTS, MCITP, RHCE and CCNP. He has published more than 80 research papers in various renowned international conferences and SCI indexed journals. He has contributed to more than 40 book chapters in various books and has edited 11 books from the most famed publishers such as Elsevier, IGI Global and CRC Press. He has served as Keynote Speaker (resource person) in numerous reputed international conferences held in different countries including India, Morocco, China, Belgium, Iraq and Bangladesh. In the past, he worked as an Assistant Professor at HMR Institute of Technology and Management, New Delhi and Network Engineer in HCL Infosystems Ltd., Noida. He is also a member of numerous renowned bodies including IEEE, IAENG, CSTA, SCIEI, IAE and UACEE.

Prof. (Dr.) Nitin Rakesh is Head of Computer Science & Engineering Department for BTech/MTech (CSE/IT), BTech CSE-IBM Specializations, BTech CSE-I Nurture, BCA/MCA and BSc/MSc-CS at School of Engineering and Technology, Sharda University, India. He received his PhD degree in Computer Science & Engineering with Network Coding as his specialization. He received Master of Technology degree in Computer Science & Engineering and Bachelor of Technology degree in Information Technology. He is having 100+ research publications in reputed SCI or Scopus indexed Journals and International Conferences. Currently, he is guiding eight PhD students from various Universities and Industries. His research outlines emphasis on Network Coding, Interconnection Networks & Architecture and Online Phantom Transactions. Dr. Nitin has been accorded several other awards for Best Paper Published, Session Chairs, Highest Cited author, Best Students Thesis Guided and many others. He is a recipient of IBM Drona Award and Top 10 State Award Winner. He is an active member of professional societies like IEEE (USA), ACM, SIAM (USA), Life Member of CSI and other professional societies.

Prof. (Dr.) Yousef Farhaoui is Professor at Moulay Ismail University, Faculty of Sciences and Techniques, Morocco and Local Publishing and Research Coordinator, Cambridge International Academics in United Kingdom. He obtained his PhD degree in Computer Security from Ibn Zohr University of Science.

His research interests include learning, e-learning, computer security, big data analytics and business intelligence. Farhaoui has published three books in computer science. He is a Coordinator and Member of the organizing committee, a Member of the scientific committee of several international congresses and also a Member of various international associations. He has authored four books and many book chapters with reputed publishers such as Springer and IGI. He is served as a Reviewer for IEEE, IET, Springer, Inderscience and Elsevier journals. He is also the Guest Editor of many journals with Wiley, Springer, Inderscience, etc. He has been the General Chair, Session Chair and Panellist in Several Conferences. He is Senior Member of IEEE, IET, ACM and EAI Research Group.

Parma Nand Astya is Dean at School of Engineering Technology, Sharda University Greater Noida. He has more than 26 years of experience in teaching, industry and research. He has expertise in Wireless and Sensor Network, Cryptography, Algorithm and Computer Graphics. He has earned his PhD from IIT Roorkee, MTech and BTech in Computer Science & Engineering from IIT Delhi. He has been Ex-President of National Engineers Organization. He is senior member of IEEE (USA). He is a Member of Executive Council of IEEE UP section (R10), Executive Committee IEEE Computer and Signal Processing Society, Executive of India Council Computer Society and Executive Council Computer Society of India, Noida section and has acted as an observer in many IEEE conferences. He has delivered many invited/keynotes talks at International & National Conferences/Workshops/Seminars in India and abroad. He has published more than 85 papers in peer-reviewed international/national journals and conferences. He is also having active memberships of ACM, CSI, ACEEE, ISOC, IAENG and IASCIT. He is a lifetime member of Soft Computing Research Society (SCRS) and ISTE.

Prof. (Dr.) Bhuvan Unhelkar (BE, MDBA, MSc, PhD; FACS; PSM-I, CBAP®) is an accomplished IT Professional and Professor of IT at the University of South Florida, Sarasota-Manatee (Lead Faculty). He is also Founding Consultant at Method Science and a Co-Founder/Director at PlatiFi. He has mastery in Business Analysis & Requirements Modelling, Software Engineering, Big Data Strategies, Agile Processes, Mobile Business and Green IT. His domain experience is banking, financial, insurance, government and telecommunications. Bhuvan is a Thought-Leader and a Prolific Author of 25. He is the winner of the Computerworld Object Developer Award (1995), Consensus IT Professional Award (2006) and IT Writer Award (2010). He has a Doctorate in the area of "Object Orientation" from the University of Technology, Sydney, in 1997. Bhuvan is Fellow of the Australian Computer Society, IEEE Senior Member, Professional Scrum Master, Life member of Computer Society of India and Baroda Management Association, Member of SDPS, Past President of Rotary Sarasota Sunrise (Florida) & St. Ives (Sydney), Paul Harris Fellow (+6), Discovery Volunteer at NSW parks and wildlife and a previous TiE Mentor. He also chaired the Business Analysis Specialism Group of the Australian Computer Society.

Contributors

Faris. A. Almalki
Department of Computer Engineering,
  College of Computers and
  Information Technology
Taif University
Taif, Saudi Arabia

R. Anuradha
School of Business and Management
CHRIST (Deemed to be University)
Bangalore, India

W. Basmi
Computer Sc. Dept.
FSTM, Hassan II University of
  Casablanca
Casablanca, Morocco

Abhishek Bhardwaj
School of Engineering and
  Technology (SET)
Sharda University
Greater Noida, India

Trisha Bhowmik
School of Engineering and
  Technology (SET)
Sharda University
Greater Noida, India

Bharat Bhushan
School of Engineering and
  Technology
Sharda University
Greater Noida, India

A. Boulmakoul
Computer Sc. Dept.
FSTM, Hassan II University of
  Casablanca
Casablanca, Morocco

Aarthy Chellasamy
School of Business and Management
CHRIST (Deemed to be University)
Bangalore, India

Prince Chitopho
Department of Electronics and
  Telecommunications Engineering,
  Faculty of Computer Engineering,
  Informatics and Communications
University of Zimbabwe
Harare, Zimbabwe

Chamitha de Alwis
Department of Electrical and
  Electronic Engineering
University of Sri Jayewardenepura
Nugegoda, Sri Lanka

K.A. Fasila
Department of Computer Science and
  Engineering
Muthoot Institute of Technology and
  Science
India

Raghav Gupta
School of Computing and Information
  Technology
Manipal University Jaipur
Jaipur, India

A.K.M. Bahalul Haque
Department of Software Engineering
LENS, LUT University
Lappeenranta, Finland

Md. Rifat Hasan
Department of Electrical and
    Computer Engineering
North South University
Dhaka, Bangladesh

Tabassum Jahan
School of Engineering and
    Technology (SET)
Sharda University
Greater Noida, India

Garima Jain
Computer Science and
    Engineering
Noida Institute of Engineering and
    Technology
Greater Noida, India

Ankush Jain
Bennett University
Greater Noida, India

Biswabandhu Jana
Advanced Technology Development
    Centre
IIT Kharagpur
Kharagpur, India

Anshuman Kalla
Centre for Wireless Communications
University of Oulu
Oulu, Finland

L. Karim
LISA Lab. ENSA Berrechid
Hassan 1st University
Casablanca, Morocco

Snigdha Kashyap
School of Engineering and
    Technology (SET)
Sharda University
Greater Noida, India

Ila Kaushik
Department of Information
    Technology
Krishna Institute of Engineering &
    Technology
Ghaziabad, India

Jacek Klich
Cracow University of Economics
Kraków, Poland

Avinash Kumar
School of Engineering and
    Technology (SET)
Sharda University
Greater Noida, India

Chaitanya Kumar Dixit
Department of Botany, School of Life
    Sciences
Dr. Bhimrao Ambedkar
    University
Agra, India

P.R. Mahalingam
Department of Computer Science and
    Engineering
Muthoot Institute of Technology and
    Science
India

Ayasha Malik
Department of Information
    Technology
Noida Institute of Engineering
    Technology (NIET)
Greater Noida, India

Halima Mhamdi
MACS Research Laboratory, National
    Engineering School of Gabes
University of Gabes
Gabes, Tunisia

Tawanda Mushiri
Department of Industrial and
    Mechatronics Engineering,
    Faculty of Engineering & the Built
    Environment
University of Zimbabwe
Harare, Zimbabwe

Surekha Nayak
School of Business and Management
CHRIST (Deemed to be University)
Bangalore, India

Ahmed J. Obaid
Faculty of Computer Science and
    Mathematics
Kufa University
Kufa, Iraq

Kavitha Rajamohan
School of Sciences
CHRIST (Deemed to be University)
Bangalore, India

Sangeetha Rangasamy
School of Business and Management
CHRIST (Deemed to be University)
Bangalore, India

Hedi Sakli
MACS Research Laboratory, National
    Engineering School of Gabes
Gabes University
Gabes, 6029, Tunisia
EITA Consulting 5 Rue du Chant des
    Oiseaux
Montesson, France

Muzafer Saracevic
Department of Computer Sciences
University of Novi Pazar
Novi Pazar, Serbia

Nikhil Sharma
Department of Computer Science &
    Engineering
Delhi Technological University
Delhi, India

Adarsh Singh
School of Computing and Information
    Technology
Manipal University Jaipur
Jaipur, India

Ananya Smirti
School of Computing and Information
    Technology
Manipal University Jaipur
Jaipur, India

Ben Othman Soufiene
PRINCE Laboratory Research,
    ISITcom, Hammam Sousse
University of Sousse
Tunisia

Jaya Srivastava
Department of Information
    Technology
Noida Institute of Engineering
    Technology (NIET)
Greater Noida, India

Shadreck N. Tasiyana
Department of Industrial and
    Mechatronics Engineering,
    Faculty of Engineering & the Built
    Environment
University of Zimbabwe
Harare, Zimbabwe

Tanmayee Prakash Tilekar
Digital Forensics Analyst
ISAC India
Noida, India

Vishakha
Tata Consultancy Services
Gurugram, India

Neha Yadav
Department of Information
   Technology
Babasaheb Bhimrao Ambedkar
   University (A Central University)
Lucknow, India

Abid Yahya
Botswana International University of
   Science & Technology

Palapye, BotswanaMd.
Oahiduzzaman Mondol Zihad
Department of Electrical and
   Computer Engineering
North South University
Dhaka, Bangladesh

Ahmed Zouinkhi
MACS Research Laboratory, National
   Engineering School of Gabes
University of Gabes
Gabes, 6029, Tunisia

1 Blockchain for Securing Internet of Things – A Layered Approach

AKM Bahalul Haque
LUT University

Md. Oahiduzzaman Mondol Zihad and Md. Rifat Hasan
North South University

CONTENTS

DOI: 10.1201/9781003224075-1

1.1 INTRODUCTION

The introduction of the Internet of Things (IoT) in communication and data processing changes the application of technologies worldwide [1]. More people are now indulged in the internet, while IoT uses the medium to interact directly or indirectly with the user. The things can interact with each other, and by things, we mean billions of unique devices. It is estimated that by 2025 IoT devices will cross 21 billion [2]. They are more like watching, speaking, and listening to us. These things work under a small domain, but a ubiquitous implementation can execute numerous applications. Transforming these traditional purpose devices into smart devices, IoT provides the ground for vast computation, big data processing, and real-life services. Applications such as smart homes, smart transportation, smart power system, industrial ecosystems, and many more can come to practice with the power of IoT [3,4]. Generally, IoT devices use different types of networks like cloud, edge, fog computing, and their IP address [5,6]. Moreover, for the massive heterogeneity of the connected devices, they use different types of data processing mechanisms. So, major issues regarding security, privacy, data management, data transmission, etc. have been raised. Furthermore, using these security gaps, intruders can get the advantage and alter information creating a hazard in the whole system. A lot of work has been conducted by the researchers to find solutions for such instances. Blockchain is the latest and one of the most fruitful generalized additions to these solutions [7,8].

The blockchain concept is relatively old, but its recent practical implementation in cryptocurrency has created an immense opportunity for data management and communication. The drawbacks of IoT networks are mainly due to the centralized processing mechanism and lack of homogenous computation characteristics among the devices [9]. It increases the cost and reduces trust compromising the security of data. Blockchain, on the other hand, introduces a decentralized system that can ensure security in a trustless environment. Moreover, it can provide efficient authentication and access control policy against security threats [10]. The user's anonymity, the robust consensus protocol for data validation, and the use of public-key cryptography mechanism in transaction procedure initiate a strong urge to research on blockchain to resolve the IoT security issues [11].

Considering the facts mentioned above, IoT security issues need to be solved with utmost importance. Since data security is a great concern and blockchain is known for providing data integrity, security, and transparency, it can be a potential leveraging technology. For this reason, there needs to be a study that addresses the security issues of IoT and explores the potential feasibility of blockchain for addressing those issues.

This chapter explains the crucial security issues of the IoT ecosystem and their solution with the blockchain integrated system. The domain can be extended to the IoT perspective for the vast application of blockchain technology. The outline of the contributions of this work can be briefed as follows:

- The concept of blockchain and its evolution are concisely discussed.
- Blockchain architecture is explained along with the latest classification.

- Blockchain characteristics are evaluated that make it efficient for IoT infrastructure.
- System design for blockchain transactions is discussed in easy steps.
- Five-layered architecture for IoT has been speculated for its relevance in Industrial Internet of Things (IIoT).
- Major components that build the IoT system are described briefly.
- Crucial shortcomings in security and cyberattacks at each layer are analyzed in detail.
- State-of-the-art solutions for IoT security issues using blockchain are discussed.
- A step ahead to point the challenges that blockchain will face to secure an IoT environment for future research directions is discussed.

The rest of the chapter is structured as follows. Section 1.2 provides an overview of blockchain principles elaborating structure, characteristics, and transaction process. Section 1.3 details the IoT fundamentals explaining layered architecture and components. Section 1.4 shows significant security issues and attacks at each of the layers. Section 1.5 illustrates recent blockchain-based solutions to mitigate certain security cases. Finally, Section 1.6 highlights the challenges for blockchain to comply with IoT security inspiring future research, followed by a conclusion in Section 1.7.

1.2 BLOCKCHAIN PRINCIPLES

Blockchain was first popularized with the application in Bitcoin proposed by Satoshi Nakamoto in 2008 [12]. Blockchain comes with the idea of a decentralized ledger introducing more secured transactions. Blockchain, used in the transaction of digital currencies from 2009 to 2013, was known as blockchain 1.0 [13]. Later, the utilization of Smart Contracts introduced blockchain 2.0 in 2015 providing better authentication and tamperproof transaction process [14]. Ethereum platform comes with the idea of DApps and introduces blockchain 3.0 [15]. Today, we live in the era of blockchain 4.0 that brings forward its application in business and industries [16].

1.2.1 OVERVIEW

Blockchain can be discussed by dividing into three main sections: block, chain, and network.

- **Block**: Block holds the data in an encrypted form for the transaction. It uses information like nonce, Merkle root hash, timestamp, and previous and current hash information to encrypt the data. These blocks are immutable and divided into two parts – "head" and "body" [17]. The type of the blockchain determines its functions and characteristics like size and execution procedure.

- **Chain**: Blockchain is like a linked list where blocks are chained together.
- **Network**: Blockchain is built on the concept of the decentralized network. It ensures that no single actor or entity can control the transaction or verification of blocks. It establishes a P2P network, but the blocks containing information are processed and stored by peers called miners [18].

Generally, blockchain can be of two types: Public and Private. In Public blockchain, users can join in a permissionless ledger, i.e., they have the options of both reading and writing [19]. The participants can make their identity anonymous, but security is ensured by the valid block mining and public-key cryptosystem. Although the blocks are tamperproof, the execution and transaction are slower than private blockchain [20]. On the other hand, private blockchain restricts participants and allows only selected miners to read or write. The concept of decentralization is a little compromised here, but the efficiency is very high ensuring all other characteristics of blockchain [21]. There is another type of blockchain named Consortium or Hybrid blockchain. It comprises both the conditions of public and private blockchains following the desired outcome.

1.2.2 CHARACTERISTICS

In addition to its use in cryptocurrency, blockchain has a versatile application for its characteristics like:

- **Decentralization**: Blockchain ensures that no single entity or third-party organization can control the network. Miners need to mine blocks following consensus algorithm ensuring the authenticated transaction [22].
- **Immutability**: Once the block is added to the network, no one can change the information inside it or delete it [23].
- **Anonymity**: Even if all the miners will have a copy of each block, the data cannot be extracted except the one with the key [24]. Moreover, the individual information participating in a transaction will also be unknown to all as they will use a generated address for each time.
- **Auditability**: Using the hash function, each block will have the previous block's information [25]. So, transparency and audibility will be maintained.
- **Security and Privacy**: The most important characteristic of blockchain is that it offers a great deal of security and privacy. The use of public-key cryptosystem, consensus protocol, digital signature, peer-to-peer networks, and the latest addition like Ethereum strengthens blockchain even more from malicious activity and cyberattacks [26].

1.2.3 TRANSACTION PROCESS

1. **Requesting Transaction**: A user encrypts the data using a private key generating a unique hash value along with a digital signature and requests to add it to the peer-to-peer network [27].

2. **Authenticating Transaction**: The transaction is authenticated using public-key cryptography and the network validates the request.
3. **Block Validation**: Using the authentic hash value, nonce, timestamp, etc., the block is validated by the miners and considered for appending to the network.
4. **Addition to Blockchain**: Finally, the block is assembled into the blockchain network, complying with the consensus protocols like PoW or PoS. The block is non-removable and non-changeable henceforth [28].

1.3 IOT FUNDAMENTALS

IoT is spreading its domain of linked sensors and devices continuously, making the system more complex than ever before. So, to efficiently execute the benefits of IoT, a different architecture of IoT is proposed [29]. Keeping the growing industrial use and application of blockchain and IoT in mind, we will discuss the five-layered approach that is gaining popularity day by day. The five-layered architecture includes

1. Objects Layer
2. Network Layer
3. Service Management Layer
4. Application Layer and
5. Business Layer

1.3.1 OBJECTS LAYER

The Objects or Perception layer works as a data gathering and processing layer. It uses IoT sensors and devices to collect information like humidity, location, temperature, vibration, and weight [30]. Later, it is transmitted to the Network layer to create the communication process. This layer uses secure channels and transmits big data.

1.3.2 NETWORK LAYER

The Network layer or Object Abstraction layer serves to transfer the gathered information from the Objects Layer to Service Management Layer. It utilizes technologies like GSM, RFID, Wi-Fi, WiMAX, 3G, 4G, Satellite, Bluetooth, and infrared to transfer the data [31]. Moreover, tasks like data management and cloud computing are maintained by this layer [32].

1.3.3 SERVICE MANAGEMENT LAYER

The Service Management or Middleware layer's purpose is to connect services among different types of IoT devices. The devices create a request with their address and names and the Middleware layer manages the service request and stores information from a lower layer. This layer also participates in decision-making and delivers the computational results to devices [33].

1.3.4 APPLICATION LAYER

The Application layer connects with the user directly. It delivers generated or collected information like temperature or humidity from the previous layers to the end-customer [34]. Some examples of this layer are smart home, smart transportation, smart governance, and smart identification.

1.3.5 BUSINESS LAYER

The Business or Management layer represents the aggregated performance or analysis of the system. It can generate graphs, flowcharts, or models based on received and transmitted data. Hence, it provides a complete efficiency of the layers and devices that are used in the architecture. Furthermore, it can also improve the performance by comparing the expected and achieved output of each layer [35].

Other proposed architectures of IoT like the three-layered model or middleware model are also effective for some instances. Nevertheless, not all layers can utilize all types of technologies and data transfer processes. For example, SOA-based architecture has a Service Composition layer that takes much time in data execution and transfer [36]. On the other hand, this five-layered model can generate an analysis of the architecture and also tends to improve the performance. The Business layer can use a big load of data and perform complex computation on powerful devices. So, to meet the present need for big data and faster transmission, the five-layered model is one of the preferable architectures.

1.3.6 IoT COMPONENTS

Generally, an IoT system is structured with five major components [37]:

1. **Sensors**: IoT system uses many sensors to identify, collect, and transfer data. There are different types of sensors according to the diverse kind of data.
2. **Computation**: There are nodes containing processors to process information collected by sensors. These nodes are used to perform certain computations to further secure and transfer the received data.
3. **Receiver**: It works like a transceiver that transmits the messages from one node to another. It usually connects the local and remote nodes and collects their computed data.
4. **Activator**: It generates the signal for the requested service according to the received and computed data from the previous components. Functions of the IoT devices are activated to trigger the aimed device.
5. **Device**: After triggering the function, devices connected to the IoT system execute the desired function.

1.4 SECURITY ISSUES OF IOT

IoT systems, along with their different types of communicating devices, have several security issues. Researchers are trying to find solutions to the security risks and propose multiple architectures to address them. However, still, there is no single architecture that can be considered to function in every kind of situation. Five-layered architecture is proposed as a generalized solution to these security issues, but some are still unaddressed [38]. Here, we will discuss the security issues of the five-layered model of IoT in detail.

1.4.1 SECURITY ISSUES OF OBJECTS LAYER

The objects or perception layer faces issues mostly in its sensors and data collection process. Crucial security issues in this layer are as follows:

- **Node Hijack**: Node hijack or capture attack is a dangerous attack on the perception layer. It happens in the WSN (wireless sensor network) [39]. The intruder can replace a wireless sensor in the system taking place of another. So, the information that needed to be gathered or transferred goes to another source. It can even change the information creating an overall miscalculation. Moreover, taking over a node of the whole system, an intruder can leak the data, which makes the system's security more vulnerable. The attacker can also try to infer keys from the sender and receiver that can be used later to extract information and memory of their communication [40].
- **Eavesdropping**: In this attack, the intruder listens or sees the information exchanged between a sender and a receiver without any trace [41]. Attackers try to find information like pictures, messages, and voice calls. Although attackers cannot change any information transmitted in a network, they can gather and record secret data shared only with the selected participants.
- **Replay Attack**: One of the most common attacks is to play the "fake sender" role or playback attack. In this attack, the intruder enters the communication channel secretly. Then collects the sender's message. Rather than changing it, the attacker creates a new message just like the sender with lookalike authentication and identity [42]. It seems valid to the receiver but as soon as he enters the encrypted message from the attacker, all the information of the victim goes to the attacker [43].
- **Timing Attack**: All the sensors in an IoT system collect and process data with varying computation times. This computation time varies due to the size of data processed and the use of the cryptographic algorithm. Furthermore, intruders can observe the execution time of various sensors for specific requests or queries. An attacker can use this varying time of exchanged messages or signatures to exploit the cryptosystem [44].
- **Malicious and Fake Node**: An attacker can also add a sensor as a node in the system that only he can control. Using this fake node, an attacker

can inject malicious data or files into the system [45]. It works exactly like all other nodes but transfers the secret information of the sender and receiver to the attacker. It also has the power to destroy the whole system consuming a great deal of energy [46].

1.4.2 SECURITY ISSUES OF NETWORK LAYER

The layer that ties the perception layer to the application layer is the network layer. It refers to the communication channel among the devices or sensors or smart things. So, intruders like to attack especially this layer. Security issues that make it vulnerable are as follows:

- **Man in the Middle Attack**: In this attack, the intruder stays in the middle of the communication channel between two sides [47]. The attacker uses different types of fraudulent sensors or devices to remain unknown. He can alter the messages in real time, while the actual sender and receiver could not configure who are they communicating with [48].
- **Exploit Attack**: The attacker uses the security gap of software or hardware used in the IoT device to intercept malicious data or commands and extract essential data from the network. Again, the attacker can use the IP address of devices to get access and thrust contaminated data into the system [49].
- **Denial of Service (DoS) Attack**: This attack makes specific nodes or devices unavailable to service, creating a massive amount of traffic or messages that slow down the network and make the network unavailable or even crash the system [50].
- **Sybil Attack**: A device is used to replicate several devices with genuine addresses and infringe the information of the network. The replicated device (Sybil device) with a false identity can also bring other security threats like a DoS attack, phishing if the device is put forward with all the traffic in one route [51].
- **Sinkhole and Wormhole Attack**: This attack generates false traffic and routing data to other devices so that the packets generated by the WSN cannot reach the destination. Instead, they are dropped in fake routes. It can further increase combining two fraudulent devices connected with a private link that is only useful to the attacker. Other devices then use this link (wormhole tunnel) as their routing path and the attacker can extract information from it [52].

1.4.3 SECURITY ISSUES OF MIDDLEWARE LAYER

The middleware or processing layer filters the data to separate critical data needed for specific devices. It eradicates extra information that is unnecessary for certain operations. Some of the critical attacks on this layer are as follows:

- **Virus Attack**: The attacker uses contents, files, or executable code to enter the system [53]. This attack comprises viruses, Trojan horses, spyware, malware, adware, etc. to get information about the user.
- **Exhaustion**: Exhaustive attacks can hamper the devices and networks physically. It can happen due to other types of attacks. For example, a DoS attack can generate a lot of traffic and eventually make the device exhaust wasting memory, database resources, or power system [54].

1.4.4 SECURITY ISSUES OF APPLICATION LAYER

The application layer is the output tier of the whole structure from where users receive the final service. According to its service and implementation differences, different security issues arise. Some of the significant security issues of the application layer are as follows:

- **Data Hamper**: The attacker can send false information to the base station resulting in a miscalculation. Moreover, he can take advantage of gaps in service management among the IoT devices to leak data [55].
- **Phishing Attack**: The attacker can use phishing links or websites or email malicious files and require the user to click on them [56]. Private information of users like password, date of birth, and ID can be hacked easily and attackers can get access to the victim's credentials.
- **Malicious Scripts and Trojan Horse**: IoT applications are very prone to attacks like a virus or Trojan Horse. The intruder injects malware that can generate duplicates and gradually move to destroy the victim's environment. This malicious code attack is very hard to prevent with only anti-virus software. The malicious scripts can also change the fundamental commands of installed software in a device [57]. An attacker can extend this attack after a certain portion of the system is affected with HTML, script injection, and worms. It also creates the scope for other attacks like phishing, DoS, and buffer overflow.
- **Software and Firmware Uncertainty**: With the different applications of IoT devices, there come different types of software and different types of firmware to run them [58]. But for the lack of standardization and proper review, it becomes hard to create secure code. Moreover, failure to regular security updates to the devices increases vulnerability. The attacker can also hamper the synchronization process of IoT devices with other devices manipulating clock time. Eventually, it becomes easier for the intruder to exploit the backend code and change the code for pre-allocated memory [59].
- **XMPPilot Attack**: In order to eavesdrop on the communication channel between the sender and receiver, the attacker uses XMPPilot. He writes code to hamper XMPP connection and confines the encryption process at receiver side communication [60].

- **Credibility Issues**: Lack of authentication standards or authorized party to maintain security ease the attack for the intruders [61]. They can use the update file to inject their own manipulated script. Again, it is necessary to authenticate end-to-end encryption in communication.

1.4.5 SECURITY ISSUES OF BUSINESS LAYER

The business layer is the latest addition to the IoT structure that enables the system to be more productive and easier to use. Not many threats to this layer are still found but attackers can manipulate the previous layer attacks. Some possible security issues in this layer are as follows:

- **Zero-Day Attack**: A Zero-Day attack is an attack pointing to certain security weaknesses of a software or application that is discovered by the developer but not yet mitigated. It can occur the same day the developer found the weakness. Usually, this type of attack exploits security holes without the vendor having any kind of knowledge of it [62].
- **Logic Attack**: The business layer uses a lot of logic to compute the data and generate necessary graphs or decisions. Mistakes in the logic while programming initiates certain threats while computing these outcomes [63]. Again, shortcomings in the algorithm of password recovery or authentication, encryption, input validation, etc. can poise some security threats on the business layer too.

There are other approaches to discover the security gaps of IoT and classification for possible threats. But the five-layered architecture holds almost all the crucial attacks that are common in all the IoT ecosystems.

1.5 BLOCKCHAIN-BASED SOLUTION

Blockchain can offer improved solutions in different domains of IoT. IoT devices need to deal with a lot of private data. Permissioned blockchain can be an excellent solution to avoid exposing user data [64]. Direct communication eliminating the use of central authority can handle the increasing traffic of exponentially growing IoT devices. It can also decrease the load on a cloud server for storing data. Strengthening the infrastructure, blockchain can further contribute to the prevention of data manipulation and numerous cyberattacks.

Several approaches have been taken in the previous years to solve the issues of IoT. The researchers propose different architectures and system designs. Table 1.1 represents some recent works on blockchain solutions aiming to solve issues in security as well as IoT architecture and data management.

The above table henceforth shows that blockchain has a huge scope in improving IoT security issues. But more studies are needed to conduct on finding the efficiency and simplicity of blockchain applications.

TABLE 1.1

State-of-the-Art IoT Security Solutions with Blockchain

Attack Name	Effect	Blockchain Solutions	References
Eavesdropping	Transmitted data loses privacy	• Divides blockchain into two parts: off-blockchain and on-blockchain to process data in three steps each.	[65]
Timing attack	Subject to side-channel attack exposing the cryptosystem	• Combines blockchain with a domestic commercial cryptographic algorithm. • A probabilistic model is applied in blockchain framework for data collection.	[66,67]
Node Hijack	Hampers data collection or transfers to attacker	• Proposes a signature scheme of permissioned blockchain. • Introduces a blockchain-based framework in the unmanned aerial vehicles network.	[68,69]
Replay attack	Destroys private data security	• Blockchain-based logistics system with special monitoring sensors. • Two-way authentication in a blockchain scheme. • BSS (blockchain enabled security system) scheme with the batch system.	[70–72]
Malicious and fake node	Consumes energy	• RSA (Rivest–Shamir–Adleman) signature-based authentication in a blockchain network. • Manage identity authentication with lightweight blockchain. • Hyperledger Fabric private blockchain-based framework.	[73–75]
Sybil attack	Corrupts data acquisition	• SSDT (Blockchain-Based Sybil-Secure Data Transmission) framework based on blockchain. • Blockchain-based detection mechanism for UWSN	[76,77]
Black hole and gray hole attack	Network latency	• Coded blockchain-based energy-efficient mechanism • Efficient lightweight integrated blockchain (ELIB) model for public blockchain	[78,79]
Exploitation	Contaminates network/IP address	• Hybrid blockchain based on DPoA (Delegated Proof of Authority)	[80]
Man in the middle attack	Network security, key management	• Seed-based blockchain scheme for key generation and management • Blockchain-based architecture for CAV (connected and autonomous vehicles)	[81,82]

(Continued)

TABLE 1.1 (*Continued*)
State-of-the-Art IoT Security Solutions with Blockchain

Attack Name	Effect	Blockchain Solutions	References
DoS/DDoS	Network unavailability, system crash	• Hybrid blockchain for IIoT. • Private blockchain using Ethereum platform. • Blockchain framework using smart contract and LSTM (long short-term memory) for access control	[83–85]
Virus attack	Dara/System disruption	• Proposed consortium blockchain-based recovery service. • Detection mechanism using blockchain in distributed database.	[86,87]
Exhaustion	Decay memory/ resources	• Proposed a blockchain-based data edge verification system. • Lightweight blockchain for IIoT. • Hybrid model of public and local blockchain for authentication.	[88–90]
Phishing attack	Credentials' security	• Blockchain and Zero Trust-based framework.	[91]
Logic attack	Runtime error	• Hyperledger Fabric for verification and access control	[92]
Zero-day attack	Network security, zero knowledge	• Detection mechanism with deep blockchain framework. • Blockchain-based authentication mechanism	[93,94]
Sniffing attack	Unauthorized access	• Blockchain-based event log security mechanism. • GADV in blockchain encryption scheme.	[95,96]
Routing attack	Deteriorates network efficiency, DoS	• Blockchain-based framework using smart contract to identify tampered sensor nodes.	[97]

1.6   CHALLENGES AND FUTURE WORK

The main drawback of implementing blockchain in the IoT ecosystem is that there is no general methodology or system architecture to combine these systems as per demand. Blockchain has its issue with scalability in consensus protocol and big data handling. These concerns create some challenges that need more attention.

1.6.1   Heterogeneity of Devices

IoT ecosystem deals with low-level devices to high-end servers. They compute data in multiple layers each with its mechanism [98]. So, a general framework for security enabling the devices to adapt to the security requirement at each layer dynamically needs to be introduced.

1.6.2 HARDWARE AND FIRMWARE VULNERABILITIES

With the increased demand, IoT devices tend to be more low cost and low power-consuming. It makes the system user-friendly at the cost of low-quality hardware or firmware [99]. Aside from the physical disturbance, software-related problems like malware and routing problems may also occur. So, a standard system is required to monitor these issues.

1.6.3 SCALABILITY

IoT devices are used to work with big data collected by billions of devices. Blockchain takes a good amount of computation time when processing this data. Again, the IoT devices themselves have certain limitations to synchronize and transmit decisions based on this massive chunk of data. So, a scalable generalized mechanism is yet to be found to work with IoT and blockchain simultaneously [100].

1.6.4 LIMITATIONS IN IoT-FRIENDLY CONSENSUS MECHANISM

IoT devices mostly perform a real-time interaction. It collects, processes, transfers, and synchronizes at a fast speed to provide essential services. The consensus protocols recently being followed with most of the proposals like PoW, PoET, and PoC are used in the public blockchain. Their computation time is considerable and results in a time delay in producing quick responses. So, a more IoT-centric consensus mechanism is needed to work for blockchain more efficiently [101].

Along with these issues, blockchain and the IoT ecosystems need more impactful works in data integrity, communication protocol, and ubiquitous integration of future IoT devices to mitigate the security issues.

1.7 CONCLUSION

In this chapter, we present a comprehensive study on IoT security issues and their solution based on blockchain. Fundamental properties and terminologies of blockchain technology and IoT architecture are also mentioned for better insight. The five-layer architecture can be very fruitful for the implementation of industrial sectors and smart city concepts. By combining blockchain technology, the whole ecosystem can be more effective and intact. The security issues we have pointed are very common and IoT devices are much prone to fall for them. The network and middleware layer is very crucial to maintain communication among devices. The attackers get an advantage in finding the entry point to these layers and generate cyberattacks easily. Its own mechanism to restrict unauthorized access or detect an intruder is still a work in progress. Blockchain becomes the most promising technology in this regard. We hope these findings will help to get a good understanding of the whole system and inspire us to work on the existing security issues of IoT devices as well as upcoming IoT applications.

REFERENCES

1. Andrade, T., & Bastos, D. (2019, June). Extended reality in IoT scenarios: concepts, applications and future trends. In *2019 5th Experiment International Conference (exp. At'19)* (pp. 107–112). IEEE. Funchal, Portugal.
2. Sami, N., Mufti, T., Sohail, S. S., Siddiqui, J., & Kumar, D. (2020). Future Internet of Things (IOT) from cloud perspective: aspects, applications and challenges. In: Alam, M., Shakil, K., & Khan, S. (eds) *Internet of Things (IoT)* (pp. 515–532). Springer, Cham.
3. Goyal, S., Sharma, N., Bhushan, B., Shankar, A., & Sagayam, M. (2020). IoT enabled technology in secured healthcare: applications, challenges and future directions. *Cognitive Internet of Medical Things for Smart Healthcare*, 25–48. Doi: 10.1007/978-3-030-55833-8_2.
4. Sethi, R., Bhushan, B., Sharma, N., Kumar, R., & Kaushik, I. (2020). Applicability of industrial IoT in diversified sectors: evolution, applications and challenges. *Studies in Big Data Multimedia Technologies in the Internet of Things Environment*, 45–67. Doi: 10.1007/978-981-15-7965-3_4
5. ur Rehman, M. H., Yaqoob, I., Salah, K., Imran, M., Jayaraman, P. P., & Perera, C. (2019). The role of big data analytics in industrial Internet of Things. *Future Generation Computer Systems*, 99, 247–259.
6. Dai, H. N., Wang, H., Xu, G., Wan, J., & Imran, M. (2020). Big data analytics for manufacturing Internet of Things: opportunities, challenges and enabling technologies. *Enterprise Information Systems*, 14(9–10), 1279–1303.
7. Wu, M., Wang, K., Cai, X., Guo, S., Guo, M., & Rong, C. (2019). A comprehensive survey of blockchain: from theory to IoT applications and beyond. *IEEE Internet of Things Journal*, 6(5), 8114–8154.
8. Bhushan, B., Sahoo, C., Sinha, P., & Khamparia, A. (2021). Unification of blockchain and Internet of Things (BIoT): requirements, working model, challenges and future directions. *Wireless Networks*, 27(1), 55–90.
9. Christidis, K., & Devetsikiotis, M. (2016). Blockchains and smart contracts for the Internet of Things. *IEEE Access*, 4, 2292–2303.
10. Haque, A. B., & Bhushan, B. (2021). Emergence of blockchain technology: a reliable and secure solution for IoT systems. In: Sharma, S. K., Bhushan, B., Khamparia, A., Astya, P. N., & Debnat, N. C. (eds), *Blockchain Technology for Data Privacy Management* (pp. 159–183). CRC Press, London.
11. Xiao, Y., Zhang, N., Lou, W., & Hou, Y. T. (2020). A survey of distributed consensus protocols for blockchain networks. *IEEE Communications Surveys & Tutorials*, 22(2), 1432–1465.
12. Berentsen, A. (2019). Aleksander Berentsen recommends "Bitcoin: a peer-to-peer electronic cash system" by Satoshi Nakamoto. In: Frey, B., & Schaltegger, C. (eds) *21st Century Economics* (pp. 7–8). Springer, Cham.
13. Padmavathi, U., & Rajagopalan, N. (eds). (2021). Concept of blockchain technology and its emergence. In: *Blockchain Applications in IoT Security* (pp. 1–20). IGI Global, Hershey, PA.
14. Yiu, N. C. (2021). Toward blockchain-enabled supply chain anti-counterfeiting and traceability. *Future Internet*, 13(4), 86.

15. AlShamsi, M., Salloum, S. A., Alshurideh, M., & Abdallah, S. (2021). Artificial intelligence and blockchain for transparency in governance. In: Hassanien, A., Bhatnagar, R., & Darwish, A. (eds), *Artificial Intelligence for Sustainable Development: Theory, Practice and Future Applications* (pp. 219–230). Springer, Cham.

16. Wang, W., Hoang, D. T., Hu, P., Xiong, Z., Niyato, D., Wang, P., … Kim, D. I. (2019). A survey on consensus mechanisms and mining strategy management in blockchain networks. *IEEE Access, 7*, 22328–22370.

17. Kumar, A., Abhishek, K., Bhushan, B., & Chakraborty, C. (2021). Secure access control for manufacturing sector with application of ethereum blockchain. *Peer-to-Peer Networking and Applications.* Doi: 10.1007/s12083-021-01108-3.

18. Bhushan, B., Sahoo, C., Sinha, P., & Khamparia, A. (2020). Unification of blockchain and Internet of Things (BIoT): requirements, working model, challenges and future directions. *Wireless Networks.* Doi: 10.1007/s11276-020-02445-6.

19. Bhushan, B., Khamparia, A., Sagayam, K. M., Sharma, S. K., Ahad, M. A., & Debnath, N. C. (2020). Blockchain for smart cities: a review of architectures, integration trends and future research directions. *Sustainable Cities and Society, 61,* 102360. Doi: 10.1016/j.scs.2020.102360.

20. Saxena, S., Bhushan, B., & Ahad, M. A. (2021). Blockchain based solutions to Secure IoT: background, integration trends and a way forward. *Journal of Network and Computer Applications,* 103050. Doi: 10.1016/j.jnca.2021.103050.

21. Bhushan, B., Sinha, P., Sagayam, K. M., & J, A. (2021). Untangling blockchain technology: a survey on state of the art, security threats, privacy services, applications and future research directions. *Computers & Electrical Engineering, 90,* 106897. Doi: 10.1016/j.compeleceng.2020.106897.

22. Li, C., & Palanisamy, B. (2020, September). Comparison of decentralization in DPoS and PoW blockchains. In *International Conference on Blockchain* (pp. 18–32). Springer, Cham.

23. Yaqoob, I., Salah, K., Jayaraman, R., & Al-Hammadi, Y. (2021). Blockchain for healthcare data management: opportunities, challenges, and future recommendations. *Neural Computing and Applications*, Special Issue: Healthcare Analytics, 1–16.

24. Wang, W., Huang, H., Xue, L., Li, Q., Malekian, R., & Zhang, Y. (2021). Blockchain-assisted handover authentication for intelligent telehealth in multi-server edge computing environment. *Journal of Systems Architecture, 115,* 102024.

25. Ahmad, R. W., Hasan, H., Jayaraman, R., Salah, K., & Omar, M. (2021). Blockchain applications and architectures for port operations and logistics management. *Research in Transportation Business & Management, 61,* 100620.

26. Guha Roy, D., & Srirama, S. N. (2021). A blockchain-based cyber attack detection scheme for decentralized Internet of Things using software-defined network. *Software: Practice and Experience, 51*(7), 1540–1556.

27. Chelladurai, U., & Pandian, S. (2021). A novel blockchain based electronic health record automation system for healthcare. *Journal of Ambient Intelligence and Humanized Computing, 12,* 1–11.

28. Al-Rakhami, M. S., & Al-Mashari, M. (2021). A blockchain-based trust model for the Internet of Things supply chain management. *Sensors, 21*(5), 1759. Doi: 10.3390/s21051759.

29. Hadzovic, S., Mrdovic, S., & Radonjic, M. (2021). Identification of IoT actors. *Sensors, 21*(6), 2093.

30. Al-Fuqaha, A., Guizani, M., Mohammadi, M., Aledhari, M., & Ayyash, M. (2015). Internet of Things: a survey on enabling technologies, protocols, and applications. *IEEE Communications Surveys & Tutorials, 17*(4), 2347–2376.

31. Hu, B., Chen, Y., Yu, H., Meng, L., & Duan, Z. (2021). Blockchain enabled data sharing scheme for consumer IoT applications. Early Access, March 2021. *IEEE Consumer Electronics Magazine*. Doi: 10.1109/MCE.2021.3066793.
32. Yang, Z., Yue, Y., Yang, Y., Peng, Y., Wang, X., & Liu, W. (2011, July). Study and application on the architecture and key technologies for IOT. In *2011 International Conference on Multimedia Technology* (pp. 747–751). Hangzhou, China, IEEE.
33. Vashi, S., Ram, J., Modi, J., Verma, S., & Prakash, C. (2017, February). Internet of Things (IoT): a vision, architectural elements, and security issues. In *2017 International Conference on I-SMAC (IoT in Social, Mobile, Analytics and Cloud) (I-SMAC)* (pp. 492–496), Palladam, India, IEEE.
34. Ghotbou, A., & Khansari, M. (2021). Comparing application layer protocols for video transmission in IoT low power lossy networks: an analytic comparison. *Wireless Networks*, 27(1), 269–283.
35. Khan, R., Khan, S. U., Zaheer, R., & Khan, S. (2012, December). Future internet: the Internet of Things architecture, possible applications and key challenges. In *2012 10th International Conference on Frontiers of Information Technology* (pp. 257–260), Islamabad, Pakistan, IEEE.
36. Kakkar, L., Gupta, D., Saxena, S., & Tanwar, S. (2021). IoT architectures and its security: a review. In *Proceedings of the Second International Conference on Information Management and Machine Intelligence* (pp. 87–94). Springer, Singapore.
37. Chegini, H., Naha, R. K., Mahanti, A., & Thulasiraman, P. (2021). Process automation in an IoT–fog–cloud ecosystem: a survey and taxonomy. *IoT*, 2(1), 92–118.
38. Lombardi, M., Pascale, F., & Santaniello, D. (2021). Internet of Things: a general overview between architectures, protocols and applications. *Information*, 12(2), 87.
39. Kumar, C., & Prakash, S. (2021). Routing protocols: key security issues and challenges in IoT, ad hoc, and sensor networks. In: Sharma, S. K., Bhushan, B., & Debnath, N. C. (eds) *Security and Privacy Issues in IoT Devices and Sensor Networks* (pp. 105–132). Academic Press. Cambridge, MA.
40. Bharathi, M. V., Tanguturi, R. C., Jayakumar, C., & Selvamani, K. (2012, December). Node capture attack in wireless sensor network: a survey. In *2012 IEEE International Conference on Computational Intelligence and Computing Research* (pp. 1–3). Coimbatore, India, IEEE.
41. Chen, Q., Li, M., Yang, X., Alturki, R., Alshehri, M. D., & Khan, F. (2021). Impact of residual hardware impairment on the IoT secrecy performance of RIS-assisted NOMA networks. *IEEE Access*, 9, 42583–42592.
42. Qi, M., & Chen, J. (2021). Secure authenticated key exchange for WSNs in IoT applications. *The Journal of Supercomputing*, 77(12), 1–14.
43. Puthal, D., Nepal, S., Ranjan, R., & Chen, J. (2016). Threats to networking cloud and edge data center in the IoT. *IEEE Cloud Computing*, 3(3), 64–71.
44. Palop, J. J., Mucke, L., & Roberson, E. D. (2010). Quantifying biomarkers of cognitive dysfunction and neuronal network hyperexcitability in mouse models of Alzheimer's disease: depletion of calcium-dependent proteins and inhibitory hippocampal remodeling. In: Roberson, E. (eds), *Alzheimer's Disease and Frontotemporal Dementia*, (pp. 245–262). Humana Press, Totowa, NJ.
45. Attarian, R., & Hashemi, S. (2021). An anonymity communication protocol for security and privacy of clients in IoT-based mobile health transactions. *Computer Networks*, 190, 107976.
46. Burhan, M., Rehman, R. A., Khan, B., & Kim, B. S. (2018). IoT elements, layered architectures and security issues: a comprehensive survey. *Sensors*, 18(9), 2796.

47. Perti, A., Singh, A., Sinha, A., & Srivastava, P. K. (2021). Security risks and challenges in IoT-based applications. In *Proceedings of International Conference on Big Data, Machine Learning and their Applications* (pp. 99–111). Springer, Singapore.
48. Chen, K., Zhang, S., Li, Z., Zhang, Y., Deng, Q., Ray, S., & Jin, Y. (2018). Internet-of-things security and vulnerabilities: taxonomy, challenges, and practice. *Journal of Hardware and Systems Security, 2*(2), 97–110.
49. Mukaddam, A., Elhajj, I., Kayssi, A., & Chehab, A. (2014, May). IP spoofing detection using modified hop count. In *2014 IEEE 28th International Conference on Advanced Information Networking and Applications* (pp. 512–516), Victoria, BC, IEEE.
50. Al-Hadhrami, Y., & Hussain, F. K. (2021). DDoS attacks in IoT networks: a comprehensive systematic literature review. *World Wide Web, 24*(1), 1–31.
51. Deogirikar, J., & Vidhate, A. (2017, February). Security attacks in IoT: a survey. In *2017 International Conference on I-SMAC (IoT in Social, Mobile, Analytics and Cloud) (I-SMAC)*, Palladam, India, (pp. 32–37). IEEE.
52. Al-Maslamani, N., & Abdallah, M. (2020, February). Malicious node detection in wireless sensor network using swarm intelligence optimization. In *2020 IEEE International Conference on Informatics, IoT, and Enabling Technologies (ICIoT)*. (pp. 219–224). Doha, Qatar, IEEE.
53. Meziane, H., Ouerdi, N., Kasmi, M. A., & Mazouz, S. (2021). Classifying security attacks in IoT using CTM method. In:Ben Ahmed, M., Mellouli, S., Braganca, L., Anouar Abdelhakim, B., & Bernadetta, K. A. (eds), *Emerging Trends in ICT for Sustainable Development* (pp. 307–315). Springer, Cham.
54. Ashraf, Q. M., & Habaebi, M. H. (2015). Autonomic schemes for threat mitigation in Internet of Things. *Journal of Network and Computer Applications, 49*, 112–127.
55. Frustaci, M., Pace, P., Aloi, G., & Fortino, G. (2017). Evaluating critical security issues of the IoT world: present and future challenges. *IEEE Internet of Things Journal, 5*(4), 2483–2495.
56. Tsiknas, K., Taketzis, D., Demertzis, K., & Skianis, C. (2021). Cyber threats to industrial IoT: a survey on attacks and countermeasures. *IoT, 2*(1), 163–188.
57. Pusuluri, R., Kalaiarasan, K., & Yogaraj, A. (2021). Software-defined networking and architecture of IoT with security, challenges and applications: a survey. In: Suresh, P., Saravanakumar, U., & Hussein Al Salameh, M. (eds), *Advances in Smart System Technologies* (pp. 519–531). Springer, Singapore.
58. Hernández-Ramos, J. L., Baldini, G., Matheu, S. N., & Skarmeta, A. (2020, June). Updating IoT devices: challenges and potential approaches. In *2020 Global Internet of Things Summit (GIoTS)* (pp. 1–5). Dublin, IEEE.
59. Ahemd, M. M., Shah, M. A., & Wahid, A. (2017, April). IoT security: a layered approach for attacks & defenses. In *2017 International Conference on Communication Technologies (ComTech)* (pp. 104–110). Rawalpindi, Pakistan, IEEE.
60. Billure, R., Tayur, V. M., & Mahesh, V. (2015, June). Internet of Things-a study on the security challenges. In *2015 IEEE International Advance Computing Conference (IACC)* (pp. 247–252). Banglore, India,IEEE.
61. Wang, E. K., Sun, R., Chen, C. M., Liang, Z., Kumari, S., & Khan, M. K. (2020). Proof of X-repute blockchain consensus protocol for IoT systems. *Computers & Security, 95*, 101871.
62. Bilge, L., & Dumitraş, T. (2012, October). Before we knew it: an empirical study of zero-day attacks in the real world. In *Proceedings of the 2012 ACM Conference on Computer and Communications Security* (pp. 833–844). Raleigh, NC, ACM.

63. Alkatheiri, M. S., Sangi, A. R., & Anamalamudi, S. (2020). Physical unclonable function (PUF)-based security in Internet of Things (IoT): key challenges and solutions. In: Gupta, B., Perez, G., Agrawal, D., & Gupta, D. (eds) *Handbook of Computer Networks and Cyber Security* (pp. 461–473). Springer, Cham.
64. Chen, C. M., Deng, X., Gan, W., Chen, J., & Islam, S. H. (2021). A secure blockchain-based group key agreement protocol for IoT. *The Journal of Supercomputing*, 77(2), 1–23.
65. Yang, D., Yoo, S., Doh, I., & Chae, K. (2021). Selective blockchain system for secure and efficient D2D communication. *Journal of Network and Computer Applications, 173*, 102817.
66. Zhang, L., & Ge, Y. (2021, January). Identity authentication based on domestic commercial cryptography with blockchain in the heterogeneous alliance network. In *2021 IEEE International Conference on Consumer Electronics and Computer Engineering (ICCECE)* (pp. 191–195). Guangzhou, China. IEEE.
67. Tahir, M., Sardaraz, M., Muhammad, S., & Saud Khan, M. (2020). A lightweight authentication and authorization framework for blockchain-enabled IoT network in health-informatics. *Sustainability, 12*(17), 6960.
68. Li, T., Wang, H., He, D., & Yu, J. (2020). Permissioned blockchain-based anonymous and traceable aggregate signature scheme for Industrial Internet of Things. *IEEE Internet of Things Journal, 8*(10), 8387–8398.
69. Qiao, G., & Zhuang, Y. (2020, December). A blockchain-based reconstruction framework for UAV network. In *International Conference on Security, Privacy and Anonymity in Computation, Communication and Storage* (pp. 301–311). Springer, Cham.
70. Chen, C. L., Deng, Y. Y., Weng, W., Zhou, M., & Sun, H. (2021). A blockchain-based intelligent anti-switch package in tracing logistics system. *The Journal of Supercomputing, 77*(7), 7791–7832.
71. Vangala, A., Sutrala, A. K., Das, A. K., & Jo, M. (2021). Smart contract-based blockchain-envisioned authentication scheme for smart farming. *IEEE Internet of Things Journal, 8*(13), 10792–10806.
72. Vishwakarma, L., & Das, D. (2020, November). BSS: blockchain enabled security system for Internet of Things applications. In *2020 IEEE 19th International Symposium on Network Computing and Applications (NCA)* (pp. 1–4), Cambridge, MA, IEEE.
73. Nesarani, A., Ramar, R., & Pandian, S. (2020). An efficient approach for rice prediction from authenticated Block chain node using machine learning technique. *Environmental Technology & Innovation, 20*, 101064.
74. Mukhandi, M., Andrade, E., Damião, F., Granjal, J., & Vilela, J. P. (2020, November). Blockchain-based scalable authentication for IoT. In *Proceedings of the 18th Conference on Embedded Networked Sensor Systems*, Japan, (pp. 667–668). ACM.
75. Seshadri, S. S., Rodriguez, D., Subedi, M., Choo, K. K. R., Ahmed, S., Chen, Q., & Lee, J. (2020). IoTCop: a blockchain-based monitoring framework for detection and isolation of malicious devices in Internet-of-Things systems. *IEEE Internet of Things Journal, 8*(5), 3346–3359.
76. Kumar, S., Das, A. K., & Sinha, D. (2021). Blockchain-Based Sybil-Secure Data Transmission (SSDT) IoT framework for smart city applications. In: Bhateja, V., Peng, S. L., Satapathy, S. C., Zhang, Y. D. (eds),*Evolution in Computational Intelligence* (pp. 355–370). Springer, Singapore.
77. Arifeen, M. M., Al Mamun, A., Ahmed, T., Kaiser, M. S., & Mahmud, M. (2021). A blockchain-based scheme for sybil attack detection in underwater wireless sensor

networks. In *Proceedings of International Conference on Trends in Computational and Cognitive Engineering* (pp. 467–476). Springer, Singapore.

78. Tariq, N., Asim, M., Khan, F. A., Baker, T., Khalid, U., & Derhab, A. (2021). A blockchain-based multi-mobile code-driven trust mechanism for detecting internal attacks in Internet of Things. *Sensors, 21*(1), 23.

79. Mohanty, S. N., Ramya, K. C., Rani, S. S., Gupta, D., Shankar, K., Lakshmanaprabu, S. K., & Khanna, A. (2020). An efficient lightweight integrated blockchain (ELIB) model for IoT security and privacy. *Future Generation Computer Systems, 102*, 1027–1037.

80. Maselli, G., Piva, M., & Restuccia, F. (2020, September). HyBloSE: hybrid blockchain for secure-by-design smart environments. In *Proceedings of the 3rd Workshop on Cryptocurrencies and Blockchains for Distributed Systems* (pp. 23–28).

81. Choi, J., Shin, W., Kim, J., & Kim, K. H. (2020, January). Random seed generation for IoT key generation and key management system using blockchain. In *2020 International Conference on Information Networking (ICOIN)* (pp. 663–665), London, IEEE.

82. Gupta, R., Kumari, A., & Tanwar, S. (2021). A taxonomy of blockchain envisioned edge-as-a-connected autonomous vehicles. *Transactions on Emerging Telecommunications Technologies, 32*(6), e4009.

83. Rathee, G., Ahmad, F., Sandhu, R., Kerrache, C. A., & Azad, M. A. (2021). On the design and implementation of a secure blockchain-based hybrid framework for Industrial Internet-of-Things. *Information Processing & Management, 58*(3), 102526.

84. Kruthik, J. T., Ramakrishnan, K., Sunitha, R., & Honnavalli, B. P. (2021). Security model for Internet of Things based on blockchain. In: Raj, J. S., Iliyasu, A. M., Bestak, R., & Baig, Z. A. (eds), *Innovative Data Communication Technologies and Application* (pp. 543–557). Springer, Singapore.

85. Chen, M., Tang, X., Cheng, J., Xiong, N., Li, J., & Fan, D. (2020, July). A DDoS attack defense method based on blockchain for IoTs devices. In *International Conference on Artificial Intelligence and Security* (pp. 685–694). Springer, Singapore.

86. Lei, I. S., Tang, S. K., & Tse, R. (2020). Integrating consortium blockchain into edge server to defense against ransomware attack. *Procedia Computer Science, 177*, 120–127.

87. Gupta, S., Thakur, P., Biswas, K., Kumar, S., & Singh, A. P. (2021). Developing a blockchain-based and distributed database-oriented multi-malware detection engine. In: Maleh, Y., Shojafar, M., Alazab, M., & Baddi, Y. (eds), *Machine Intelligence and Big Data Analytics for Cybersecurity Applications* (pp. 249–275). Springer, Cham.

88. Zhang, W., Wang, J., Han, G., Huang, S., Feng, Y., & Shu, L. (2020). A data set accuracy weighted random forest algorithm for IoT fault detection based on edge computing and blockchain. *IEEE Internet of Things Journal, 8*(4), 2354–2363.

89. Zhang, W., Wu, Z., Han, G., Feng, Y., & Shu, L. (2020). LDC: a lightweight dada consensus algorithm based on the blockchain for the industrial Internet of Things for smart city applications. *Future Generation Computer Systems, 108*, 574–582.

90. Cui, Z., Fei, X. U. E., Zhang, S., Cai, X., Cao, Y., Zhang, W., & Chen, J. (2020). A hybrid blockchain-based identity authentication scheme for multi-WSN. *IEEE Transactions on Services Computing, 13*(2), 241–251.

91. Dhar, S., & Bose, I. (2021). Securing IoT devices using zero trust and blockchain. *Journal of Organizational Computing and Electronic Commerce, 31*(1), 18–34.

92. Hang, L., & Kim, D. H. (2020). Reliable task management based on a smart contract for runtime verification of sensing and actuating tasks in IoT environments. *Sensors, 20*(4), 1207.

93. Alkadi, O., Moustafa, N., Turnbull, B., & Choo, K. K. R. (2020). A deep blockchain framework-enabled collaborative intrusion detection for protecting IoT and cloud networks. *IEEE Internet of Things Journal, 8*(12), 9463–9472.

94. Salem, M. (2020, March). Blockchain-based authentication approach for securing transportation system. In *International Symposium on Intelligent Computing Systems* (pp. 55–64). Springer, Cham.

95. Kłos, M., & El Fray, I. (2020, October). Securing event logs with blockchain for IoT. In *International Conference on Computer Information Systems and Industrial Management* (pp. 77–87). Springer, Cham.

96. Zhang, X., Liu, C., Chai, K. K., & Poslad, S. (2021). A privacy-preserving consensus mechanism for an electric vehicle charging scheme. *Journal of Network and Computer Applications, 174*, 102908.

97. Sahay, R., Geethakumari, G., & Mitra, B. (2020). A novel blockchain based framework to secure IoT-LLNs against routing attacks. *Computing, 102*, 2445–2470.

98. Abbasi, M. A., Memon, Z. A., Durrani, N. M., Haider, W., Laeeq, K., & Mallah, G. A. (2021). A multi-layer trust-based middleware framework for handling interoperability issues in heterogeneous IoTs. *Cluster Computing, 24*, 2133–2160, 1–28.

99. Tang, Q., & Du, F. (2021). Analysis of firmware vulnerabilities. In: Tang, Q. & Du, F. (eds) *Internet of Things Security: Principles and Practice* (pp. 121–197). Springer, Singapore.

100. Iqbal, U., & Mir, A. H. (2020). Secure and scalable access control protocol for IoT environment. *Internet of Things, 12*, 100291.

101. Salimitari, M., Chatterjee, M., & Fallah, Y. P. (2020). A survey on consensus methods in blockchain for resource-constrained IoT networks. *Internet of Things, 11*, 100212.

2 A Novel Framework for Robust Data Collection in Industrial IoT Based on Proof-of-Stake Algorithm

P.R. Mahalingam and K.A. Fasila
Muthoot Institute of Technology and Science

CONTENTS

2.1 INTRODUCTION: INDUSTRIAL INTERNET OF THINGS

Industrial Internet of Things (IIoT) is a booming domain in today's era of automation. IIoT refers to the application of Internet of Things (IoT) to improve operational efficiency in industries. Information Technology (IT) and Operational Technology (OT) are converged in IIoT, to enable industries to improve their performance [1,2]. The convergence of IT and OT helps organizations to integrate automation, optimization, data analysis, etc. The IoT ecosystem consisting of smart sensors and actuators will make the monitoring and control of machines and other infrastructures easier. An abstract view of IIoT is given in Figure 2.1.

The architecture given in Figure 2.1 incorporates a layered view of the model. The bottom layer forms the "edge", which is made up of tangible components like sensors and gateways. This is connected to the "network" layer, which forms the bridge between compute infrastructure and gateways. The topmost layer forms

DOI: 10.1201/9781003224075-2

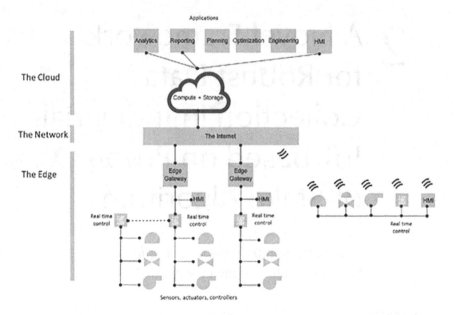

FIGURE 2.1 IIoT architecture. (Courtesy: The Future of Industrial Automation by Paul McLaughlin and Rohan McAdam.)

the "cloud" part, which contains the processing unit on the cloud, and various applications like dashboards and analytics.

IIoT forms an autonomous environment and hence, security features are to be addressed seriously. With the tremendous increase in the use of IIoT applications, cyber security threats have also increased. In an autonomous connected environment like IIoT, multiple vulnerabilities may arise and such attacks will compromise the reliability of the system. There are several issues while considering the security challenges in an IIoT ecosystem. One major issue is the lack of risk mitigation. This means, the operators in the OT section may not have a deep understanding of principles, which are handled by IT specialists. So, even though several mitigation techniques are present, only a few are being utilized effectively. Other issues are lack of proper security updates, impact of attacks, lack of end component visibility, etc.

Another major issue is the vulnerability in system components involved. Since industrial equipment were designed to be used in closed environments, the security issues were not considered then. The security risks associated with the IIoT devices include device management, patch management, use of the same authentication credentials, and returning wrong data. IIoT depends on a vast array of sensors, processing elements, and actuators to automate data collection, processing, and response. Reliability in an IoT ecosystem depends on several phases of implementations such as device reliability, communication reliability, network reliability, and application reliability [3].

The device layer in an IoT system contains electromagnetic devices, which are called sensors and actuators. Once these resource-constrained sensor devices are deployed on a large scale, at various locations, it is difficult to monitor and ensure accurate data delivery from them. One of the major challenges that is faced in the stage of data collection is the accuracy given by electromechanical devices. Performance of sensors may degrade because of several reasons such as device failure, environmental factors, and lack of firmware updates. This work proposes a blockchain-based algorithm to improve sensor reliability in the data collection phase of IIoT applications. The scope for this was originally explored in [4].

The rest of the chapter is organized as follows. Section 2.2 talks about how IoT can be deployed on an industrial scale to obtain IIoT. Section 2.3 deals with Blockchain, in general, and gives an introduction to the proof-of-stake (PoS) algorithm. Section 2.4 describes how IIoT and blockchain can be combined, with a focus on PoS. Section 2.5 introduces an algorithm that has been proposed based on the concept of stake that ensures the reliability of sensors. Section 2.6 discusses a simulation of the algorithm and evaluates its performance. The chapter comes to a close with concluding remarks in Section 2.7.

In the rest of this chapter, the terms device, node, and sensor will be used interchangeably. Even though they are different in the real world, the current focus is on the algorithm, and the underlying hardware can be abstracted out to any of these terms.

2.2 IIOT – USE CASES

IIoT, also known as Industry 4.0, has several applications. Every industrial sector like retail, healthcare, manufacturing, education, oil and gas, transportation, and energy have several benefits from using IIoT. Other use cases like smart cities and agriculture are also benefited from IIoT. The key benefits of using IIoT are improved device connectivity, M2M communication, improved efficiency, increased profit, industrial safety, etc. In addition to these points, other benefits like the development of new services, business models, and innovations are in the goal sets of industries. Table 2.1 gives a summary of some major industrial organizations that have been working based on IIoT and reaping benefits from it. As the most important use case, IIoT is used for automation, which is popularly implemented using wireless sensor networks [5].

The examples mentioned in Table 2.1 give an idea of how diverse IIoT can be implemented. With the advent of Industry 4.0 and beyond, the scope of IoT is at an all-time high [6]. Senathipathi et al. [7] described the prospective applications of IIoT with blockchain.

2.3 BLOCKCHAIN AND PROOF-OF-STAKE ALGORITHM

Blockchain was envisaged as a distributed ledger that can replace the centralized record keeping models existing today. It was introduced as the platform on which Bitcoin, the first accepted cryptocurrency, ran. Blockchains generally work on

TABLE 2.1

Industry Use Cases

Organization	Area/Major Benefits
ABB	Using predictive maintenance for smart robotics
Boeing	To improve manufacturing efficiency
Bosch	Used IoT methods to track and trace tools, which helped the workers to save a lot of time
Caterpillar	Heavy equipment maker company that uses IoT and augmented reality (AR) applications to give an at-a-glance view of everything, to the machine operators
Stanley Black & Decker	Smart factory, Construction IoT

the concept of distributed consensus, which ensures that a ledger entry is added only if a majority agree to the authenticity of the same. This is the responsibility of validators. Transactions are stored on a chain of entries, each holding the hash of the previous entry in the chain. This makes blockchains inherently immutable, since any changes done on the blockchain after a transaction will cause the hash to change, thereby invalidating all entries after that. The basic components and aspects of a blockchain as described in [8] are as follows:

- **Transactions**: Transactions are the fundamental units of a blockchain. In order to perform a transaction, the source address, source digital signature, transaction information, and destination address are used.
- **Miner**: Miner is a consensus participant in the blockchain network, which ensures that all transactions are validated. Each transaction is validated and added with other transactions into a block. If successful, it is broadcast to all other nodes for verification and marked as the latest block.
- **Hash Pointer**: This is created by hash functions to map the contents of the block to the hash pointer. It is normally created by taking the hash of the previous block and adding it as an entry to the current block. This makes any tampering evident by ensuring that any change in the previous data will result in a different hash value in the next block, and it can be traced back to the genesis block, i.e., the first block of the chain.
- A block can also contain additional data depending on the requirements of different consensus mechanisms. To reduce storage space, the transactions in a block can be stored in the form of a Merkle tree.

These concepts make the blockchain decentralized, transparent, immutable, secure, and private. They are decentralized because miners work independently, and only broadcast the success of each process. The transaction is transparent to all participants since they carry all necessary identifiers. The hash pointer makes it impossible to modify any specific part of the chain, since hashes are one-way, and cryptography-grade hashes like SHA-256 and SHA-512 have nearly zero collision. Cryptographic security and privacy can be easily incorporated on top of the existing chains.

The base concept has been extended subsequently by enabling lightweight algorithms to run on the chain, using concepts like smart contracts. Different implementation flavours of the concept exist today, with the most popular ones being Hyperledger (using the original concept) and Ethereum (using smart contracts).

Like any other multi-agent system in a distributed environment, blockchain also has to ensure overall system reliability. Hence, all the coordinating processes will have to reach an agreement which is called consensus. It is a fault-tolerant mechanism used between distributed nodes to reach a common state. This mechanism ensures the synchronization between nodes and agreement on the transactions added to the blockchain. Commonly used consensus mechanisms in blockchain are Proof of Work (PoW) and PoS [8]. PoW requires the validators to have enough computational power to verify transactions. In PoS, the validators are selected based on their holdings or stakes. PoS requires the validators to have a minimum quantity of stakes. So, a malicious node will have to acquire enough computational power or stakes in PoW and PoS, respectively, in order to become a validating node. Among these two mechanisms, PoS is more energy efficient. In addition, [8] specifies that PoS has negligible energy consumption, which is ideal for low-power devices like in IIoT. In addition, no additional hardware is needed, and the processing is fast.

2.4 INTEGRATING PROOF-OF-STAKE MODEL INTO IIOT

The concept of including blockchain platforms with the IoT has been explored by a number of researchers [9–14]. Miller [15] explored the possibility of adapting the same to IIoT. But the common factor among available research is that they try to adapt the platform of blockchain directly onto IoT implementations, enabling decentralized processing. But these implementations will carry the overhead of more powerful edge nodes, which have storage and computing capabilities at their disposal. In addition, security and scalability are of utmost importance in existing research.

In this chapter, the focus is no longer on the security and scalability of IoT using blockchain. The application domain shifts to how the reliability of sensors can be ensured using concepts from blockchain. Fortino et al. [16] proposed a reputation-based model using blockchain for ensuring reliability in IIoT. Kang et al. [17] proposed an incentive-based model for proper consensus propagation, and Yang et al. [18] proposed adding a downgrade mechanism to PoS for easier isolation of malicious nodes. These concepts can be adapted easily to implement an algorithm that eliminates the need of blockchain, but retains the capability of isolating malicious nodes. The restriction placed in the absence of stored chains is that all processing should be done real time, and it can be either centralized or decentralized.

Two aspects of the PoS model can be directly integrated to manage reliability in IIoT,

1. Selection of contributors and validators,
2. Transfer of stake and fee.

The fundamental principle behind this integration is on how to effectively penalize erring sensors, while keeping them within the ecosystem. It also aims at allowing sensors (or nodes) to come back to a prominent state if they restart giving proper observations. This will provide an effective mechanism for monitoring byzantine failures, and at the same time, accommodate factors like replacement of faulty equipment.

Bhushan et al. [19] describe different aspects of blockchain that enable widespread usage in today's technological domain. Bhushan et al. [20] explore the possibility of integrating blockchain and IoT further by analysing the advantages and disadvantages and observe that energy efficiency and latency are points of concern. Even though privacy and security are equally important, they are not being considered in our study since a sterile environment is being assumed. The security aspect is explored in depth by Uddin et al. [21] and Krishna et al. [22].

2.5   PROPOSED ALGORITHM

The basic algorithm for IIoT reliability with PoS is as follows. This is done at every sampling interval for the sensors.

Algorithm: pow_iiot_reliability
Inputs: stakes, observations
Outputs: accepted observation, failure status, revised stakes

1. Accept the latest set of observations from the sensors.
2. Select sensors that have stakes greater than min_stake. They form the contribution set (c_set). Others form the validator set (v_set).
3. Find the average of observations given by sensors in the c_set.
4. Find deviation of each c_set observation from the average.
5. If the smallest deviation is above min_deviation, report that the system is invalidated, and terminate. Otherwise continue.
6. Accept the observation that has minimum deviation from the average.
7. Set allow_contrib will be formed with sensors in c_set with observation deviations not greater than min_deviation. Other contributors form the set deny_contrib.
8. Take k% of stake from each element in the deny_contrib set, where k is called the "penalty score". Add all those stakes to stake_pool.
9. Evenly distribute stake_pool to all members of allow_contrib.

10. Within v_set, select observations that have deviations not greater than min_deviation and add them to fee_set.
11. Take n% of stake from each element in c_set, where n is called the "fee rate". Add all those stakes to fee_pool.
12. Evenly distribute fee_pool to all members of fee_set.

The process can be explained in easier terms. The working can be considered from multiple levels of detail. A high-level design is given in Figure 2.2.

A first-level detail can be added at this point, and the internal modules along with their interactions are depicted in Figure 2.3. This breaks the process down into five steps – selection of contributors/validators, averaging, deviation testing, fee eligibility measurement, and stake reallocation.

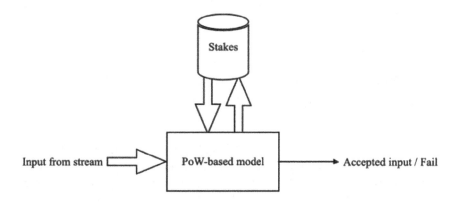

FIGURE 2.2   High-level design for the PoW-based reliability model.

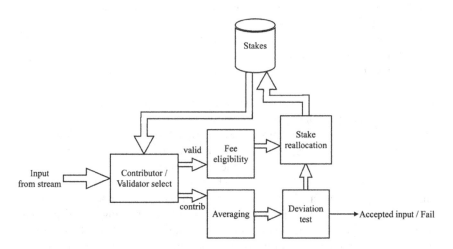

FIGURE 2.3   Modules present in the PoW-based reliability model.

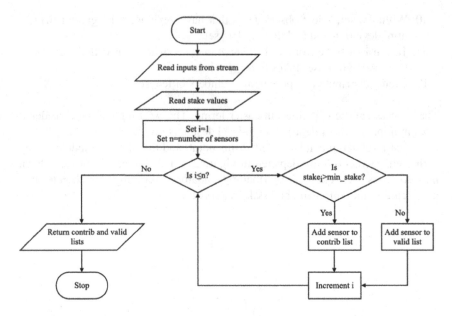

FIGURE 2.4   Contributor/validator selection module.

Whenever a new reading comes in from all sensors, the algorithm checks if all sensors have a minimum amount of stake left in them. Those nodes with a minimum stake available with them will be named "contributors", while others remain "validators". In principle, this differentiation doesn't change the behaviour of any node. It only creates a difference when the readings are accepted. This demarcation is inspired by the PoS concept, where a node will be able to execute an Ethereum transaction only if there is sufficient stake available with it. This is depicted by the flowchart in Figure 2.4.

Once contributors are selected, their readings are averaged to get an estimate of what may be the original value. This operation has an additional advantage that it is easy to identify inconsistencies using this measure. If the distribution of readings has a high variance, it means that sensors have picked up a fair amount of noise (it is highly unlikely that the same ecosystem will contain largely varying readings). Considering that, every reading is cross-checked with the average, to find the deviation. Those readings violating a threshold set for the deviation will be out of contention, keeping the assumption that they are erroneous. The reading closest to the average value is taken as the accepted value.

While taking the mean value, there can be cases where the actual value is somewhere towards the outliers. In order to keep this in check, the number of violations beyond the threshold is kept track of, and if none of the readings fall within the threshold, the algorithm will report an error and stop. This will handle issues that arise because of all readings sitting towards the extremities. In any other case, the variance will be less enough to account for the error between actual and expected

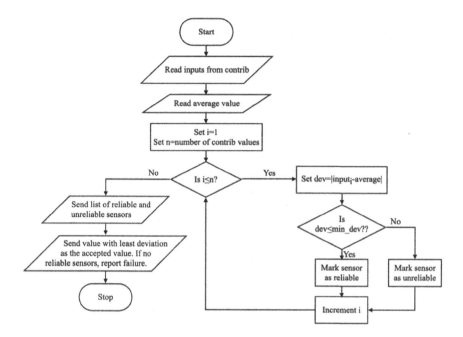

FIGURE 2.5 Deviation test module.

values. Depending on the critical nature of the application, the threshold can be modified appropriately, with those applications requiring stringent quality control having tighter thresholds. But care should be taken that the number of system failures will increase with tighter thresholds, which will be better than the consequences of undetected failures. Figure 2.5 summarizes the process.

Once the set of violations has been recorded, each violator will surrender a fixed percentage of their stake, which is then evenly distributed to those who have given proper readings. This will give benefit to reliable sensors, while penalizing others. The validator set remains unaffected by all these changes.

Once the stake transfer is complete, the validator set is checked for readings that come within the threshold (even though the mean did not consider these values). If any validator was able to generate a reliable reading, they can charge a "fee" to the contributors, who then donate a fixed percentage of their available stake, evenly distributed among all eligible validators. This enables validators to return to the contributor state eventually, once they start generating good readings. Ineligible nodes will remain with their same stake and wait for proper readings to resume. This is equivalent to charging the "gas fee", which is surrendered by nodes upon execution. Figures 2.6 and 2.7 explain the process in depth.

The end result is a system that always maintains a consistent total stake, distributed appropriately among different nodes based on their reliability. Even if a node gets flagged as unreliable and moves out of contributory privilege, there remains a chance for it to resume its role.

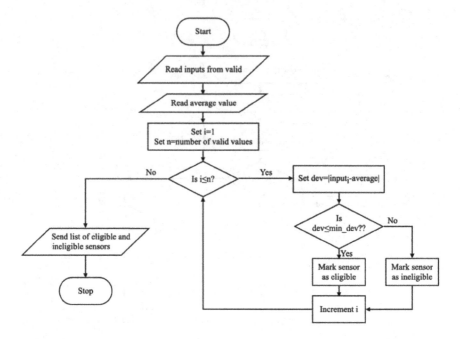

FIGURE 2.6   Fee eligibility module.

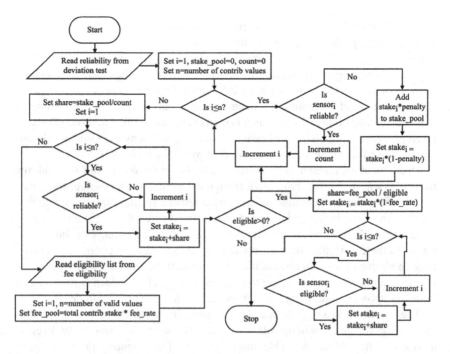

FIGURE 2.7   Stake transfer module.

2.6   SIMULATION AND RESULTS

The algorithm was simulated using Python. Randomized values were given as input to test the robustness of the algorithm, and how it behaves under different conditions. Two cases are being considered – one in which the algorithm allows the system to run as usual and one in which the algorithm terminates operations because of huge mismatches.

Case 1: System completes normal operation
The parameters for this experiment are as follows:
Number of sensors = 5, Starting stake for each sensor = 100
Minimum stake needed for contribution (min_stake) = 75
Number of iterations simulated = 20
Deviation limit (dev_limit) = 10, Stake penalty = 10%, Validation fee = 5%

The readings are taken as random numbers in the range 90–110. This is to ensure that the chance of readings going out of bounds of dev_limit is less. It simulates an ideal scenario. Tables 2.2–2.8 summarize the working of the proposed model at each iteration.
Iteration 1

TABLE 2.2
Iteration 1 (Normal Operation)

Sensor Number	1	2	3	4	5
Current stake (s)	100	100	100	100	100
Reading received (r)	92	109	104	102	102
Contributor? (s>min_stake)	True	True	True	True	True
Average reading (avg)	101.8	101.8	101.8	101.8	101.8
Deviation (d)=|avg−r|	9.8	7.2	2.2	0.2	0.2
Accepted reading				Accept	Accept
Within the deviation limit? (d<dev_limit)	Yes	Yes	Yes	Yes	Yes
Stake for transfer (10%)	0	0	0	0	0
Stake for fee (5%)	5	5	5	5	5
Revised stakes	100	100	100	100	100

Here, even though the stake was set aside for fee, there was no transfer since everyone functioned as a contributor.

Iteration 2

TABLE 2.3
Iteration 2 (Normal Operation)

Sensor Number	1	2	3	4	5
Current stake (s)	100	100	100	100	100
Reading received (r)	108	103	109	104	106
Contributor? (s>min_stake)	True	True	True	True	True
Average reading (avg)	106	106	106	106	106
Deviation (d)=|avg−r|	2	3	3	2	0
Accepted reading					Accept
Within the deviation limit? (d<dev_limit)	Yes	Yes	Yes	Yes	Yes
Stake for transfer (10%)	0	0	0	0	0
Stake for fee (5%)	5	5	5	5	5
Revised stakes	100	100	100	100	100

Iteration 3

TABLE 2.4
Iteration 3 (Normal Operation)

Sensor Number	1	2	3	4	5
Current stake (s)	100	100	100	100	100
Reading received (r)	105	97	104	108	99
Contributor? (s>min_stake)	True	True	True	True	True
Average reading (avg)	102.6	102.6	102.6	102.6	102.6
Deviation (d)=|avg−r|	2.4	5.6	1.4	5.4	3.6
Accepted reading			Accept		
Within the deviation limit? (d<dev_limit)	Yes	Yes	Yes	Yes	Yes
Stake for transfer (10%)	0	0	0	0	0
Stake for fee (5%)	5	5	5	5	5
Revised stakes	100	100	100	100	100

Iteration 4

TABLE 2.5
Iteration 4 (Normal Operation)

Sensor Number	1	2	3	4	5
Current stake (s)	100	100	100	100	100
Reading received (r)	102	94	98	95	102
Contributor? (s>min_stake)	True	True	True	True	True
Average reading (avg)	98.2	98.2	98.2	98.2	98.2
Deviation (d)=|avg−r|	3.8	4.2	0.2	3.2	3.8
Accepted reading			Accept		
Within the deviation limit? (d<dev_limit)	Yes	Yes	Yes	Yes	Yes
Stake for transfer (10%)	0	0	0	0	0
Stake for fee (5%)	5	5	5	5	5
Revised stakes	100	100	100	100	100

Iteration 5

TABLE 2.6
Iteration 5 (Normal Operation)

Sensor Number	1	2	3	4	5
Current stake (s)	100	100	100	100	100
Reading received (r)	96	97	95	96	92
Contributor? (s>min_stake)	True	True	True	True	True
Average reading (avg)	95.2	95.2	95.2	95.2	95.2
Deviation (d)=|avg−r|	0.8	1.8	0.2	0.8	3.2
Accepted reading			Accept		
Within the deviation limit? (d<dev_limit)	Yes	Yes	Yes	Yes	Yes
Stake for transfer (10%)	0	0	0	0	0
Stake for fee (5%)	5	5	5	5	5
Revised stakes	100	100	100	100	100

This continues for 15 more iterations. The result is summarized below.

Iter: Iteration number

R1–R5: Reading from sensors 1–5

A: Accepted reading

In: Within dev_limits

Out: Outside dev_limits

S1–S5: Revised stake for sensors 1–5

TABLE 2.7

Iterations 6–20 (Normal Operation)

Iter	R1–R5					A	In	Out	S1–S5				
6	103	96	98	107	108	103	All	Nil	100	100	100	100	100
7	107	108	106	91	109	106	1,2,3,5	4	102.5	102.5	102.5	90	102.5
8	94	94	98	104	101	98	All	Nil	102.5	102.5	102.5	90	102.5
9	100	101	103	92	102	100	All	Nil	102.5	102.5	102.5	90	102.5
10	101	99	91	99	90	99	All	Nil	102.5	102.5	102.5	90	102.5
11	104	103	104	99	96	103	All	Nil	102.5	102.5	102.5	90	102.5
12	101	103	106	98	98	101	All	Nil	102.5	102.5	102.5	90	102.5
13	101	103	104	98	100	101	All	Nil	102.5	102.5	102.5	90	102.5
14	101	97	101	97	105	101	All	Nil	102.5	102.5	102.5	90	102.5
15	104	93	105	105	108	104	All	Nil	102.5	102.5	102.5	90	102.5
16	105	101	95	97	109	101	All	Nil	102.5	102.5	102.5	90	102.5
17	98	101	104	108	100	101	All	Nil	102.5	102.5	102.5	90	102.5
18	101	104	100	98	109	101	All	Nil	102.5	102.5	102.5	90	102.5
19	106	106	103	98	93	103	All	Nil	102.5	102.5	102.5	90	102.5
20	101	99	90	98	95	98	All	Nil	102.5	102.5	102.5	90	102.5

The system seems highly stable, and only one case occurred when a sensor was found to misbehave, and the stake got transferred. That iteration is elaborated below.

Iteration 7

TABLE 2.8

Iteration 7 (Normal Operation)

Sensor Number	1	2	3	4	5
Current stake (s)	100	100	100	100	100
Reading received (r)	107	108	106	91	109
Contributor? (s>min_stake)	True	True	True	True	True
Average reading (avg)	104.2	104.2	104.2	104.2	104.2
Deviation (d)=lavg–rl	2.8	3.8	1.8	13.2	4.8
Accepted reading			Accept		
Within the deviation limit? (d<dev_limit)	Yes	Yes	Yes	No	Yes
Stake for transfer (10%)	0	0	0	10	0
Stake for fee (5%)	5	5	5	5	5
Revised stakes	102.5	102.5	102.5	90	102.5

Here, sensor 4 was found to give an unnaturally low reading, and it was penalized by taking 10% of its stake and giving it to others. But it was found to rectify itself, and further iterations didn't seem to further modify the stake of any sensor.

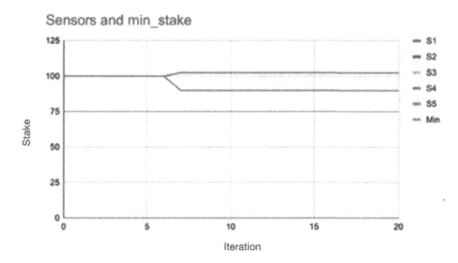

FIGURE 2.8 Change in stake of different sensors, compared to min_stake (Case 1).

Fee was not transferred in any of the cases since there were no validators (none of the nodes had a stake less than 75).

On analysing the variation in stake for each sensor, the system is seen to be extremely stable and reliable. The variation is depicted in Figure 2.8.

Case 2: System failure

The parameters for this experiment are as follows:

Number of sensors = 5, Starting stake for each sensor = 100

Minimum stake needed for contribution (min_stake) = 75

Number of iterations simulated = 20, Deviation limit (dev_limit) = 10

Stake penalty = 10%, Validation fee = 5%

Since this is a known case of system failure, all iterations are given in detail. The readings are taken as random numbers between 70 and 130. This simulates a non-ideal scenario, where the readings have a good chance of violating dev_limit. Tables 2.9–2.18 summarize the performance of the model at each iteration.

Iteration 1

TABLE 2.9
Iteration 1 (Case: System Failure)

Sensor Number	1	2	3	4	5
Current stake (s)	100	100	100	100	100
Reading received (r)	114	90	116	116	123
Contributor? (s>min_stake)	True	True	True	True	True
Average reading (avg)	111.8	111.8	111.8	111.8	111.8
Deviation (d)=|avg−r|	2.2	21.8	4.2	4.2	11.2
Accepted reading	Accept				
Within the deviation limit? (d<dev_limit)	Yes	No	Yes	Yes	No
Stake for transfer (10%)	0	10	0	0	10
Stake for fee (5%)	5	5	5	5	5
Revised stakes	106.67	90	106.67	106.67	90

During the first iteration itself, there is a variation in reading from sensor 2. This results in its stake getting reduced by 10% and distributed to others. Since there are no validators, even though the stake is set apart for fee, it is unused, and returned to the contributors. Similar behaviour is found in subsequent iterations also, with a number of sensors giving invalid output.

Iteration 2

TABLE 2.10
Iteration 2 (Case: System Failure)

Sensor Number	1	2	3	4	5
Current stake (s)	106.67	90	106.67	106.67	90
Reading received (r)	78	102	101	100	127
Contributor? (s>min_stake)	True	True	True	True	True
Average reading (avg)	101.6	101.6	101.6	101.6	101.6
Deviation (d)=|avg−r|	23.6	0.4	0.6	1.6	25.4
Accepted reading		Accept			
Within the deviation limit? (d<dev_limit)	No	Yes	Yes	Yes	No
Stake for transfer (10%)	10.667	0	0	0	9
Stake for fee (5%)	5.33	4.5	5.33	5.33	4.5
Revised stakes	96	96.56	113.22	113.22	81

Iteration 3

TABLE 2.11
Iteration 3 (Case: System Failure)

Sensor Number	1	2	3	4	5
Current stake (s)	96	96.56	113.22	113.22	81
Reading received (r)	119	123	84	95	96
Contributor? (s>min_stake)	True	True	True	True	True
Average reading (avg)	103.4	103.4	103.4	103.4	103.4
Deviation (d)=|avg−r|	15.6	19.6	19.4	8.4	7.4
Accepted reading					Accept
Within the deviation limit? (d<dev_limit)	No	No	No	Yes	Yes
Stake for transfer (10%)	9.6	9.656	11.322	0	0
Stake for fee (5%)	4.8	4.83	5.66	5.66	4.05
Revised stakes	86.4	86.9	101.9	128.51	96.29

Iteration 4

TABLE 2.12
Iteration 4 (Case: System Failure)

Sensor Number	1	2	3	4	5
Current stake (s)	86.4	86.9	101.9	128.51	96.29
Reading received (r)	119	119	89	105	129
Contributor? (s>min_stake)	True	True	True	True	True
Average reading (avg)	112.2	112.2	112.2	112.2	112.2
Deviation (d)=|avg−r|	6.8	6.8	23.2	7.2	16.8
Accepted reading	Accept	Accept			
Within the deviation limit? (d<dev_limit)	Yes	Yes	No	Yes	No
Stake for transfer (10%)	0	0	10.19	0	9.629
Stake for fee (5%)	4.32	4.35	5.09	6.43	4.81
Revised stakes	93	93.5	91.71	135.12	86.66

Iteration 5

TABLE 2.13
Iteration 5 (Case: System Failure)

Sensor Number	1	2	3	4	5
Current stake (s)	93	93.5	91.71	135.12	86.66
Reading received (r)	122	112	91	117	120
Contributor? (s>min_stake)	True	True	True	True	True
Average reading (avg)	112.4	112.4	112.4	112.4	112.4
Deviation (d)=|avg−r|	9.6	0.4	21.4	4.6	7.6
Accepted reading		Accept			
Within the deviation limit? (d<dev_limit)	Yes	Yes	No	Yes	Yes
Stake for transfer (10%)	0	0	9.171	0	0
Stake for fee (5%)	4.65	4.68	4.59	6.76	4.33
Revised stakes	95.3	95.8	82.54	137.41	88.95

Iteration 6

TABLE 2.14
Iteration 6 (Case: System Failure)

Sensor Number	1	2	3	4	5
Current stake (s)	95.3	95.8	82.54	137.41	88.95
Reading received (r)	122	129	94	78	76
Contributor? (s>min_stake)	True	True	True	True	True
Average reading (avg)	99.8	99.8	99.8	99.8	99.8
Deviation (d)=|avg−r|	22.2	29.2	5.8	21.8	23.8
Accepted reading			Accept		
Within the deviation limit? (d<dev_limit)	No	No	Yes	No	No
Stake for transfer (10%)	9.53	9.58	0	13.741	8.895
Stake for fee (5%)	4.77	4.79	4.13	6.87	4.45
Revised stakes	85.77	86.22	124.29	123.67	80.06

Iteration 7

TABLE 2.15
Iteration 7 (Case: System Failure)

Sensor Number	1	2	3	4	5
Current stake (s)	85.77	86.22	124.29	123.67	80.06
Reading received (r)	84	78	115	99	122
Contributor? (s>min_stake)	True	True	True	True	True
Average reading (avg)	99.6	99.6	99.6	99.6	99.6
Deviation (d)=|avg−r|	15.6	21.6	15.4	0.6	22.4
Accepted reading				Accept	
Within the deviation limit? (d<dev_limit)	No	No	No	Yes	No
Stake for transfer (10%)	8.577	8.622	12.429	0	8.006
Stake for fee (5%)	4.29	4.31	6.22	4.95	4.003
Revised stakes	77.2	77.6	111.86	161.3	72.05

At the end of iteration 7, the stake of sensor 5 has reduced below 75, because of repeated invalid readings. Hence, from the next iteration, it will assume only the role of the validator. Even if it generates a value, it will not be taken into account for acceptance.

Iteration 8

TABLE 2.16
Iteration 8 (Case: System Failure)

Sensor Number	1	2	3	4	5
Current stake (s)	77.2	77.6	111.86	161.3	72.05
Reading received (r)	114	77	126	118	85
Contributor? (s>min_stake)	True	True	True	True	False
Average reading (avg)	108.75	108.75	108.75	108.75	108.75
Deviation (d)=|avg−r|	5.25	31.75	17.25	9.25	23.75
Accepted reading	Accept				
Within the deviation limit? (d<dev_limit)	Yes	No	No	Yes	No
Stake for transfer (10%)	0	7.76	11.186	0	Validator
Stake for fee (5%)	3.86	3.88	5.59	8.07	Ineligible
Revised stakes	86.67	69.84	100.67	170.77	72.05

Sensor 5 has acted as the validator in this iteration. Stake transfers happen as usual. The stake is also kept apart for the fee, and there is a validator available for receiving the stake. But no transfer happens since the validator still gave a reading which is quite far from the average and doesn't seem to be reliable yet. Hence, stakes are returned. In addition, the stake for sensor 2 has moved below 75. Hence, two validators will be available in the next iteration.

Iteration 9

TABLE 2.17
Iteration 9 (Case: System Failure)

Sensor Number	1	2	3	4	5
Current stake (s)	86.67	69.84	100.67	170.77	72.05
Reading received (r)	111	106	123	92	126
Contributor? (s>min_stake)	True	False	True	True	False
Average reading (avg)	108.67	108.67	108.67	108.67	108.67
Deviation (d)=|avg−r|	2.33	2.67	14.33	16.67	17.33
Accepted reading	Accept				
Within the deviation limit? (d<dev_limit)	Yes	Yes	No	No	No
Stake for transfer (10%)	0	Validator	10.07	17.077	Validator
Stake for fee (5%)	4.33	Eligible	5.04	8.53	Ineligible
Revised stakes	108.12	87.74	86.07	146.01	72.05

In this iteration, there are two validators. Sensor 2 was able to generate a good reading in this round of execution, while sensor 5 still gave a poor reading. Hence, the stake set apart for fee is transferred completely to sensor 2, and it is able to recover from the validator state back to the contributor state.

Iteration 10

TABLE 2.18
Iteration 10 (Case: System Failure)

Sensor Number	1	2	3	4	5
Current stake (s)	108.12	87.74	86.07	146.01	72.05
Reading received (r)	124	123	89	95	83
Contributor? (s>min_stake)	True	True	True	True	False
Average reading (avg)	107.75	107.75	107.75	107.75	107.75
Deviation (d)=|avg−r|	16.25	15.25	18.75	12.75	24.75
Accepted reading	Halt	Halt	Halt	Halt	Halt
Within the deviation limit? (d<dev_limit)	No	No	No	No	No
Stake for transfer (10%)	Halt	Halt	Halt	Halt	Halt
Stake for fee (5%)	Halt	Halt	Halt	Halt	Halt
Revised stakes	Halt	Halt	Halt	Halt	Halt

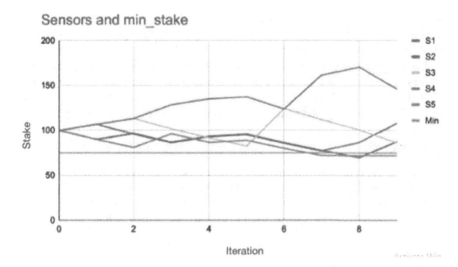

FIGURE 2.9   Variation in stake for each sensor, compared with min_stake (Case 2).

Since none of the contributors could generate a value within the deviation limit, the system is assumed to have failed. This case occurs only when sensors give radically diverging values, and that is always taken as an alert. Hence, the system shut down before completing the quota of 20 iterations it was originally designed to complete.

The graph in Figure 2.9 shows a highly erratic behaviour in terms of stakes, and two sensors breached the minimum threshold. But the algorithm was able to behave in such a way that it was able to reinstate the contribution privilege of one of the sensors as it started giving proper readings. The same can be done when faulty sensors are replaced. As the new sensor starts giving proper readings, its stake will be recovered.

2.7   CONCLUSION

The success of blockchain technology is not limited to the immutability offered by the architecture. It is also because of the variety of consensus models offered by it. This chapter explored the use of one such model – PoS, which ensures that transactions can be executed only by nodes that have enough "stake" associated with them. The stake gives the equivalence of authority, which is transferred within the blockchain as transactions proceed. This concept was adapted to ensure distributed reliability of IIoT implementations through a similar consensus mechanism.

In this implementation, consensus is reached by looking at the stake carried by each node, which is initially preset to a common value. As the node generates reliable values, the stake either remains consistent or increases. If values become unreliable, nodes end up losing their stake, and any node without enough stake cannot contribute values to the system. The algorithm also gives enough provisions for a misbehaving node to return to the contributory role.

The proposed model assumes a sterile environment in the IIoT ecosystem and ignores all security and privacy considerations. They have been abstracted out when the term "node" is used. An edge-based solution for the problem is proposed by Pavithran et al. [23], and further options are explored by Saxena et al. [24].

REFERENCES

1. Boyes, H., Hallaq, B., Cunningham, J., & Watson, T. 2018. The industrial Internet of Things (IIoT): an analysis framework. *Computers in Industry*, 101: 1–12.
2. Aziz, A., Schelén, O., & Bodin, U. 2020. A study on Industrial IoT for the mining industry: synthesized architecture and open research directions. *IoT*, 1(2): 529–550.
3. Moore, S. J., Nugent, C. D., Zhang, S., & Cleland, I. 2020. IoT reliability: a review leading to 5 key research directions. *CCF Transactions on Pervasive Computing and Interaction*, 2: 1–17.
4. Wu, Y., Dai, H. N., & Wang, H. 2020. Convergence of blockchain and edge computing for secure and scalable IIoT critical infrastructures in industry 4.0. *IEEE Internet of Things Journal*, 8(4): 2300–2317.
5. Bhushan, B., & Sahoo, G. 2020. Requirements, protocols, and security challenges in wireless sensor networks: an industrial perspective. In *Handbook of Computer Networks and Cyber Security*, 683–713. Springer, Cham.
6. Sethi, R., Bhushan, B., Sharma, N., Kumar, R., & Kaushik, I. 2021. Applicability of industrial IoT in diversified sectors: evolution, applications and challenges. In *Multimedia Technologies in the Internet of Things Environment*, 45–67. Springer, Singapore. Doi: 10.1007/978-981-15-7965-3_4.
7. Senathipathi, K., Kayalvili, S., Anitha, P., & Henna, K. C. 2021. Blockchain integrated IIoT–future of IoT. *Materials Today: Proceedings*. Doi: 10.1016/j.matpr.2020.12.1051.
8. Nguyen, C. T., Hoang, D. T., Nguyen, D. N., Niyato, D., Nguyen, H. T., & Dutkiewicz, E. 2019. Proof-of-stake consensus mechanisms for future blockchain networks: fundamentals, applications and opportunities. *IEEE Access*, 7: 85727–85745.
9. Kshetri, N. 2017. Can blockchain strengthen the Internet of Things? *IT Professional*, 19(4): 68–72. Doi: 10.1109/MITP.2017.3051335.
10. Fernández-Caramés, T. M., & Fraga-Lamas, P. 2018. A review on the use of blockchain for the Internet of Things. *IEEE Access*, 6: 32979–33001. Doi: 10.1109/ACCESS.2018.2842685.
11. Dai, H. N., Zheng, Z., & Zhang, Y. 2019. Blockchain for Internet of Things: a survey. *IEEE Internet of Things Journal*, 6(5): 8076–8094. Doi: 10.1109/JIOT.2019.2920987.
12. Conoscenti, M., Vetro, A., & De Martin, J. C. 2016. November. Blockchain for the Internet of Things: a systematic literature review. In *2016 IEEE/ACS 13th International Conference of Computer Systems and Applications (AICCSA)*:1–6. IEEE. Doi: 10.1109/AICCSA.2016.7945805.
13. Wang, X., Zha, X., Ni, W., Liu, R. P., Guo, Y. J., Niu, X., & Zheng, K. 2019. Survey on blockchain for Internet of Things. *Computer Communications*, 136: 10–29. Doi: 10.1016/j.comcom.2019.01.006.
14. Ferrag, M. A., Derdour, M., Mukherjee, M., Derhab, A., Maglaras, L., & Janicke, H. 2018. Blockchain technologies for the internet of things: research issues and challenges. *IEEE Internet of Things Journal*, 6(2): 2188–2204. Doi: 10.1109/JIOT.2018.2882794.

15. Miller, D. 2018. Blockchain and the Internet of Things in the industrial sector. *IT Professional*, 20(3): 15–18. Doi: 10.1109/MITP.2018.032501742.
16. Fortino, G., Messina, F., Rosaci, D., & Sarné, G. M. :2019. Using blockchain in a reputation-based model for grouping agents in the Internet of Things. *IEEE Transactions on Engineering Management*, 67(4): 1231–1243. Doi: 10.1109/TEM.2019.2918162.
17. Kang, J., Xiong, Z., Niyato, D., Wang, P., Ye, D., & Kim, D. I. 2018. Incentivizing consensus propagation in proof-of-stake based consortium blockchain networks. *IEEE Wireless Communications Letters*, 8(1): 157–160. Doi: 10.1109/LWC.2018.2864758.
18. Yang, F., Zhou, W., Wu, Q., Long, R., Xiong, N. N., & Zhou, M. 2019. Delegated proof of stake with downgrade: a secure and efficient blockchain consensus algorithm with downgrade mechanism. *IEEE Access*, 7: 118541–118555. Doi: 10.1109/ACCESS.2019.2935149.
19. Bhushan, B., Sinha, P., Sagayam, K. M., & Andrew, J. 2021. Untangling blockchain technology: a survey on state of the art, security threats, privacy services, applications and future research directions. *Computers & Electrical Engineering*, 90: 106897. Doi: 10.1016/j.compeleceng.2020.106897.
20. Bhushan, B., Sahoo, C., Sinha, P., & Khamparia, A. 2021. Unification of Blockchain and Internet of Things (BIoT): requirements, working model, challenges and future directions. *Wireless Networks*, 27(1): 55–90.
21. Uddin, M. A., Stranieri, A., Gondal, I., & Balasubramanian, V. 2021. A survey on the adoption of blockchain in IoT: challenges and solutions. *Blockchain: Research and Applications*, 2(2): 100006.
22. Krishna, B., Rajkumar, P., & Velde, V. 2021. Integration of blockchain technology for security and privacy in Internet of Things. *Materials Today: Proceedings*. Doi: 10.1016/j.matpr.2021.01.606.
23. Pavithran, D., Al-Karaki, J. N., & Shaalan, K. 2021. Edge-based blockchain architecture for event-driven IoT using hierarchical identity based encryption. *Information Processing & Management*, 58(3): 102528. Doi: 10.1016/j.ipm.2021.102528.
24. Saxena, S., Bhushan, B., & Ahad, M. A. 2021. Blockchain based solutions to secure IoT: background, integration trends and a way forward. *Journal of Network and Computer Applications*, 103050. Doi: 10.1016/j.jnca.2021.103050.

3 Blockchain Technology for IoT Security of Smart City Applications

W. Basmi and A. Boulmakoul
Hassan II University of Casablanca

L. Karim
Hassan 1st University

CONTENTS

3.1 INTRODUCTION

Data security has been a major concern of modern science and continues to contribute to innovation, maintaining a steady curve of making new technologies to protect all sorts of information from theft and corruption. Side by side, we are transiting to a world that operates a countless number of connected smart devices, also called "Internet of Things" or IoT in short, that work in interoperability and

DOI: 10.1201/9781003224075-3

conjunction with remote servers for various purposes in different domains (Fox et al. 2019), namely, agriculture (Puranik et al. 2019) supply chain (Pal and Kant 2018), healthcare (Al-Mahmud et al. 2020), traffic management (Akhtar et al. 2020) and the list goes on. These smart devices compose of smart phones, sensors, actuators and computer programs that constitute an ecosystem crucial to modern society's functioning. In fact, in just two decades, human societies turned from wired connected cell phones, zero to limited internet-connected machines and human-managed services, to wireless society and an uncountable number of connected devices producing a large amount of information. Yet, as formidable as it sounds, such grandiose and ubiquity is dangerous as any collateral damage to smart objects data and communication infrastructure could result in the demise of many vital services. Correspondingly, blockchain is a revolutionary technology adopted in cryptocurrencies, as the core payment network and constitutes of a decentralized ledger that holds multiple connected nodes of transactions, each works as a source of truth and forms a consensus to decide whether a transaction is eligible or not (Nakamoto 2009). While Blockchain is often employed with cryptocurrencies, it's also used in other fields and application sectors, such as digital identity (Takemiya and Vanieiev 2018), election (Cooley et al. 2018) and contract validation (Upadhyay et al. 2020). Consequently, there could possibly be a way to employ it in IoT applications and solve some of its challenges.

This chapter confers Blockchain utility as a security component of IoT applications, and how it mitigates the increasing risks of having a cyberworld made of connected objects sharing personal and non-personal data across the globe. We divided this work into four separate sections, and it is structured in the following order. In Section 3.2, we explore Blockchain as a new technology and the secrets of its reliability, additionally, we discuss its origins, its characteristics, its key components and the different protocols it uses that boosted its fame. In Section 3.3, we introduce smart cities, IoT applications concepts and how they have already become part of modern society, in a true omnipresence in our daily lives. Furthermore, we introduce the concept of complex events, and explain how they can enlarge the pool of choices to enrich the data harvest. Finally, in Section 3.4, we discuss and provide a methodical solution, in how Blockchain can be integrated into IoT applications to reinforce its security.

3.2 BLOCKCHAIN OVERVIEW

Blockchain and Bitcoin are two terms that are ubiquitous in the literature. Yet, they are both completely different, but connected, as we shall confer in the following subsection.

3.2.1 INTRODUCING BLOCKCHAIN

At the beginning of 2009, Satoshi Nakamoto created the first genesis block of Bitcoin, detonating the birth of the first original cryptocurrency Bitcoin and its backbone network technology Blockchain was brought to light (Nakamoto 2009). Blockchain refers to a series of immutable blocks data structure composed of indefinite number of blocks holding encrypted information about a specific transaction. In other words, it represents a linked list where each block has a reference to the previous one, additionally, its immutability consists of how each block cryptography information depends on the previous one; therefore, the bigger the ledger, the more difficult it becomes to corrupt its data without the right technology. The major seller point of Blockchain is how naturally it provides data security without a third party; moreover, it had attracted a lot of attention and care, which helped in its improvement. Consequently, Blockchain has been developed and transformed over the last few years since 2009 and is portrayed in three different versions.

The first version of Blockchain refers to Blockchain 1.0, a Kickstarter that was used in developing Bitcoin, which enables any computer to start a node and become part of a network that replicates the ledger – also known as full nodes, digital wallets, mining rigs and mining software. Figure 3.1 illustrates how a Bitcoin transaction is processed and the role of Blockchain in its execution. The validation is called the Proof-of-Work (PoW) consensus process and it validates the transactions that happen within the nodes network. Upon creating the transaction by a light node, it is distributed and encrypted using cryptographic hashing. Then, the nodes participate in solving a problem whose difficulty escalates with the size of the ledger. This operation is called mining and requires important physical resources and energy capacity to function. Once a miner solves the problem, the transaction is committed and broadcast to all the present nodes in the P2P network, and in return, it receives a reward as a fee for having being part of the decentralized validation of the transaction, and consequently adding the block of information to the immutable chain (Schinckus 2020). This process is called the consensus protocol and it is important to allow the P2P network to cooperate and work together trustfully.

The blockchain protocol verifies and secures the blocks introduction into the ledger.

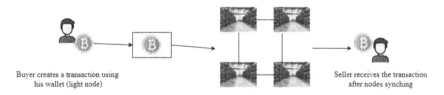

Buyer creates a transaction using his wallet (light node)

Seller receives the transaction after nodes synching

Transaction is distributed and validated using cryptographic hashing

- One Miner finds the solution
- Other miners validate the solution
- Miners are rewarded
- Transaction is committed in the blockchain and distributed over the nodes

FIGURE 3.1 Bitcoin transaction illustration.

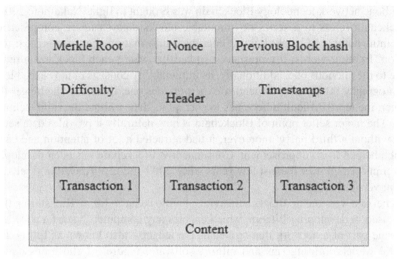

FIGURE 3.2 Blockchain block structure.

3.2.2 BLOCK STRUCTURE

The blockchain ledger functions autonomously using a P2P network and a public time-stamping server. It is made of many blocks; each block has a unique hash value representing its identifier.

The first block in the chain is the genesis block, a.k.a., the head of the ledger has no parent block, and is illustrated in Figure 3.2, its structure is split into two sections (Torky and Hassanein 2020):

- **Markle Tree Root Hash** – it is a hash used to verify all the block transactions and is made recursively as a binary tree of hash codes.
- **Timestamp** – Unix timestamp and is used to immutably track the creation and update time of the block to validate its integrity.
- **N-Bits** identifies the target threshold of hash code that specifies the valid block.
- **Nounce** is a random 4-byte number that is used in the cryptographic operations.
- **Parent Block Hash** is a 256-bit hash code that refers to the previous block.
- **Difficulty** is a 256-bit hash code that refers to the previous block.
- **Content** holds the transactions to be saved into the ledger.

3.2.3 CONSENSUS PROTOCOLS

Blockchain is a decentralized ledger made of many nodes connected in a P2P network managed by a timestamping server. In order to attach newly created blocks to the ledger, the consensus protocol aims to solve this problem: the consensus problem. The problem is equivalent to the Byzantine Generals Problem (BGP). The problem states of the generals can come to a common conclusion in the presence of traitors and miscommunications. Blockchain consensus protocols are BFT, and follow the convention Proof-of-*, in which their mechanism purpose is to decide which nodes will participate in validating the block (Panarello et al. 2018). In cryptocurrency, consensus protocols aim to increase the difficulty of the mining process in order to achieve the impenetrable layer of immutability, since each block is inter-dependent and altering the whole chain is theoretically possible, but without newer technological infrastructure (Quantum computers) (Fernández-Caramès and Fraga-Lamas 2020), this ordeal cost-wise is futile.

The PoW protocols are the first mechanisms adopted in Blockchain technology, where one party has to solve a computationally intensive mathematical problem to one party in order to prove that it has undergone an important effort. In the cryptocurrency context, the mathematical problem is a cryptographic puzzle and its difficulty scales with the size of the ledger. The efforts that PoW employs in creating the hash and verifying it are asymmetric. In fact, starting with the verification process, any small change to the block's hash will result in a negative match, since the output hash will be different. However, for the hash generation, the Blockchain network uses a cryptographic puzzle that can only be solved through a trial-and-error method, and the parameters given to these problems will always change and turns what could be possibly a generic task into an actual "work" with a cost in time. However, PoW protocols are obsolete because of their limitations in the number of transactions it can handle at one time (Nakamoto 2009), and also their energy cost that can have a negative impact on the environment if the Blockchain is public, namely, cryptocurrencies (O'Dwyer and Malone 2014).

PoW is proven to have many disadvantages, but it is still being used in Bitcoin and Ethereum as of 2021. However, the latter cryptocurrency will be switching to another consensus mechanism, which is Proof-of-Stake (PoS). It is designed mainly to face security threats that face PoW, such as the 51% attack – where malicious users take over 51% of the network majority, to corrupt voting when deciding whether a block is corrupted or not. In fact, when deciding to append a transaction to the blockchain, PoS protocols require that validator nodes must have a certain amount of blockchain tokens – coins in cryptocurrency terminology, in order to participate in the validation. Therefore, with this mechanism, the Blockchain forces the attackers to put themselves at risk in order to carry on the attack (Tasca and Tessone 2019).

A greener alternative to PoW, which is Proof-of-Space (PoS), that revolves around allocating disk space rather than computation. It's also a class of consensus mechanisms that is based on pre-requirements. In fact, instead of continuously searching and using effort to find solutions to cryptographic puzzles, before starting the nodes, store a list of possible solutions (plotting) and then use these solutions to start mining. Thus, an alternative proves to be more energy-efficient since it requires less electricity, and the prices of hard drives are cheaper than powerful processors (Dziembowski et al. 2013). The existence of PoW has led researchers to start finding alternatives that are cost-efficient, thus environment-friendly and secure to maintain the stability and the essential pillars of Blockchain.

3.2.4 SMART CONTRACTS

Blockchain is a technology that has enabled having a completely trustless system without needing the third parties to participate in a transaction between two of its users. Smart contracts are one other feature of Blockchain proposed by the lawyer and cryptographer Nick Szabo. They are simply digital forms of contract, i.e., a group of terms that needs to be met in order to execute certain tasks, such as transferring assets or doing a deposit (Alharby and van Moorsel 2017). Additionally, the essential documents are present on a public ledger and thus they also adhere to security from loss and can be backed up given there are enough nodes. Finally, smart contracts are scripted and are automatic; therefore, they don't require any intermediaries, and so they are convenient.

3.3   SMART CITY AND IOT APPLICATIONS

For a long decade, the prophecy of a world ruled by small smart devices was roaming speculator minds, then inspired many scientists and entrepreneurs to invest their resources to turn the whole world upside down with innovative technologies, which are part of our everyday lives. In the following section, we explain what sort of technology it is, and explore its magnitude in modern society.

3.3.1 GENERAL OVERVIEW

IoT plays an important role in building a space where smart things (group of physical or virtual objects connected to the internet) are connected and exchanging data either autonomously or as groups of units (Lo et al. 2019). Cloud computing, Machine learning and Data Analysis are employed in IoT construction (Panarello et al. 2018). For more than a decade, it has been a hot topic in the research field, and their textual existence has jumped over reality and has been crucial life of our lives for a long time now, and continues to cut through everything from natural, industrial to urban phenomenon. IoT has helped many cities around the world to increase their smartness spectrum, and so many of them now have been considered smart cities in newspapers headlines. Basically, a smart city is a term given to cities that make use of IoT to help decision-makers to automate urban and citizen services, bring forward facilities logistical and legislative to grow an ecosystem where small, big and large companies can thrive and contribute as well in IoT-isation of their respectful cities (Kummitha and Crutzen 2019). Moreover, the Smart city badge is a result of a bijective relationship between the city and its citizens, be they individuals or organizations as illustrated in Figure 3.3. In fact, the latter is involved in being part of decision-makers plans to generate feedback, enrich the process and optimize it up to its limits while in parallel, compacting the

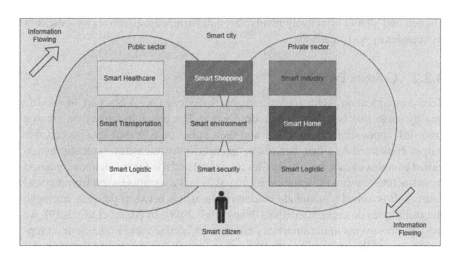

FIGURE 3.3   Smart city components.

city as a sum of its inhabitants and promoting the city's economy and the country that it takes part of (Basmi et al. 2020).

Most of human society activities' domains continued to evolve side by side since the old times. Agriculture being one of the major human technologies that helped our species thrive and multiply, went from traditional methods involving human labor, to mechanical machines controlled by humans, and it ended up now, with the combination of various devices operating autonomously to measure the environment playing factors that control the quality and characteristics of crops to meet the increasing food demand (Hsu et al. 2020). Likewise, the supply chain is one of the crucial sectors, and one of the many vital organs of an economy. Individuals and organizations alike now have become accustomed to track their goods from the provider to its destination. For this reason, many warehouse companies and factories are promoting techniques and policies ranging from ingenious to inhuman work conditions for their employees. For instance, in Huiyang, China, Alibaba's warehouse is almost completely managed by robots able to carry 500 kg of goods, they use lasers to avoid collision and are managed by a central application monitored by one single human being at once. In contrast, Amazon warehouse workers are one of the least paid in the U.S. ranging around 15 dollars per hour. Such jobs put a toll on the human body, and maybe solutions such as exoskeletons can help reduce musculoskeletal disorders (Bances et al. 2020), it is important to better come up with ergonomic solutions that don't involve individuals in repetitive tasks and can be replicated with smart devices. In a Utopian society, human resources are the most valuable asset for a society; thus, the latter infrastructure must be designed to produce individuals that are able to adapt to the fast technological leap that we are undergoing since the first industrial revolution. In fact, according to the Mckinsey Global Institute, 45 million Americans would lose their jobs by 2030 (Lund et al. 2021). Thus, IoT technologies must be aligned and should effectively revolve around being cost-effective, regardless of its complexity and creativity.

3.3.2 COMPLEX EVENTS

Telecommunication technologies and smart devices take a big part in the life quality surge that bestowed the modern world. But the cumulative data coming from IoT applications is analyzed and then either transformed into perceivable output consumed by other devices or grouped into ostensibly synthetic events called complex events. It's a higher-level concept and a software technology based on extracting relevant information from massive data streams issued from various sources. It is aimed to conclude hidden relationships between the data, although the techniques do certainly differ (Bruns et al. 2019). In Basmi et al. (2019), we use complex events in the smart city context, and define them as the abstract representation of the group of events that can occur within a smart city, for example: urban, natural or industrial events. We provided a data model that represents these events to be part of an interactive system that plays the role of a portal between sensors and actuators alike. Likewise, we have broadened the definitions of sensors and actuators, to be complex events related, and such, they correspond to any object virtual or physical that can communicate events either by observing or by receiving to transform it into an actual observable virtual or physical phenomenon. Thus, we create an environment where data circulates, but can also mature and turn into another form as shown in Figure 3.4.

To help in understanding the concepts we brought with the Complex events framework Portunus, we enriched the domain data model we presented in Basmi et al. (2020); it represents the system domain data model. In Figure 3.5, starting with the feature of interest, it represents the object that exists in the real world

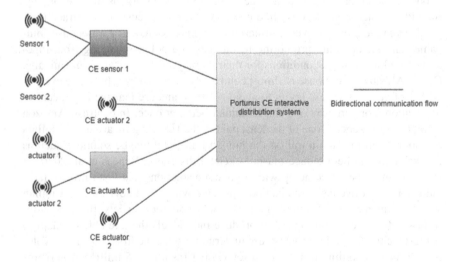

FIGURE 3.4 Complex events data distribution.

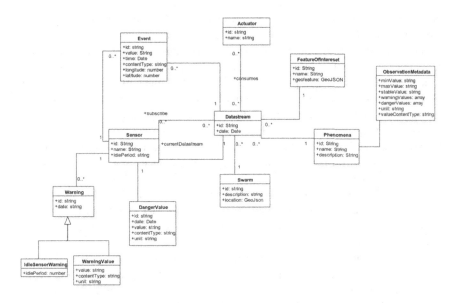

FIGURE 3.5 Portunus complex events domain data model.

and is linked to a data stream. A data stream is an object with an identifier that regroups a set of events collected by sensors that collect events related to a certain phenomenon, whose value's meta information can be found in the observation metadata data model and is later consumed by subscribed actuators. A sensor has other meta information that helps the system to recognize when any of its thresholds is attained such as the "WarningValue", "IddleSensorWarning" and "DangerValue". The data stream is the key to connect sensors and actuators interested in a certain feature of interest's phenomenon, regardless of its nature. This access opens possibilities for creating a much richer data pool and helps to expose underlying links between separate different events.

3.4 IOT AND BLOCKCHAIN INTEGRATION

After hovering over Blockchain and IoT, many flags can be raised such as the possibilities of combining these two technologies, and their benefits to promote a secure ecosystem for information circulating in the smart city sphere. Thus, we try to address these topics in the following sections.

3.4.1 IoT Security Deflation

The ubiquitous presence of IoT could be considered a blessing as it replaces manual or systematic services managed by humans with replaceable high preferment small machines. The latter communicate with a distant server or directly within its unit to achieve its task using the data they collected from the outside world: surrounding environment, inanimate objects, natural or industrial phenomenon and humans. IoT connected devices keep growing and every year predictions exceed billions of devices. Although the numbers are not precise, just 10 billion of devices if not less are exposed to the outer world and their data physically exists and represents a snapshot of part of it at a specific point of time. And much like every database or generally a system, malicious entities could prey on the data for the aim of stealing it or corrupting it and consequently inflicting real world damage.

As an example, in 2016, many major high-profile websites were shutdown using a malware called **Mirai**. The virus continuously scans the internet for the IP address of IoT devices. Mirai includes a table of IP address ranges that it will not infect, including private networks and addresses allocated to the United States Postal Service and Department of Defense. A large part of the addresses Mira was able to scrap were IoT devices, which are still mapped to their factory settings and credentials, which were part of its algorithm. It then proceeds to take control of the device, conceal itself by consuming a larger part of bandwidth, delete any sort of malware and block all administrative ports to protect itself, and finally, upon rebooting, Mirai will reinfect the device again within instants. Consequently, the virus took over what could be a large portion of the billion devices that fortifies IoT's reputation and build an army of infected devices that set GitHub, Twitter, Reddit, Netflix, Airbnb and many other services as their DDOS (Distributed Denial-of-Service) attack target and out of service for an entire day (Zhang et al. 2020).

Many similar incidents happened in the following years and will still happen. However, with the increasing years' number, the modern world is converging toward a tighter coupling and stronger dependency on IoT, and the consequences could be more serious than 5 minutes without access to your favorite search engine, taking for example, self-driving cars and urban IoT devices.

In the literature, Blockchain could be described as the Messiah of data security with its solid natural secure architecture based on anonymity, immutability and trustlessness. However, mixing these two technologies is still a problem in its infancy and is subject to many proposals and solutions in research (Tran et al. 2021). Additionally, some techniques may not be suitable for different applications and can only be applied within the context of the same or a similar scenario.

3.4.2   IoT Applications Architecture

Figure 3.6 illustrates the four stages comprising IoT applications in general. The first stage regroups the part that interacts with the outside world, covering both physical and virtual things (sensors and actuators alike). Generally, IoT devices have limited processing capabilities and restrict their tasks exclusively to creating measurements or generating an output. Any data manipulation would only be in the context of serving these purposes. The second stage represents the Internet gateway, the transmission support, the tools and programs used to transform analog measurements into their digital form, and send them over the internet or directly to other devices through Bluetooth or a similar medium. The third stage represents the technology responsible for preprocessing and transforming data

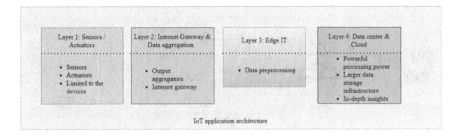

FIGURE 3.6 IoT applications architecture stages.

before being sent to the data center. The technological infrastructure present in this stage relieves the data centers from the heavy resources' usage. It is also referred to in the literature as the fog layer, which comprises technologies and techniques that ease the burden on the end devices (Bhushan et al. 2020). For example, it can play the role of data filtering using machine learning to detect anomalies, filtering abnormal transmissions, or optimization using some volatile memory to control a swarm of devices. Finally, the fourth stage represents the destination of the prepared data, where the latter is harvested and deeply analyzed, managed and stored (Fuller 2019). There are other logical architectures that resemble the four stages of IoT architecture, but apart from notations and slight differences, they remain the same. The next step is to determine the right role for Blockchain within an IoT system. We start with the least relevant possibilities and discuss the validity of their applications.

3.4.3 Blockchain as a Component in the IoT Architecture

After presenting IoT applications as complex systems with a flexible architecture, we discuss how Blockchain can be used as an efficient extension in the latter.

3.4.3.1 Blockchain as a Secure Data Store

In Tran et al. (2021), the logical position of Blockchain in an IoT system as the functional replaceable module of the system comes with the Blockchain. Although the major mainstream technologies using Blockchain such as cryptocurrencies, for example, are public, it can also be incorporated as a private solution (Bhushan et al. 2021). Although, the module varies between Access control management, Business process orchestration, data storage, authentication management, trust management system or communication channel as examples of the appliance. IoT applications are systems that generate a large amount of data in a very short amount of time, wrapping the data inside transactions to store them securely would be deterrent and will slow down the system performance with the growing blockchain transactions number being stored, given how much time and delay it takes for the blockchain nodes take to validate incoming transactions, that scales with the increasing difficulty and the network load (Cao et al. 2020). More importantly, in many use case scenarios, the output data is not important as single

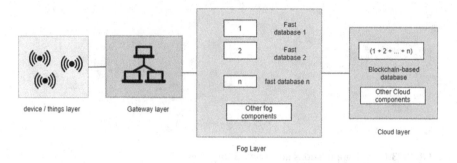

FIGURE 3.7   IoT applications architecture using Blockchain as a database.

measurements or observations regardless of their nature, but the data is important when treated as a group of large chunks segmented by intervals of timestamps or specific properties. However, it is not far from saying that the integrity and the data gathered by the devices are not important, in fact, the same statement that says how units of data are not as valuable as their sum, if most of the units are corrupt, then the operations and analysis will have to be applied on corrupted data, and as a result, the results will be nothing but misleading noise. Therefore, an IoT architecture relying on Blockchain to store its data must not compromise speed and responsiveness. Figure 3.7 features an architecture, where the data center and cloud stage provide a Blockchain database. As mentioned earlier, it would be non-optimal to store and try to read the data within systems that require high interactivity. Therefore, to compensate it, the cloud layer would provide a registry that can run batch operations to synchronize with fragments distributed over many components in the fog layer that serve as fast replicate databases.

3.4.3.2   Blockchain as an Authentication Manager

In Basmi et al. (2020), we presented an architecture for complex space time events framework, highlighting four layers \emph{(i) Data distribution layer}: it hosts components that collect complex events from sensors and distribute it to actuators. \emph{(ii) Logging Layer}: logs all system activities including errors, warnings and system information. \emph{(iii) Object data Information Layer}: provides components that take care of storing all events circulating in the system, the things that communicate with it and all the features of interest with their respective information. \emph{(iii) Authentication Layer}: holds components that control authentication and access for connected complex event objects. Designing the system as a swarm of microservices within its components provides endless possibilities to evolve the architecture physical components (database systems, decentralized system orchestration frameworks and core applications), as they are autonomous and either communicate choreographically, using request-response or both (Newman 2015). We chose to not present the inner components in detail of the distribution, logging and object data information layers to keep an emphasis on how we integrate Blockchain as an authentication manager.

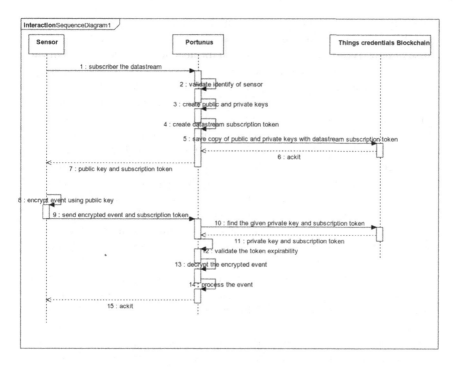

FIGURE 3.8 Saving CE sensors authentication credentials in a Blockchain database.

In the previous architecture, the authentication layer provides the possibility to verify the digital identity of sensors, by generating expirable Public-key cryptography and subscription token – the subscription token is used to connect to a specific data stream. The sensor holds the public key by which it encrypts its data and sends it with the token to save its events. Internally, the authenticator saves its data within a centralized database. By replacing the centralized database with a blockchain-based database, the whole framework would benefit from enhanced security. In Figure 3.8, we show how a sensor needs to undertake a process in which the system creates a token and couple of public and private keys for it, so it can use it to encrypt its events and send it to the system gatherer service. Portunus takes the blockchain as a database, except that it's a database that is very hard to break given how each block holds the history of the entire hashes of the previous transactions saved. If then, the retrieved token has not expired, then it proceeds to decrypt the hash using the private key as a secondary barrier, if it fails the event is rejected, but if it works then it is processed and saved in the system and distributed to the other actuators that are part of the same data stream.

3.5 CONCLUSION

With the arrival of cryptocurrencies, Blockchain has been one of the game players in technological revolution in the last decade. Thanks to its natural security, anonymity, auditability and decentralization, many cryptocurrencies value has jumped from a few hundred dollars to dozens of thousands of dollars over the course of only 6 years. Such success helped this technology to be adopted in various other domains, including IoT. IoT applications are systems that manipulate a network of sensors and actuators to exchange and operate on their data, either locally or globally. On the other hand, some cities are called Smart, when their decision-makers use IoT to improve their vital services. A Smart city involves the sum of individuals and organizations from public and private sectors to densify the amount of data circulating within its diameter and aerate its channels. Sometimes, data or specifically singular events propagating within a city can be assembled and can form what are called complex events. Furthermore, complex events do also cover up phenomenon that are other than natural, such as industrial, urban events, or basically any observable object that can emit meaningful data. In the same context, Portunus is a complex events distribution framework that provides essential components to manipulate complex events. In effect, in addition to the billions of smart devices connected to the internet, we get more additional candidates to send over an additional form of data, raising the question of whether there can be a possible way to improve IoT applications security. Hence, we found that Blockchain can be adapted intelligently to serve this purpose, as long as we don't compromise the rapid and lightning-fast interactivity of these systems. For this reason, we proposed a schema on how the integration can be accomplished, through the extension of the authenticator with Blockchain to secure cryptographic keys database.

REFERENCES

Akhtar, M., M. Raffeh, F. ul Zaman et al. (2020). Development of congestion level based dynamic traffic management system using IoT. In *2020 International Conference on Electrical, Communication, and Computer Engineering (ICECCE)*, pp. 1–6. Doi: 10.1109/ICECCE49384.2020.9179375.

Alharby, M. and A. van Moorsel (2017, 08). Blockchain based smart contracts: a systematic mapping study. In *CSIT-2017*, pp. 125–140. Doi: 10.5121/csit.2017.71011.

Al-Mahmud, O., K. Khan, R. Roy, and F. Mashuque Alamgir (2020). Internet of things (IoT) based smart health care medical box for elderly people. In *2020 International Conference for Emerging Technology (INCET)*, pp. 1–6. Doi: 10.1109/INCET49848.2020.9153994.

Bances, E., U. Schneider, J. Siegert, and T. Bauernhansl (2020). Exoskeletons towards industries 4.0: benefits and challenges of the IoT communication architecture. *Procedia Manufacturing* 42, 49–56. International Conference on Industry 4.0 and Smart Manufacturing (ISM 2019). Doi: 10.1016/j.promfg.2020.02.087.

Basmi, W., A. Boulmakoul, L. Karim, and A. Lbath (2020). Modern approach to design a distributed and scalable platform architecture for smart cities complex events data collection. *Procedia Computer Science* 170, 43–50. *The 11th International Conference on Ambient Systems, Networks and Technologies (ANT)/The 3rd International Conference on Emerging Data and Industry 4.0 (EDI40)/Affiliated Workshops*. Doi: 10.1016/j.procs.2020.03.008.

Bhushan, B., A. Khamparia, K. M. Sagayam, S. K. Sharma, M. A. Ahad, and N. C. Debnath (2020). Blockchain for smart cities: a review of architectures, integration trends and future research directions. *Sustainable Cities and Society* 61, 102360. Doi: 10.1016/j.scs.2020.102360.

Bhushan, B., C. Sahoo, P. Sinha, and A. Khamparia (2021, Jan). Unification of blockchain and Internet of Things (bIoT): requirements, working model, challenges and future directions. *Wireless Networks* 27(1), 55–90. Doi: 10.1007/s11276-020-02445-6.

Bruns, R., J. Dunkel, and N. Offel (2019). Learning of complex event processing rules with genetic programming. *Expert Systems with Applications* 129, 186–199. Doi: 10.1016/j.eswa.2019.04.007.

Cao, B., Z. Zhang, D. Feng, S. Zhang, L. Zhang, M. Peng, and Y. Li (2020). Performance analysis and comparison of PoW, PoS and DAG based blockchains. *Digital Communications and Networks* 6(4), 480–485. Doi: 10.1016/j.dcan.2019.12.001.

Cooley, R., S. Wolf, and M. Borowczak (2018). Blockchain-based election infrastructures. In *2018 IEEE International Smart Cities Conference (ISC2)*, pp. 1–4. Doi: 10.1109/ISC2.2018.8656988.

Dziembowski, S., S. Faust, V. Kolmogorov, and K. Pietrzak (2013). *Proofs of Space*. Cryptology ePrint Archive, Report 2013/796. https://ia.cr/2013/796.

Fernández-Caramès, T. M. and P. Fraga-Lamas (2020). Towards post-quantum blockchain: a review on blockchain cryptography resistant to quantum computing attacks. *IEEE Access* 8, 21091–21116. Doi: 10.1109/ACCESS.2020.2968985.

Fox, J., A. Donnellan, and L. Doumen (2019). The deployment of an IoT network infrastructure, as a localised regional service. In *2019 IEEE 5th World Forum on Internet of Things (WF-IoT)*, pp. 319–324. Doi: 10.1109/WF-IoT.2019.8767188.

Fuller, J. (2019, Feb). How to design an IoT-ready infrastructure: the 4-stage architecture. Accessed August 24, 2021.

Hsu, T.-C., H. Yang, Y.-C. Chung, and C.-H. Hsu (2020). A creative IoT agriculture platform for cloud fog computing. *Sustainable Computing: Informatics and Systems* 28, 100285. Doi: 10.1016/j.suscom.2018.10.006.

Kummitha, R. K. R. and N. Crutzen (2019). Smart cities and the citizen-driven internet of things: a qualitative inquiry into an emerging smart city. *Technological Forecasting and Social Change* 140, 44–53. Doi: 10.1016/j.techfore.2018.12.001.

Lo, S. K., Y. Liu, S. Y. Chia, X. Xu, Q. Lu, L. Zhu, and H. Ning (2019). Analysis of blockchain solutions for IoT: a systematic literature review. *IEEE Access* 7, 58822–58835. Doi: 10.1109/ACCESS.2019.2914675.

Lund, S., A. Madgavkar, J. Manyika, S. Smit, K. Ellingrud, and O. Robinson (2021, Mar). The future of work after covid-19. Accessed August 24, 2021.

Nakamoto, S. (2009, Mar.). Bitcoin: a peer-to-peer electronic cash system. *Cryptography Mailing list* at https://metzdowd.com. Doi: 10.2139/ssrn.3440802.

Newman, S. (2015). *Building Microservices Designing Fine-Grained Systems*. O'Reilly Media, Inc., Sebastopol, CA.

O'Dwyer, K. J. and D. Malone (2014). Bitcoin mining and its energy footprint. In *25th IET Irish Signals Systems Conference 2014 and 2014 China-Ireland International Conference on Information and Communications Technologies (ISSC 2014/CIICT 2014)*, pp. 280–285. Doi: 10.1049/cp.2014.0699.

Pal, A. and K. Kant (2018). IoT-based sensing and communications infrastructure for the fresh food supply chain. *Computer* 51(2), 76–80. Doi: 10.1109/MC.2018.1451665.

Panarello, A., N. Tapas, G. Merlino, F. Longo, and A. Puliafito (2018). Blockchain and IoT integration: a systematic survey. *Sensors* 18(8). Doi: 10.3390/s18082575.

Puranik, V., Sharmila, A. Ranjan, and A. Kumari (2019). Automation in agriculture and IoT. In *2019 4th International Conference on Internet of Things: Smart Innovation and Usages (IoTSIU)*, pp. 1–6. Doi: 10.1109/IoT-SIU.2019.8777619.

Schinckus, C. (2020). The good, the bad and the ugly: an overview of the sustainability of blockchain technology. *Energy Research & Social Science* 69, 101614. Doi: 10.1016/j. erss.2020.101614.

Takemiya, M. and B. Vanieiev (2018). Sora identity: secure, digital identity on the block-chain. In *2018 IEEE 42nd Annual Computer Software and Applications Conference (COMPSAC)*, 02, 582–587. Doi: 10.1109/COMPSAC.2018.10299.

Tasca, P. and C. J. Tessone (2019, Feb.). A taxonomy of blockchain technologies: principles of identification and classification. *Ledger* 4. Doi: 10.5195/ledger.2019.140.

Torky, M. and A. E. Hassanein (2020). Integrating blockchain and the Internet of Things in precision agriculture: analysis, opportunities, and challenges. *Computers and Electronics in Agriculture* 178, 105476. Doi: 10.1016/j.compag.2020.105476.

Tran, N. K., M. Ali Babar, and J. Boan (2021). Integrating blockchain and Internet of Things systems: a systematic review on objectives and designs. *Journal of Network and Computer Applications* 173, 102844. Doi: 10.1016/j.jnca.2020.102844.

Upadhyay, K., R. Dantu, Z. Zaccagni, and S. Badruddoja (2020). Is your legal contract ambiguous? Convert to a smart legal contract. In *2020 IEEE International Conference on Blockchain (Blockchain)*, pp. 273–280. Doi: 10.1109/blockchain50366.2020.00041.

Zhang, X., O. Upton, N. L. Beebe, and K.-K. R. Choo (2020). IoT botnet forensics: a comprehensive digital forensic case study on Mirai botnet servers. *Forensic Science International: Digital Investigation* 32, 300926. Doi: 10.1016/j.fsidi.2020.300926.

4 Cryptocurrency Revolution

Bitcoin Time Forecasting & Blockchain Anomaly Detection

Vishakha
Tata Consultancy Services

Nikhil Sharma
Delhi Technological University

Ila Kaushik
Krishna Institute of Engineering & Technology

Bharat Bhushan
Sharda University

Chaitanya Kumar Dixit
Dr Bhimrao Ambedkar University

CONTENTS

DOI: 10.1201/9781003224075-4

4.1 INTRODUCTION

A few days ago, one headline is creating a lot of buzz in the market "The ICICI Bank became the first Indian bank to utilise blockchain for settlements. They are currently in the testing phase". Now a question arises that what is blockchain? Blockchain is simply a distributed database and P2P ledger [1]. Ledger is basically a registry of transactions. The database is shared, replicated and synchronised among members of the decentralised network. Each participant governs and consensus on the updates to the record in the ledger [2]. Every record consists of a timestamp and unique cryptographic signature, which makes the ledger immutable and auditable. Hacking is unfeasible in this layout. It can transfer any item of value across participants. It is an underlying technology behind bitcoin [3]. It is said to be distributive because everyone is an authority which makes it unsusceptible to collapses. As no intermediary is required, the overall cost is reduced. The concept of blockchain came into existence after the 2008 financial crisis [4]. It was known as the largest recession since 1929. Reasons for the 2008 financial crisis were as follows: inefficient and corrupted financial systems, the economic market was crashed in a domino effect and several investment banks went bankrupt resulting in several bailouts.

After effects of the economic crisis include the lost faith of people in existing financial systems, which results in the mass withdrawal from the banks. This results in the evolution of bitcoin [5]. It was invented by a person named Satoshi Nakamoto in 2008 to serve as the community deal or business registry of bitcoin. Bitcoin generally known as BTC [6] is completely digital in nature and operates like any independent currency. It is an open-source P2P money with data stored on multiple vertices simultaneously [7]. It offers a high level of privacy as the transactions are anonymous. It is immutable, cheaper, secured and deflationary. It is also fiat in nature as it is not backed by a tangible substance [8]. Here some concepts of machine learning and deep learning algorithms [9] are presented to work upon the bitcoin dataset and hence the time prediction of bitcoin prices and trend is proposed. For forecasting time series, two types of algorithms can be used: (1) white box algorithms such as Auto Regressive Integrated Moving Average (ARIMA) [10], ARMA and AR, (2) black box algorithms such as long short-term memory (LSTM) [11], Recurrent Neural Network (RNN), CNN and NNETAR and some supervised learning concepts such as support vector machine [12]. Time series can be forecasted with different models. Some of them are as follows: Naïve, Seasonal decomposition (+ any model), ARIMA, GARCH, Prophet, NNETAR and LSTM.

The prediction of the number of anomalies in a dataset using K-means clustering [13] is done to detect the anomaly in the bitcoin transaction process. As blockchain is a digitalised process, it is very much susceptible to fake transactions and anomalies [14]. To overcome this situation, first the chances and areas of anomalies in a transaction should be predicted. Blockchain anomaly detection [15] helps to construct the model of standard behaviour and then make predictions on a new dataset (test data) for divergence from such base model. The key concept of blockchain technology underlies within two principal components: Hash Tree and Timestamp. Merkle Tree (Hash Tree): It was proposed in 1979 by R. Merkle. The apex of leaf is marked by a hash of data and the apex of non-leaf is marked with a deciphered hash of tag and its child vertex. If we change the data or hash, it will result in mismatch with the root hash. Hence, it is very difficult to tamper with [16].

This paper introduces a comprehensive approach for predicting the time series nature of the processes in a bitcoin and automatic recognition of anomalies in the blockchain system using various machine learning algorithms. In the present dataset, chances of anomaly occurrence are high at weighted price and volume of bitcoin; hence after date-time conversion of timestamp, we plotted the graph of weighted price and volume of bitcoin with that of timestamp, respectively. Further, the paper discusses various challenging outcomes of the implementations with the possible solutions. The major contribution of this work is summarised as below.

- A systematic detailed study of machine learning algorithms such as ARIMA, LSTM and XGBoost is presented.
- In this work, the forecasting of bitcoin trend using ARIMA, LSTM and XGBoost is presented. Further, the output graphs show that the ARIMA model yields the best prediction trend as compared to other models.
- Anomaly detection is also studied via implemented procedure using K-means clustering. Here, the timestamping concept is used to avoid tampering and single fault failure in any situation.
- The graph of weighted price and volume of bitcoin with respect to the timestamp is shown.

The remainder of the paper is organised as follows. Section 4.2 presents the background of time series forecasting and anomaly detection models. Section 4.3 presents the related work. Section 4.4 highlights the design and implementation of ARIMA model, XGBoost model and anomaly detection model. The performance evaluation of these models is presented in Section 4.5. Finally, the paper concludes itself and outlines several future research trends in Section 4.6.

4.2 BACKGROUND

The bitcoin is a cryptocurrency and it is used to exchange digital assets online. Blockchain is the mainstay of digital cryptocurrency bitcoin. It is a distributed software network, which serves two cardinal functions [17]. The first one being, to serve as a digital ledger and another being a mechanism that allows to transfer

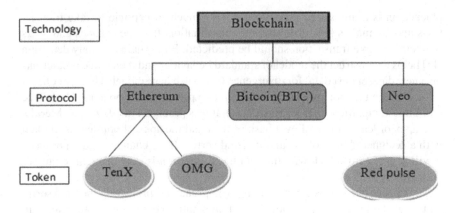

FIGURE 4.1   Difference between blockchain and bitcoin.

assets without any intercessor, securely. Many people get confused with the concepts of blockchain and bitcoin. Blockchain is a technology, whereas Ethereum [18], bitcoin and Neo are its protocols. Ethereum is an internet that built the money and payments called cryptocurrency. Neither the other applications steal your data nor they can spy. It provides an accessible economic system to everyone. It came into the concept in 2015 and is still the world's leading computerised blockchain. Ether is the native currency of Ethereum and is the same as bitcoin in many aspects. Many decentralised applications are made on Ethereum, which signifies that no single entity can control it. Figure 4.1 shows the difference in blockchain with that of bitcoin and Ethereum.

In its simplest sense, Blockchain is a P2P (Peer to Peer) ledged data structure. The contents of this data structure are blocks, for example, bitcoin transactions. This data structure also has a header, which contains data about the block, a reference of the previous block and a fingerprint, known as hash for referring to the next block. Block's fingerprint is used to reference the desired block [19]. These block fingerprints are generated using an algorithm and are used to validate the data. Every transaction is validated with 51% majority. Every participant has a complete version of the database. Some of the top investors in blockchain are as follows: Mitsubishi UFJ Capital, Andreessen Horowitz, Greylock partners, Xapo, Ripple labs, Coinbase, etc. Table 4.1 shows the comparison between Cascading Style Sheets (CSS) System and P2P System.

Time series forecasting and anomaly detection can be studied with different machine learning concepts as follows:

4.2.1 ARIMA

ARIMA represents a class of prototypes that apprehends a suite of dissimilar conventional temporal configurations in time sequence statistics [21]. Quintessence or intrinsic nature of the model is captured itself. AR stands for Autoregression,

TABLE 4.1

Difference between CSS System and P2P System [20]

Criteria	Client Server System	P2P System
Definition	Several clients connected to a server	Every node can anytime become a client or server
Provision of service	Client makes a request for service to a server	Every node can request or provide a service
Focussed on	Information sharing	Interconnections
Data storage	Centralised	On each peer node
Request handling at server	Bottleneck and single point of failure for more requests	Not applicable
Cost	High end servers, costly and scalable	Made from Chain of Things and hence cheaper

a model that uses the reliant association between actual and few lagging observations. I stand for Integrated, the utilisation of anticipation of factual raw observations (such as subtracting a latter observation from former observation) to make the time sequence consistent. MA stands for Moving Average, a model that utilises the association of observation with remaining inaccuracies of a mobilised mean model which is further applied with delayed observations. In Python, ARIMA-based forecasting prototype can be designed either utilising Auto ARIMA (Pyramid ARIMA) or Stats Model [22]. Models are further fitted into time sequence dataset to forecast the succeeding points in sequence.

4.2.2 RNN

RNN is a classification of Artificial Neural Network (ANN) where the dependency between vertices forms a pointed trace with a profane series and thus enables it to exhibit temporal dynamic performance [23]. The phrase "recurrent neural network" is employed randomly to say two extensive groups of networks with an identical common construction, out of which one is limited instinct and the other is boundless instinct. Both groups of networks represent profane dynamic conduct. A finite impulse or instinct recurrent network could also be a pointed acyclic trace, which can be unfold and restored by factually feed forward network of artificial neurons, while a boundless impulse recurrent network may be a pointed cyclic trace which will not be unfold [24]. Here, in this chapter, LSTM is implemented which is a classification of RNN.

4.2.3 PROPHET

Forecasting is used as an adviser to strategy maker or business companies and hence exhibits a significant role in moulding the business decisions [25]. Prophet is a public domain software for business forecasting, which is released by the data

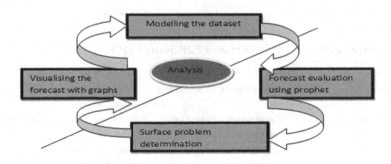

FIGURE 4.2 Prophet model.

science team of Facebook. It is based on an additive representation where irregular trends are trained to be fitted with seasonality. Figure 4.2 shows the prophet model. The general equation of prophet is given as

$$z(t)=j(t)+r(t)+h(t) + €n \quad (4.1)$$

j(t) defines the model trend of a long-term increase or decrease in the data. Prophet combines two trend representations depending on the type of forecasting problem: saturating growth model and piecewise linear model. r(t) describes how the dataset is strained by seasonal aspects such as the duration of the year basically it models the seasonality with Fourier series. h(t) models the consequences of holidays or large events that can have an adverse or favourable impact on business time series, €n represents an irreducible error term. Table 4.2 shows comparisons between various types of time series forecasting.

4.2.4 CLUSTERING

Clustering is one of the most accepted probing data evaluation approaches, which is used to obtain an instinct about the configuration of the data [28]. It can be described as recognising the subgroups in the dataset so that data points in the same cluster or subgroup are very similar while data points in dissimilar clusters or subgroups are very dissimilar. Clusters can be similar or dissimilar based upon the Euclidean distance or correlation distance. K-means clustering focuses on the division of t observations into K number of clusters. Here every observation possesses only one cluster with the nearest average value. Hence, the partition of the data space into Voronoi cells takes place.

4.2.5 XGBOOST

XGBoost fills in the missing values with zeroes or previous values. Some of the characteristics of eXtreme Gradient Boosting package are as follows: speed and performance, as it is comparatively much faster than other ensemble classifiers.

TABLE 4.2

Difference between Various Types of Time Series Forecasting [26,27]

Criteria	ARIMA	Prophet	RNN
Definition	Works on the basis of regression analysis.	It is a public domain software for business forecasting based on an additive model.	It stands for recurrent neural network, which is a classification of artificial neural network.
Base	Based on analysis of linear time sequence.	Based on Bayesian curve fitting.	Previous observations are used as input in the current step and depict the relation between past and present observations.
Users	Used by trained professionals	Used by unprofessional generally non-statisticians.	As it is a deep learning concept it is used by well-trained experts.
Advantages	It does not require tuning of hyperparameters.	Recognises complex seasonal design in an efficient way.	As compared to ARIMA, take more lags in time sequence, also very flexible in nature.
Consequences	Data needs to be continuously fed for further forecast and stationary data should be used.	Time sequence model having powerful random constituent cannot be forecasted appropriately using Prophet.	Vanishing and gradient exploding issue. Also, it takes a longer time to be trained.

The Core algorithm is parallelizable as it can harness the power of multi-core. It consistently shows better performance than other algorithm methods. A wide variety of tuning parameters are regularisation, cross validation, tree parameters, missing values and scikit-learn. XGBoost belongs to a family of uplifting algorithms and uses the gradient boosting (GBM) framework at its core. Figure 4.3 shows the XGBoost model and Table 4.3 shows the comparison between XGBoost Model and clustering.

4.3 LITERATURE REVIEW

Many research studies have already conducted price prediction using RNN and ARIMA models. Researchers are coming up with the solutions to detect anomalies and thus working in the area to prevent them. Researches are going on to maximise the throughput, bandwidth and size. To provide a low level of latency in bitcoin transaction block and to enhance the security in blockchain, more time has to be spent on a particular transaction block. So, a technique is to build to make a block and confirming its transaction within seconds by not interfering with its security model. Researchers are trying to add more levels of security to the hash function. The bitcoin application programming interfaces (APIs) are difficult to use; hence, a developer-friendly API is needed to predict better results. In countries like South Korea, blockchain is used for issuing bonds. Blockchain has

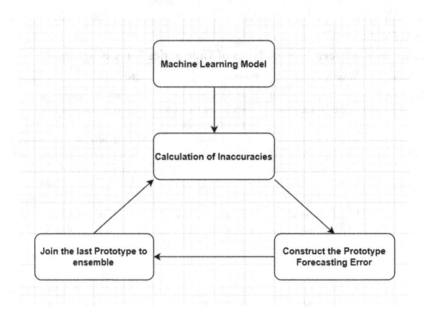

FIGURE 4.3   XGBoost model.

TABLE 4.3

Difference between XGBoost and Clusters [29,30]

XGBoost	Clustering
It is an ensembling technique and is also known as gradient boosting.	It is an unsupervised algorithm that groups data in distinct clusters so that observations within each group are similar and among other clusters it is mutually exclusive.
It indicates a group of models that have a diverse insight into specific issues and combines multiple models.	This algorithm makes sense when there is a diverse data.
In real-world issues, ensembling is performed more frequently as compared to the individual clustering.	Clustering ensembling gives better outcomes as compared to individual clusterings.
It is used for forecasting.	This approach is used for the anomaly detection.

been used to block the fake news. India is soon going to develop a blockchain voting system instead of Ethereum Virtual Machine. UAE government switched to blockchain for making their healthcare data tamper proof. Time series forecasting is already being used to simplify, observe and predict some of the causality conduct of the trends. It basically allows us to find how did the past outcomes of a dataset influence the future.

Several applications of time series forecasting are business, finance, science, engineering and health domain. In the business domain, it is been widely used in supply chain, booking, monitoring the web traffic, etc. It can effectively predict the forthcoming developments in the business regarding revenue policies, sales, taxes and demand for various resources and deliverables. Based on the historic dataset, the corporate world can predict the future outcomes and thus plans budgets and funds accordingly and can allocate their resources properly. It also affects in decision making of the strategies so as to adopt the best method for continuous growth. It is utilised for predicting the trends and prices of stock market, money exchange and econometrics and in astronomy prediction, weather forecasting, earthquake and natural disaster prediction. It is widely used in sensors and processing of control signals. It is used in the medical diagnosis of diseases and biomedical monitoring. Time series prediction can be successfully implied to predict the mortality rate, progress of a disease and accordingly predict the various risks that can occur in the future time.

Anomaly detection is widely used in protecting web-based retail businesses, finance sector, detection of intrusion and fraud activities, fault detection, monitoring of healthcare facilities, event detection in sensor networks and control signals and detecting environment disturbances. Anomaly detection using machine learning algorithms is one of the most important activities, which is carried out in almost every sector nowadays. There are many proposed research studies in the field of blockchain, which are giving new directions to the crypto world. SreeragIyer et al. [31] proposed that tokens also called assets in Hyperledger Composer (a set of tools that provide various developers and businessmen to fabricate blockchain utilisation directed towards solving business issues), which can be issued to commerce's and industries on the basis of their contribution in wastewater management. The foremost effective industry is that who features a zero percent water releasing policy in water bodies and complete re-utilisation of wastewater generated by the company for its own procedures and operations. The worst corporate is the one which throws whole wastewater in the surrounding habitat or territory without considering its after effect and did not consider it to be a reusable component. Thus, tokens are distributed by keeping both quality and quantity of wastewater reused in mind. If the corporate surpasses the defined threshold value, then it can sell tokens to other corporates that have not reached their thresholds. The number of tokens generated is directly proportional to the higher purity of reused water. Rules and regulations for issuing and trading of those tokens or assets are called smart contract [32]. Many corporates can make this an illicit means to gain bitcoin by tampering the information based on which these assets are awarded. Thus, anomaly detection algorithms are utilised in this proposed system to predict the potential scams or anomalies which can happen with an Internet of things (IoT) meter.

Various clustering algorithms such as K-means clustering and density-based spatial clustering were studied. Spatial clustering is also referred to as DBSCAN. Other algorithms from deep learning domain for anomaly detection studied were auto-encoder and LSTM. Storing data and information on a blockchain makes it an unchangeable scrutinise trail, and also give an automatic analysing system in accordance with smart contracts [33]. To make the prototype firmer and more robust, supervised and unsupervised algorithms are executed to configure out any change in IoT meters that supplies statistics on wastewater recycle from a corporate. K-means clustering specified the number of clusters to be formed beforehand by studying the elbow graph and determining the inflection points, DBSCAN algorithm forms clusters depending on its input variables. Here Hyperledger Fabric uses Kafka-based consensus mechanism unlike Ethereum or bitcoin which uses expensive Proof-of-Work. This proposed system features a control figure that supplies assets and check anomalies or fraud, hence doesn't need Proof-of-Work [34], as identification of the suppliers and borrowers need to be known.

MarwaKeshk et al. [35] proposed a solitude-safeguarding architecture that depends on blockchain and various deep learning algorithms, so as to confide the datasets of smart power grids and hence can perceive probable strikes on data in future. The architecture consists of two levels of security mechanisms. The first level defines an ePoW method for confirming information probity, while the second level comprises a variational auto encoder technique to conceal the data and rework it to a replacement configuration. The utilisation of two steps of security attains superior achievement as compared with contemporary methodologies, and it is also very efficacious in avoiding the dataset adulterine and inference strikes from exploiting native data lodge of smart power grids. One of the anomalies' observing methods is LSTM, which is applied on the data before and after performing the two-step security techniques [36]. The outcomes obtained showed that the proposed technique outshines the other proposed techniques in terms of precision rate and warning rate. Upcoming extensions of this research consist of implementing the architecture on various real-time data from smart power grids, so as to gauge its extensibility, feasibility, and profitability. The modernisation of power grids is of utmost curiosity especially to the leading advanced nations in technology such as U.S. and Australia as smart power systems have the ability to maximise the consumption of energy and supply the best solutions. Cyber-physical systems as depicted in Figure 4.4 show that how individual units of cost-per-clicks can be merged to determine smart power grids that combine

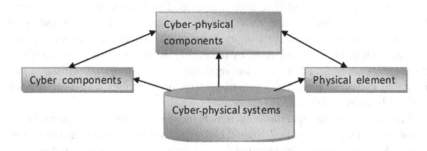

FIGURE 4.4   Block diagram of the cyberphysical system.

physical and information transmission automations and respective components to extend the ability and productivity of power grids [37].

Atzei et al. [38] proposed a classification of program pitfalls of general smart contract and noticed the various criticisations in counter with the smart contract and provide a taxonomy of common smart contract programming pitfalls. Anh et al. [39] emphasised on the concept of private blockchain with reference to the data processing view. Instead of emphasising blockchain technology, Tschorsch et al. [40] proposed a practical survey on distributed digital money. Holub et al. [41] went through more than 1,200 papers on bitcoin and differentiated them into six categories. Mingli Wu et al. [42] differentiated the blockchain technology into four layers and forwarded extensive research on the various applications of blockchain especially in the field of IoT, the network and the consensus mechanism for transaction. From version 1.0 to recent version 3.0, blockchain is continuously evolving. Version 1.0 represents the bitcoin generation, version 2.0 defines the smart contracts and version 3.0 is currently in an observation state with decentralised applications, also known as DApps. In context to the future of the financial systems, Vigna et al. [43] analysed the consequences of blockchain applications on the global commercial zone. Peters et al. [44] explore the safety attack surface of blockchain including selfish-mining, block forks and shared denial of service attacks. Swan et al. [45] proposed that the upcoming Blockchain 3.0 era is going to create many new prospects in privacy management, voting structure and IoT. Kosba et al. [46] analysed different prospects of smart contract system involving culprit smart contracts. McNally et al. [47] used the Bitcoin price index to predict the bitcoin price using machine learning and deep learning concepts, achieving an accuracy of 52% using LSTM networks. Jang et al. [48] used Bayesian neural networks with other linear and non-linear prototypes to explain the volatility of bitcoin, hence improving the predictive performance.

4.4 DESIGN AND IMPLEMENTATION

In the time sequence analysis approach, initially the data is pre-processed and transformed into a suitable form. Based on various approaches, the best model is found out and thus applied to the testing dataset. This architecture can be finely used with the real-time dataset by importing it from Google APIs. The architecture of time sequence analysis is presented in Figure 4.5.

Simple K-means clustering is implemented on the dataset in which the mean or ensemble of every individual cluster is calculated and thus differentiated the dataset points based upon the similarities or dissimilarities with the specific cluster values. Figure 4.6 shows the K-means clustering model.

The dataset consists of eight columns consisting of timestamps, open price, closing price, maximum and minimum price of each day named as High and Low, Volume_(BTC), Volume_(Currency) and Weighted price [49]. For time series forecasting, a total of 1,048,576 data entries were observed and to detect the anomalies over the same dataset we take 19,999 data entries into account to showcase the prototype.

Time sequence analysis:

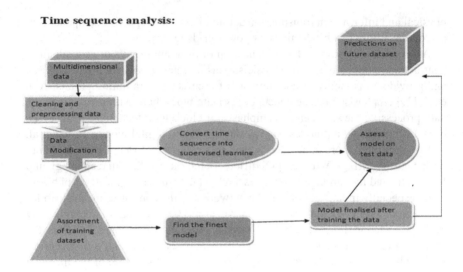

FIGURE 4.5   Architecture showing the flow of time analysis.

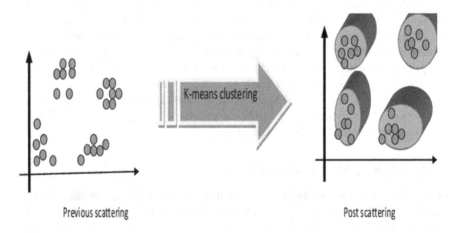

FIGURE 4.6   K-means clustering.

4.4.1   ARIMA MODEL

During the analysis of time series forecasting, the following results are obtained after implementing the steps of ARIMA models as shown in Table 4.4. Figures 4.7–4.9 represent the results obtained using ARIMA Model Predictions.

Figure 4.7 shows the analysis of decomposition of bitcoin price according to originality, trend, seasonal and residual. In general, trend is a structured linear element that varies with time and as depicted by Figure 4.7 never replicates. There is only one difference between seasonality and trend that seasonality changes with time and do repeat itself after the specified interval. Residual depicts whether

TABLE 4.4
Steps of ARIMA Model

1. START
2. Adjust the timestamp in date and time format
3. Plot the data and notice the unusual observations
4. Replace the *NaN* values with 0 or previously defined values.
5. Transform the sequence into motionless or still sequence.
6. Decompose the model to find trend, seasonal change and residuals.
7. Model the data on statsmodel.graphics.tsaplots.
8. Plot ACF models and find the best solution.
9. Build auto ARIMA model.
10. Make predictions and compare the expected and actual outcomes.
11. END

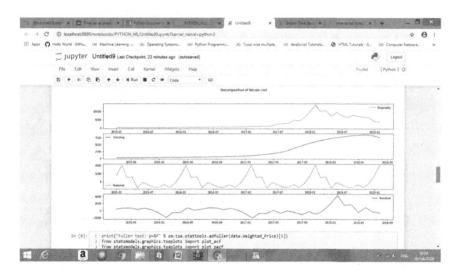

FIGURE 4.7   Analysis of decomposition of bitcoin price.

an applied model apprehended the information in the dataset perfectly or not. Non-zero residual shows that forecasting is biased.

Figure 4.8 shows the autocorrelation and partial correlation. Autocorrelation shows the degree of resemblance between an original time sequence and a lagged version of the same over consecutive intervals. It depicts the connection between current and past values of a variable whereas partial correlation depicts the connection between two random instances.

Figure 4.9 represents the LSTM, which is a classification of RNN. It mainly consists of four gates: input, output, forget gate and state of the neural cell. The cell recalls the values over random time intervals and the other gates manage the movement of information inside and outside of the cell.

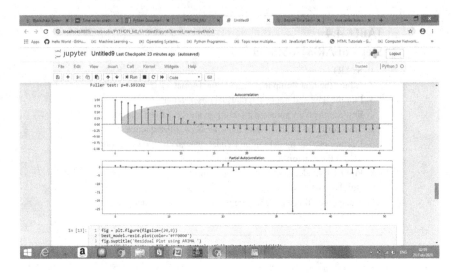

FIGURE 4.8   Analysis of autocorrelation and partial correlation.

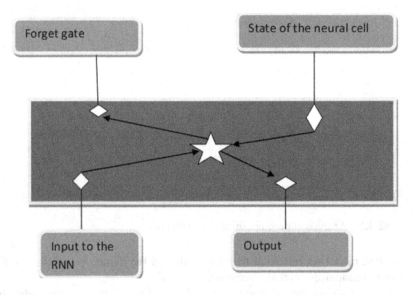

FIGURE 4.9   LSTM (long short-term memory).

Figures 4.10–4.12 represent the outputs of LSTM prediction. Figure 4.10 shows the bitcoin price variation in the time period of 4 years (2015–2018) using and at each point mentions the opening price, closing price and weighted average of bitcoin.

Figure 4.11 shows the scatter plot of bitcoin which shows the dependency of the volume of bitcoin on weighted price. A scatter plot indicates up to which extent one variable is going to be affected by the other variable.

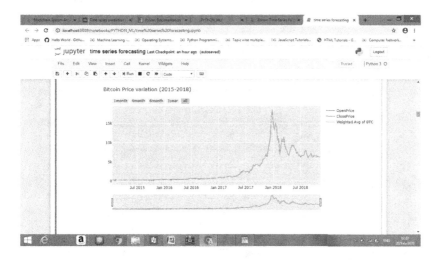

FIGURE 4.10 Bitcoin price variation from 2015 to 2018.

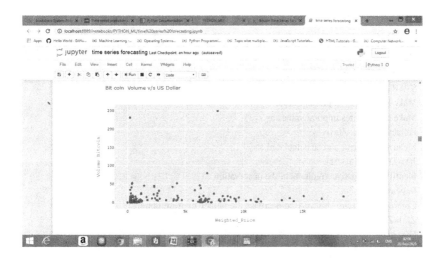

FIGURE 4.11 Scatter plot of bitcoin.

Figure 4.12 shows the comparison of predicted and actual forecasts of the data. It is clearly visible that the entire model is overfitted. The overfitted model refers to the prediction that corresponds exactly the same to a pre-defined trend or specified set of data and in future may fail to predict the additional observations genuinely.

4.4.2 XGBoost Model

Another model used for forecasting is XGBoost, which uses the gradient boosting framework and fills the missing values with those of previous values or zero. It

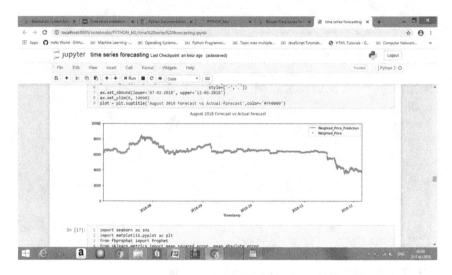

FIGURE 4.12   Comparison of predicted and actual forecast.

TABLE 4.5

Steps of XGBoost Model

1. START
2. Make a set of actual predictions as Y[a].
3. Make a set of presumption values as Z[a].
4. Fallacy=P(Y[a], Z[a])
5. Mean square error can be calculated as
   J() =Σ(Y[a]–Z[a]) ^2
6. Identify the negative gradients in the observation
7. Repeat:
8. Continuously try to shift Z[a] to decrease the fallacy in presumptions.
   Z[a]=Z[a]+γH[a]
9. H[a] is nearly approximated to ▼P(Y[a], Z[a])
10. END

works on the technique of ensembling. Table 4.5 shows the steps of the XGBoost Model.

Figure 4.13 shows the prediction of the weighted price of bitcoin hourly depicted by XGBoost modelling. For dividing the training and testing dataset, we use "25 June 2018" as the split date because there was a significant downfall in bitcoin prices during the period of June 10, 2018 to July 20, 2018. The above figure shows that the market hits the highest price of 20K in December 2017, but after that also came to the low marked price range of $5,970–$5,980 in the mid of year 2018 and could not recover till the end of the year.

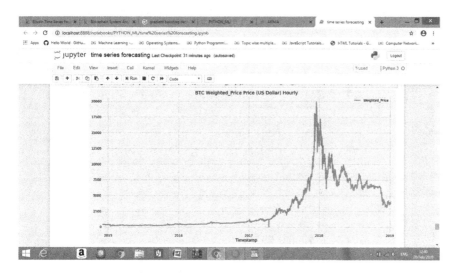

FIGURE 4.13 Prediction of weighted price of bitcoin hourly.

TABLE 4.6

Steps of K-Means Clustering Model

1. START
2. Input
   Z ← Number of clusters to be formed
   R ← Set of lift proportions
3. Randomly select Z objects from R as the starting cluster centres
4. Repeat:
   {
   4.1 Elevate each article to the cluster to which it is highly similar in configuration.
   4.2 Determine the mean or average value of the articles for individual cluster
   4.3 Till any change arrives
   }
5. END

4.4.3 ANOMALY DETECTION

For Anomaly Detection, many Machine Learning algorithms can be used such as Isolation Forest, K-nearest neighbour and K-means clustering. Here, in this chapter, K-means clustering is implemented to find the anomalies in the bitcoin dataset. Table 4.6 shows the steps of K-means clustering for Anomaly Detection.

Figure 4.14 represents the analysis of timestamp of bitcoin. Timestamp refers to the present time of an event maintained by a computer through different processes such as Network Time Protocol. The time maintained by a computer is calibrated to minute fractions of a second to provide accuracy.

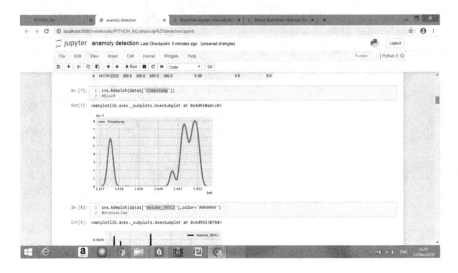

FIGURE 4.14   Analysis of timestamp of bitcoin for anomaly detection.

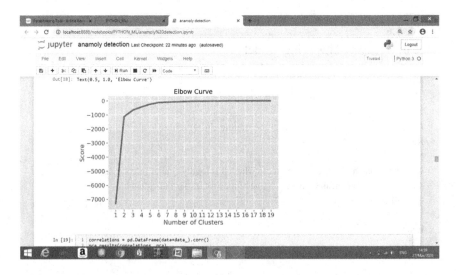

FIGURE 4.15   Elbow curve derived for the bitcoin dataset.

Figure 4.15 shows that the best possible results will be shown by the k-means cluster where the value k lies between $3 \leq k \leq 5$. The point of inflection either upward or downward called "elbow" represents the best value of "k". Where there is a strong point of inflection, the underlying model fits the best at that particular point.

Out of 3-means, 4-means, and 5-means, the best results were drawn with a plot with four clusters so we will proceed further with 4-means clustering. Figure 4.16

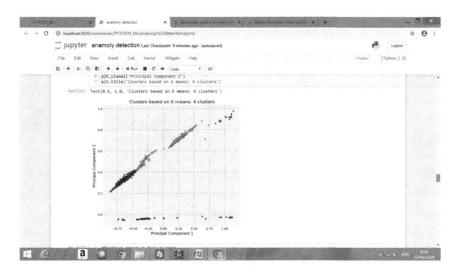

FIGURE 4.16 Clustering based on 4-means clusters.

represents the clustering of anomalies from testing dataset using 4-means cluster which provides a better and clear way for representing the various groups.

4.5 PERFORMANCE EVALUATION

After the processing of datasets, machine learning approaches are implemented one by one for time series forecasting and various outputs are already shown in the previous figures. In the anomaly detection process, as indicated from elbow curve, 4-means clustering shows the best result and hence the anomalies will be predicted based on the same. At last, the detection of anomaly is to be predicted in the weighted price and volume of bitcoin because these two attributes have the highest chances of anomaly occurrence.

Figure 4.17 shows the comparison between predicted and actual bitcoin prices using the ARIMA model, which is representing quite close approximation with the actual values.

From the analysis done so far, the ARIMA model shows the closest approximation to the actual value in time series forecasting as depicted by the output graphs. According to the results obtained, it's concluded that ARIMA is a better model for studying forecasting than LSTM and XGBoost Model.

Figure 4.18 represents that there are 999 anomalies predicted by K-means algorithm in the last 2-year records consisting of 19,999 entries. Anomalies are represented by red dots. Now, similarly plot the outlier anomaly with respect to volume and weighted price.

Figure 4.19 represents the anomalies in the volume of bitcoin. Here the red dot shows the abnormal behaviour of bitcoin volume in the transaction process. The

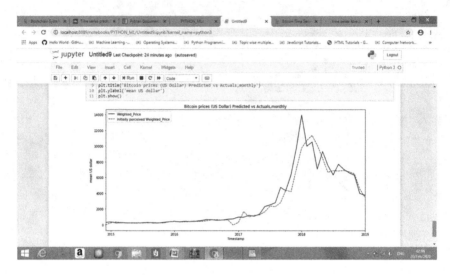

FIGURE 4.17   Comparison of actual and predicted bitcoin price in US dollars.

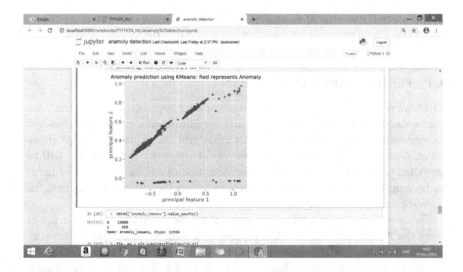

FIGURE 4.18   Clustering of the anomalies from testing dataset.

graph is plotted between volume_ BTC in the y-axis and timestamp in date-time format in the x-axis.

Figure 4.20 represents the anomalies in the weighted price. Here the red dot shows the abnormal behaviour in the transaction process. The anomaly detection tool can be constructively used to make the blockchain domain safer and stronger by automatically analysing, acknowledging and separating out the abnormalities.

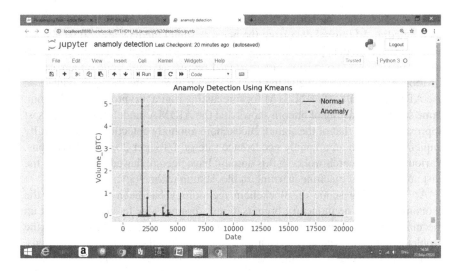

FIGURE 4.19   Anomaly in the volume of bitcoin prices.

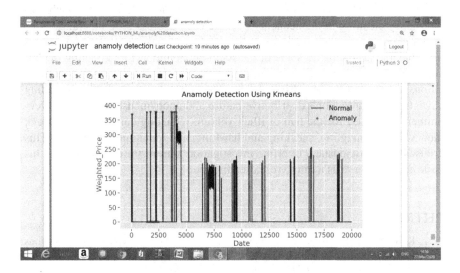

FIGURE 4.20   Anomaly in the weighted price of bitcoin prices.

4.6   CONCLUSION AND FUTURE SCOPE

Time series forecasting has indeed revolutionised the business domain as it predicts the future outcomes in advance so that the strategies can be made accordingly. For processing the blockchain database, machine learning algorithms are the most logical and superior approach. Recent researches show that the trends in the bitcoin are susceptible to inaccurate measures because the Bitcoin prices are very volatile and very random, and are often influenced by external factors (or news) such as cryptocurrency regulations, investments or simple rumours on social media. Additional data from the news or social media sites will be needed to make these models perform better and accurately. Albeit forecasting is often contemplated as a subdivision of supervised regression class, still some particular tools are mandatory due to the time-related nature of the datasets; hence, we use ARIMA, XGBoost and LSTM for forecasting digital cryptocurrency bitcoin. Time series forecasting of bitcoin shows that the ARIMA model shows the closest approximation to that of the actual. Blockchain anomaly detection is successfully implemented with an anomaly occurrence rate of 4.9% per 20,000 transactions. Various latest research works in this domain have been reviewed, which gives the vast application of machine learning in blockchain technology.

An astounding scope of Blockchain technology has been perceived in the economic field. The monetary organisations were not able to sufficiently lift up the massive workload after the 2016 demonetisation and thus brought out the problems of having a centralised authority for handling the financial transactions. Integrating blockchain with financial settlements gives out amazing benefits, such as a notable amount of time and capital could be saved, including a drastic depletion in time needed for processing and authenticating transactions. Blockchain will also aid in compressing the flow of dark-money and dealing with the substantial money cleaning in the economy because each address used for transactions is stored constantly and regularly on the databases, making all the transactions provable and accountable. Some of the socio-economic factors affecting the bitcoins are demand and supply fluctuations, banking blockades, market manipulation, price irregularities, drivers of interest (silk route), etc. Bitcoin's leading advantage of transaction's distributive nature and anonymousness made it a recommended money for the hub of illicit venture including concealment of black money, drug smuggling, sneaking and hawking, and munitions acquisition. This aroused the consciousness of crime investigation administrations. Investing this issue can also serve as a future research direction.

REFERENCES

1. K. R. Choo, S. Gritzalis and J. H. Park. (2018, Aug). Cryptographic solutions for industrial Internet-of-Things: research challenges and opportunities. *IEEE Transactions on Industrial Informatics*, 14(8), 3567–3569.
2. S. Wang, L. Ouyang, Y. Yuan, X. Ni, X. Han and F. Wang. (2019). Blockchain-enabled smart contracts: architecture, applications, and future trends. *IEEE Transactions on Systems, Man, and Cybernetics: Systems*, 1–12.
3. V. K. Aggarwal, N. Sharma, I. Kaushik and B. Bhushan. (2021). Integration of blockchain and IoT (B-IoT): Architecture, solutions, & future research direction. In *IOP Conference Series: Materials Science and Engineering*, 1022, 012103. Doi: 10.1088/1757-899x/1022/1/012103.
4. S. R. Niya, S. S. Jha, T. Bocek and B. Stiller. (2018). Design and implementation of an automated and decentralized pollution monitoring system with blockchains, smart contracts, and LoRaWAN. In *NOMS 2018-2018 IEEE/IFIP Network Operations and Management Symposium*, Taipei, 1–4.

5. C. H. Liu, Q. Lin and S. Wen. (2018). Blockchain-enabled data collection and sharing for industrial IoT with deep reinforcement learning. *IEEE Transactions on Industrial Informatics*, 15, 3516–3526.

6. B. Coma-Puig, J. Carmona, R. Gavald, S. Alcoverro and V. Martin. (2016). Fraud detection in energy consumption: a supervised approach. In *2016 IEEE International Conference on Data Science and Advanced Analytics (DSAA)*, Montreal, QC, 120–129.

7. E. Androulaki, A. Barger, V. Bortnikov, C. Cachin, K. Christidis, A. De Caro, D. Enyeart, C. Ferris, G. Laventman, Y. Manevich, S. Muralidharan, C. Murthy, B. Nguyen, M. Sethi, G. Singh, K. Smith, A. Sorniotti, C. Stathakopoulou, M. Vukoli, S. W. Cocco and J. Yellick. (2018). Hyperledger fabric: a distributed operating system for permissioned blockchains. In *Proceedings of the Thirteenth EuroSys Conference (EuroSys '18)*. ACM, New York, Article 30, 15 p.

8. D. K. Soni, H. Sharma, B. Bhushan, N. Sharma and I. Kaushik. (2020). Security Issues & Seclusion in Bitcoin System. In *2020 IEEE 9th International Conference on Communication Systems and Network Technologies (CSNT)*, IEEE, 223–229. Doi: 10.1109/csnt48778.2020.9115744.

9. R. Deng, G. Xiao, R. Lu, H. Liang, and A. V. Vasilakos. (2016). False data injection on state estimation in power systems—attacks, impacts, and defense: a survey. *IEEE Transactions on Industrial Informatics*, 13(2), 411–423.

10. B. Li, R. Lu, W. Wang, and K. R. Choo. (2017). Distributed host-based collaborative detection for false data injection attacks in smart grid cyber-physical system. *Journal of Parallel and Distributed Computing*, 103, 32–41.

11. M. Keshk, N. Moustafa, E. Sitnikova, and G. Creech. (2017). Privacy preservation intrusion detection technique for SCADA systems. In *2017 Military Communications and Information Systems Conference (MilCIS)*, IEEE, Canberra, ACT, 1–6.

12. K. Gai, Y. Wu, L. Zhu, M. Qiu, and M. Shen. (2019). Privacy-preserving energy trading using consortium blockchain in smart grid. *IEEE Transactions on Industrial Informatics*, 15, 3548–3558.

13. P. Kaur. (2016). Outlier detection using K means and fuzzy min max neural network in network data. In *2016 8th International Conference on Computational Intelligence and Communication Networks (CICN)*, Tehri, 693–696.

14. M. S. Rahman, I. Khalil, A. Alabdulatif, and X. Yi. (2019). Privacy preserving service selection using fully homomorphic encryption scheme on untrusted cloud service platform. *Knowledge-Based Systems*, 180, 104–115.

15. M. Shen, X. Tang, L. Zhu, X. Du, and M. Guizani. (2019). Privacy preserving support vector machine training over blockchain-based encrypted IoT data in smart cities. *IEEE Internet of Things Journal*, 6, 7702–7712.

16. J. Huang, L. Kong, G. Chen, M.-Y. Wu, X. Liu, and P. Zeng. (2019). Towards secure industrial IoT: blockchain system with credit-based consensus mechanism. *IEEE Transactions on Industrial Informatics*, 15, 3680–3689.

17. P. Gope and B. Sikdar. (2019). An efficient privacy-preserving authentication scheme for energy internet-based vehicle-to-grid communication. *IEEE Transactions on Smart Grid*, 10, 6607–6618.

18. B., Bhushan and N. Sharma. (2020). Transaction privacy preservations for blockchain technology. In *Advances in Intelligent Systems and Computing International Conference on Innovative Computing and Communications*, 377–393. Doi: 10.1007/978-981-15-5148-2_34.

19. D. Puthal, N. Malik, S. P. Mohanty, E. Kougianos and C. Yang. (2018). The blockchain as a decentralized security framework [future directions]. *IEEE Consumer Electronics Magazine*, 7(2), 18–21.

20. A. Zohar. (2015, Aug). Bitcoin. *Communications of the ACM*, 58(9), 104–113.
21. R. Petersen. (2016). Data mining for network intrusion detection: a comparison of data mining algorithms and an analysis of relevant features for detecting cyber-attacks. DIVA. Retrieved January 2, 2022, from http://www.diva-portal.org/smash/record.jsf?pid=diva2%3A939697&dswid=1013
22. M. A. Ambusaidi, X. He, P. Nanda and Z. Tan. (2016). Building an intrusion detection system using a filter-based feature selection algorithm. *IEEE Transactions on Computers*, 65(10), 2986–2998.
23. T. Pham and S. Lee (2016, Nov). Anomaly detection in bitcoin network using unsupervised learning methods. *Computation Research Repository*, abs/1611.03941, 1–5.
24. S. T. Ali, P. McCorry, P. H.-J. Lee, F. Hao. (2015). *ZombieCoin: Powering Next-Generation Botnets with Bitcoin*. Berlin, Heidelberg: Springer Berlin Heidelberg, 34–48.
25. N. Atzei, M. Bartoletti and T. Cimoli (2017, Apr). A survey of attacks on ethereum smart contracts (SoK). In *International Conference on Principles of Security and Trust*, 164–186, Springer, Berlin, Heidelberg.
26. M. Signorini, M. Pontecorvi, W. Kanoun and R. D. Pietro. (2018, Aug). BAD: blockchain anomaly detection. *CoRR*, abs/1807.03833.
27. Goyal, S., Sharma, N., Kaushik, I., Bhushan, B. and Kumar, A. (2020). Blockchain as a lifesaver of IoT. *Security and Trust Issues in Internet of Things*, 209–237. Doi: 10.1201/9781003121664-10.
28. K. R. Choo, S. Gritzalis and J. H. Park. (2018, Aug). Cryptographic solutions for industrial Internet-of-Things: research challenges and opportunities. *IEEE Transactions on Industrial Informatics*, 14(8), 3567–3569.
29. E. Heilman, A. Kendler, A. Zohar and S. Goldberg. (2015). Eclipse attacks on bitcoin's peer-to-peer network. In *24th {USENIX} Security Symposium {USENIX} Security*, USENIX Association, Berkeley, CA, 129–144.
30. P. T. Pham and S. Lee. (2017). Anomaly detection in bitcoin network using unsupervised learning methods. NASA/ADS. Retrieved January 2, 2022, from https://ui.adsabs.harvard.edu/abs/2016arXiv161103941P/abstract
31. S. Iyer, S. Thakur, M. Dixit, R. Katkam, A. Agrawal and F. Kazi. (2019). Blockchain and anomaly detection based monitoring system for enforcing wastewater reuse. In *2019 10th International Conference on Computing, Communication and Networking Technologies (ICCCNT)*. Doi: 10.1109/icccnt45670.2019.8944586.
32. M. Signorini, M. Pontecorvi, W. Kanoun and R. D. Pietro. (2020). BAD: A blockchain anomaly detection solution. *IEEE Access*, 8, 173481–173490. https://doi.org/10.1109/access.2020.3025622
33. S. Goyal, N. Sharma, I. Kaushik, and B. Bhushan. (2021). Blockchain as a solution for security attacks in named data networking of things. *Security and Privacy Issues in IoT Devices and Sensor Networks*, 211–243. Doi: 10.1016/b978-0-12-821255-4.00010-9.
34. V. Gramoli. (2016). On the danger of private blockchains. In *Proceeding of Workshop on Distributed Cryptocurrencies and Consensus Ledgers (DCCL 2016)*, CSIRO University of Sydney, IBM.
35. M. Keshk, B. Turnbull, N. Moustafa, D. Vatsalan and K.-K. R. Choo. (2019). A privacy-preserving framework based blockchain and deep learning for protecting smart power networks. *IEEE Transactions on Industrial Informatics*, 1–1. Doi: 10.1109/tii.2019.2957140.
36. M. Apostolaki, A. Zohar and L. Vanbever. (2017). Hijacking bitcoin: routing attacks on cryptocurrencies. In *IEEE SP*, San Jose, CA.
37. D. T. T. Anh, W. Ji, C. Gang, L. Rui, O. B. Chin and T. Kian-Lee. (2017, May). BLOCKBENCH: a framework for analyzing private blockchains. In *Proceedings of the International Conference on Management of Data*, 1085–1100.

38. N. Atzei, M. Bartoletti and T. Cimoli. (2017). A survey of attacks on ethereum smart contracts (sok). In *International Conference on Principles of Security and Trust*, Springer, Berlin, Heidelberg, 164–186.
39. T.T. Dinh, R. Liu, M. Zhang, G. Chen, B.C. Ooi and J. Wang. (2017). Untangling blockchain: a data processing view of blockchain systems. *IEEE Transactions on Knowledge and Data Engineering*, 30, 1366–1385.
40. F. Tschorsch and B. Scheuermann. (2016). Bitcoin and beyond: a technical survey on decentralized digital currencies. *IEEE Communications Surveys & Tutorials*, 18, 2084–2123.
41. M. Holub and J. Johnson. (2018). Bitcoin research across disciplines. *The Information Society*, 34(2), 114–126.
42. M. Wu, K. Wang, X. Cai, S. Guo, M. Guo and C. Rong. (2019). A comprehensive survey of blockchain: from theory to IoT applications and beyond. *IEEE Internet of Things Journal*, 6, 8114–8154.
43. P. Vigna and M. J. Casey. (2016). *The Age of Cryptocurrency: How Bitcoin and the Blockchain Are Challenging the Global Economic Order*. New York: Macmillan. [Online]. Available: https://goo.gl/tTJN2j
44. G. W. Peters and E. Panayi. (2016). Understanding modern banking ledgers through blockchain technologies: future of transaction processing and smart contracts on the internet of money. In *Banking Beyond Banks and Money*. New York: Springer, 239–278.
45. M. Swan. (2015). *Blockchain: Blueprint for a New Economy*, 1st ed. Sebastopol, CA: W O'Reilly Media, Inc. [Online].Available: https://goo.gl/7wck2T.
46. A.E. Kosba, A. Miller, E. Shi, Z. Wen and C. Papamanthou. (2016). Hawk: the blockchain model of cryptography and privacy-preserving smart contracts. In *2016 IEEE Symposium on Security and Privacy (SP)*, IEEE, San Jose, CA, 839–858.
47. S. Mcnally, J.T. Roche and S. Caton. (2018). Predicting the price of bitcoin using machine learning. In *2018 26th Euromicro International Conference on Parallel, Distributed and Network-based Processing (PDP)*, IEEE, Cambridge, 339–343.
48. H. Jang and J. Lee. (2018). An empirical study on modeling and prediction of bitcoin prices with Bayesian neural networks based on blockchain information. *IEEE Access*, 6, 5427–5437.
49. https://www.kaggle.com/mczielinski/bitcoin-historical-data.

5 Applications of AI, IoT, and Robotics in Healthcare Service Based on Several Aspects

Garima Jain and Ankush Jain
Noida Institute of Engineering and Technology

CONTENTS

5.1 INTRODUCTION: BACKGROUND

Current technological advancements are rapidly converting businesses into digital enterprises that will experience the world in ways we have yet to imagine. Artificial intelligence (AI), natural language processing (NLP), blockchain (BC), cloud computing, the Internet of Things (IoT), and virtual and augmented reality are just a few of the technologies driving this transformation. Nowadays, a

DOI: 10.1201/9781003224075-5

good percentage of the world's population is rapidly aging and comorbidities. Economically connected lifestyles will continue to result in mass growth – developments like smoking, obesity, harmful alcohol consumption, malaise diet, and sedentary lifestyle. Healthcare is the prevention, diagnosis, treatment, recovery, or treatment of illness, injury, and other physical and mental disabilities to maintain or improve people's health. Healthcare professionals and related industries provide healthcare. It encompasses work in primary, secondary, and tertiary care, as well as public health.

In the healthcare industry, the advantages of a linked, constantly monitored, automated, and machine learning world are obvious and enormous in the healthcare industry. The data capture or "listening" component of healthcare is pretty well established in the Internet of Healthy Things (IoHT) arena. The ability to grasp an individual's status by "capturing" and interpreting information is vital to healthcare, whether it's a parent listening to a child's sneeze or a doctor using a metronome to a patient's heartbeat. Works in primary care, secondary care, tertiary care, and public health are all included. IoT startups are increasingly finding new uses in healthcare and benefiting from enhanced sensors. In the healthcare industry, the IoT is becoming more common. Materials management, digitalization of medical information, and digitization of medical procedures are three of the most common IoT applications in intelligent medicine. Until the IoT, the only way for doctors and patients to communicate was through visits, texts, and telecommunications. There were no methods that allowed doctors to screen or monitor their patients and make appropriate recommendations continuously. However, the rise of IoT in the healthcare sector has drastically altered the scene. Clinicians have been able to provide better care by deploying IoT-enabled gadgets to monitor patients remotely. Furthermore, as patient connection with doctors has grown more comfortable and efficient, IoT has raised patient satisfaction ratings. The IoT has inadvertently changed the health sector and is extremely good for health.

Connected devices can gather valuable clinical and health-related information with constant observation through a smart clinical device associated with a cell phone application. The associated IoT gadget picks and transfers data about well-being, such as internal temperature, pulse, oxygen, glucose levels, weight, and electrocardiogram (ECG). The information is put away in the cloud and imparted to the approved individual as indicated by the sharing authority. The individual might be a doctor, a health firm, or a specialist, and this will permit them to see the information gathered regardless of their area and time.

Figure 5.1 demonstrates that before the invention of IoT in healthcare, it was always difficult for a patient to check body temperature by themselves through a normal thermometer. At that time, the patients did not interact directly with the doctors, and they had to go to the hospital and then take medicine for any disease and areas of interest.

Figure 5.2 demonstrates that it is easier to examine the body temperature after the invention of IoT in healthcare. To measure the accurate temperature of the individual's body, we use a temperature cover. The smartphones receive the data at regular time intervals from the antennas, and from here, the data is collected. The

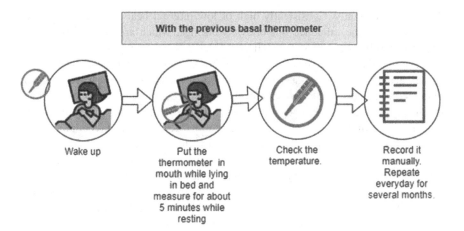

FIGURE 5.1   Healthcare without IoT.

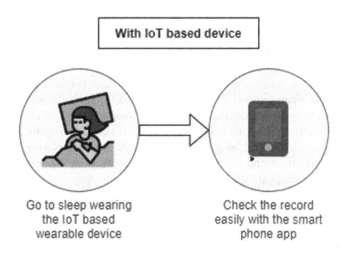

FIGURE 5.2   IoT-based healthcare.

expert advises the medicine after analyzing the data in real time. Diseases are easily identified by the graph of temperature versus time graph. Now the patient connects directly with the doctors, and there is no need to go to the hospital and take medicine after the doctor's advice. IoT has made human life easier. The application incorporates health reports for distant diagnosis, provides warnings for temperature range, plans alarms for medicine, and plans specialist visits. IoT is liable for each actual device with the opportunity to see and hear the others and to "talk" so they can share their data [1–9]. Metal Oxide Semiconductor chip has planned IoT-based equipment and programming for medical care frameworks that help healthcare departments screen their patients' medical-related problems through the Internet distantly. Consistently high or low internal heat levels throughout a specific timeframe influence our body's workings, which are controlled by the day-by-day schedule, and make medical problems, thus promoting changes in prescription with the assistance of a specialist. For instance, the bacterial disease can cause variation in internal heat levels. Indeed, it is one of the most well-known reasons for changes in internal heat levels. Since infections and microbes struggle to survive at temperatures over the body's ordinary temperature, it automatically increases its climate and the body's capacity to battle disease if it recognizes bacterial contamination. It isn't unusual to raise the internal heat level by 3°F–5°F to battle an infection. Since infections and microbes struggle to survive at temperatures over the body's ordinary temperature, it automatically increases its climate and the body's capacity to battle disease if it recognizes bacterial contamination.

It isn't unusual to raise the internal heat level by 3°F–5°F to battle an infection. Since the increased internal heat level likewise harms the body, it would prefer not to permit high temperatures to go untreated for long. Bluetooth capacity can associate with accessible cell phones. It is a low-power innovation that interacts with remote media with a temperature sensor.

For medical care-related specialist employees, IoT underpins the personalization of medical care related items utilizing timely essential information using wearable gadgets, For healthcare-related service providers, IoT supports the personalization (improvement of added value) of healthcare-related products using timely vital data to be obtained with a wearable device, and for companies who promote health management, it provides health management support for female employees as part of the benefits package, and supports the application to data health. It is healthcare equipment for supporting self-health management. The IoT connects our world as much as possible. Nowadays, we have internet infrastructure almost anywhere, and we can use it whenever we want. The main applications of IoT in intelligent medicine include

- Materials management.
- The digitization of medical information.
- The digitization of medical procedures.

This wearable gadget is certifiably not a clinical thermometer (clinical instrument). IoT refers to a preparation of interconnected, web-associated things that can gather and transfer information over a small group without human intervention. IoT attempts to set up upgraded availability (with Internet access) between gadgets (clinical sensors, wellness trackers, and so forth) or constructs computerization in all regions, gradually in the order of frameworks or administrations. Associated innovation is one of the essential utilizations of IoT in medical care. Such gadgets are utilized to screen the patient, take readings, see designs, and devices are used to monitor the patient, take tasks, see patterns, and notify patients in case of pattern imperfections.

Likewise, this procedure is utilized to continuously check patients, settle on educated choices, and forestall trauma center visits. The decrease in visits to trauma centers has additionally strengthened the commonality in clinical administration. Organizations are creating imaginative programming projects to address different issues in medical services. For example, to address the emergency department waiting time issue, GE Healthcare developed a software program, auto, that helps reduce patients' waiting times, requiring a patient bed. These advancements can help medical care associations tap into the capability of an undeniably interconnected and responsive world. If the business can produce more noteworthy interconnectivity in a solitary environment, there will be huge advantages to patients, doctors, payers, and medication engineers.

IoT gadgets, for example, smart pills, wearable screens, and sensors, permit medical care specialists to gather information ceaselessly. AI frameworks can help break down this information to distinguish changes in a patient's condition, propose therapy alternatives, recognize patterns, support patient adherence, improve patient results, and quicken the revelation of and admittance to new therapies [10–12].

The Internet will allow robots to interface this present reality to the virtual world. On the off chance that arising robots are considered, with the working framework system, communication with the Internet through Bluetooth requires one bunch of uses the programming interface (Application Program Interface) call appeared in Figure 5.3 which portrays the development of medical care (with IoT). Robots of things to come will turn out to be essential for IoT and will have the option to have consistent correspondence with the cloud. These robots will have the capacity of keen portability and contextual registering with the Internet logically with the physical encompassing their climate. A robot can likewise interface, utilizing cloud arrangement and informing with any assistance, business cycle, or gadget associated with the cloud. Discussion can be either unusual or simultaneous with the cloud (a robot holds up feedback before continuing with the following activity), mounted on the cloud-dependent on uncovered web administrations.

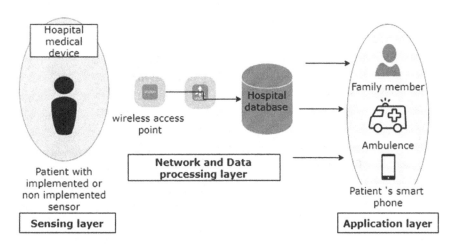

FIGURE 5.3 Development of medical care with IoT.

The IoT has immense potential in the field of clinical data on the board. The interest for clinical data on the board in emergency clinics is predominantly in the accompanying angles: distinguishing proof, example acknowledgment, and clinical record ID. Determining evidence incorporates tolerant ID, doctor ID, test ID (counting drug ID), clinical gadget ID, lab ID, and clinical record ID (counting indications and infection ID). The multiplication of medical care explicit IoT items opens up huge chances. Also, the sheer volume of information created by these associated gadgets can change medical care. It is a vast improvement in industry and humankind as reinforcing network safety has been a key concern. Creating AI aptitudes joined with related systems is promising to convey brilliant administrations and foundations. On the other hand, the wellbeing-related bundle was diminishing in the IoT nature since wearable ascertaining and procedures, which were among the most thoughtful ones by the finish of 2015, have declined in fame [13–16].

IoT has a four-stage design that is essentially arranged in a cycle. Figure 5.4 portrays the IoT with robots in medical services. Each of the four stages is associated such that the information is prepared or handled in one step and acquires the incentive in the following stage. Coordinated qualities carry instinct to the cycle and convey dynamic business possibilities.

Stage 1: The principal stage includes the organization of interconnected gadgets, which incorporate sensors, actuators, screens, finders, camera frameworks, and so on. These gadgets gather information.

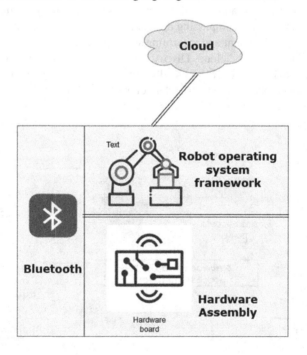

FIGURE 5.4　IoT with robots.

Stage 2: Typically, information got from sensors, and different gadgets are in a simple structure, gathered, and changed into a mechanical design for information handling.

Stage 3: Once the information is digitized and gathered, it is pre-handled, normalized, and moved to the server farm or cloud.

Stage 4: Management and examination of factual information are done at the necessary level. The progressed investigation, applied to this information, carries significant business experiences to settle on powerful choices.

Medical care is being rethought thanks to the IoT, which ensures better consideration, better therapy results, lower costs for patients, enhanced cycles and work processes, enhanced execution, and a better patient experience for medical care providers. These sensors form a network of intelligent sensors capable of gathering, preparing, moving, and dissecting crucial data in various situations, such as connecting home monitoring devices to clinic-based frameworks. From start to finish, check your health. IoT phases are also available for receiving wires and more established patients to address health-related illnesses and repeat medications. IoT-based frameworks demonstrate discipline, as well as the ability to adapt to a patient's conditions. The flare-up of COVID-19 has pushed interest in wearable gadgets, which track wellbeing and wellness, area-related data, and can be incorporated with devices, for example, workstations and cell phones. The main advantage of IoT Healthcare are as follows:

- Reduced clinical treatment costs
- Better treatment results
- Better sickness the executives
- Reduced mistakes
- Enhancing persistent experience
- Advanced Management of Medicines

Medical service frameworks characterized by the IoT stage depend on different components checking persistent illnesses, thinking about old patients, and wellbeing of the board frameworks. For example, persistent medical issues, stoutness, malignant growth, and joint pain influence many individuals. For individuals with ongoing illnesses, medical services are an everyday concern. Patients require disease the executive's devices daily, not just when they visit the specialist. Specialists receive regular health updates that enable them to use IoT devices to detect infection across the board. IoT has the potential to increase patients' overall strength and perhaps reduce the need for medical practice. IoT assumes a significant function in medical care. The fundamental of IoT permits us to facilitate a modest measure of information about a patient's sickness and wellbeing, which would take a long time to file physically. It is likewise in two sections for better understanding:

a. application-based and
b. administration-based.

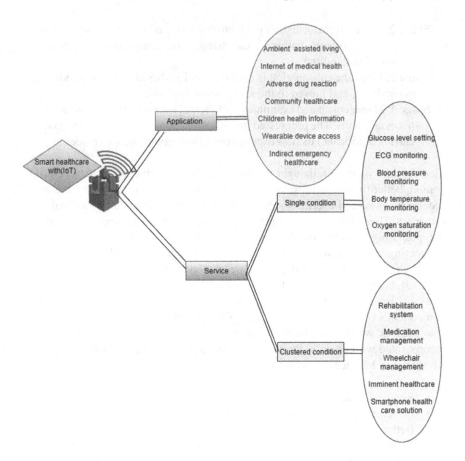

FIGURE 5.5   Impact of IoT in healthcare.

Further, application-based is separated into single status-based and bunch status-based. A solitary position alludes to explicit sicknesses, while group status appears with numerous illnesses in Figure 5.5. It depends on the present IoT medical services framework, which has a powerful nature to add single or bunch status-based infections in the future.

Different regions need more doctors, clinics, and other medical service assets to give quality consideration to the entire populace. IoT takes into account simpler correspondence among specialists and patients when they can't meet face to face. Specialists can utilize IoT-associated gadgets to screen tolerant information. Joined with video conferencing, specialists can help patients practically with a few wellbeing concerns. This framework doesn't generally supplant face-to-face visits; however, it can significantly improve openness for country networks. Telehealth is the conveyance of medical care administration and clinical data to far-off areas. It offers types of assistance like Telemedicine, Telemonitoring, Telesurgery, Remote clinical instruction, and Telehealth information administration.

Advantages of Telehealth Administrations:

- Prompt clinical consideration, particularly during seasons of health-related crisis and catastrophic events. No requirement for holding up in long lines to see a doctor
- Reduced documentation and administrative work
- Less costly
- Equal and complete medical care arrangements to everybody by taking out geological obstructions
- Better correspondence with specialist
- Expanded reach to different wellbeing specialist cooperatives.

5.1.1 OUTLINE

The remaining paper is organized as follows. Section 5.2 briefs about the related work. Section 5.3 provides a detailed analysis of some theories and concepts of Robot in Healthcare. Section 5.4 explains AI in healthcare interaction on which our future implementation will based on. Section 5.5 explains the combined concept of AI, IoT, and Robot in Healthcare protection overview with further divided into types of robots with IoT framework. Section 5.6 explains in detail about the Internet of Healthcare with its security, application, and advantages. Section 5.7 is followed by a conclusion and some suggestions for further research and areas of interest.

5.2 LITERATURE SURVEY

As per Patel et al. [17]. The author drawn-out favorable circumstances of humans in clinical administrations fragment, wellbeing-related emergencies, e-prosperity, etc., using progressed mechanics and IoT. Furthermore, the time of assignment, affiliation, challenges for the future is to be analyzed. Medical services will become more sophisticated and less expensive in the coming years, and the clinical area will be more accessible. Numerous associations and scientists include satisfying IoT challenges, appropriation issues, foundation improvement, and normalization, advancing and getting some great outcomes worldwide in the not-so-distant future.

As Guntur et al. [18] indicated, Robotics innovation is one of the most remarkable and rising advances in the field of prescription. Electronic sensors combined with a blend of control into mechanical systems fundamentally improve the presentation and versatility of structures. The mechanical advancement used to strengthen arms was not exact and unable to send the particular unmistakable analysis, clear turn of events, and arranging. With the advances in gear, programming, and control programming structures, extensive computerization is being utilized to work with more degrees of chance than individuals under many conditions. Robotics advancements are launched in various areas, which unmistakably influence patient perception and mind. Progressed mechanics advancement in the drug is the prime point of convergence of the clinical administration's organizations in

ICUs, available rooms, and operation room, which lessens chances for patients, subject matter experts and it is also utilized in labs to accumulate the models followed by transportation of tests at whatever point required, researching, and sparing them for long stretch amassing.

As indicated by Islam et al. [19], the IoT makes awesome articles definitive structure blocks to improve digital actual shrewd inescapable systems. The IoT has an assortment of utilization spaces, including medical services. The IoT unrest is updating present-day medical care with promising innovative, financial, and social possibilities. This chapter studies IoT-based medical care advances and surveys the advanced network structures/stages, applications, and modern patterns in IoT-based medical care arrangements. Moreover, this chapter examines specific IoT security and protection highlights, including security necessities, danger models, and assault scientific classifications from the medical care perspective.

As indicated by Grieco et al. [20], the author examines the advancing in surgency of the IoT, alongside creating scattering of robots in various activities of reliable life, making IoT-upheld progressed mechanical technology applications a generous reality of our impending future. As such, new advanced organizations, considering the trade among robots and "things," are being envisioned in aiding individuals. Coincidentally, the route to a creative improvement of IoT-helped progressed mechanics applications requires a couple of vital issues to be clarified, plan procedures to be blended, and strong plan choices to be inspected. Their chapter analyzes advanced mechanics suggestions, open issues, and target applications in the IoT-helped mechanical technology innovation zone. In particular, the current responsibility is four-fallen.

As per Sivaparthipan et al. [21], the author clarified huge information had collected a tremendous proportion of set aside data for applications, including mechanical innovation, a web of things (IoT), and clinical consideration system. Notwithstanding how the IoT-based clinical consideration structure accepts a vital capacity in the colossal data industry, the identification may be difficult to envision the specific result for some circumstances. The proposed design with man-created awareness and IoT for Parkinson's contamination can improve the walk execution greatly. This assessment portrays the capacity of robots in Parkinson's affliction and how they partner with enormous information examination.

As indicated by Chae et al. [22], examine the investigation of computerized advancement perspective on IoT in both academic networks and industry. Surviving examinations have reviewed the subject of IoT using different techniques. This assessment takes a modernized improvement viewpoint on IoT as an astounding climate of developments, industry applications, thoughts, methods, and social establishments, which is momentarily extraordinary and progresses after some time.

As per Yoon et al. [23], the creator clarifies that advancement-based help experience has gotten essential thought with improved development, especially computerized reasoning robots, in the clinical consideration industry. In the advancement-based help insight, the development as an expert community expects a fundamental part in succeeding the organization experience. The purpose behind this examination is to develop a structure for the accomplishment factors of an advancement-based assistance involvement with the clinical consideration industry. Elements of subjects (human and advancements) and accomplishment factors in the experience are reviewed and proposed.

As indicated by Tian [24], with the advancement of data innovation, the idea of keen medical services has slowly gone to the front. Shrewd medical services utilize another age of data advances, for example, the web of things (IoT), enormous information, distributed computing, and artificial brainpower, to change the conventional clinical framework in an overall manner, making medical services more productive, more helpful, and more customized with the point of presenting the idea of competent medical care, in this audit, the first rundown the key advances that help keen medical care and explain the current status of savvy medical services in a few significant fields.

Dimitrov [25] indicated that the creator characterizes different advances that can reduce overall costs for the expectation or the leading body of incessant diseases. These fuse contraptions ceaselessly screen prosperity markers, devices that auto-control medicines, or devices that track consistent prosperity data when a patient self-administers a treatment. Since they have extended induction to quick Internet and Personal Digital Assistants, various patients have started to use flexible (applications) to manage diverse prosperity needs. These devices and convenient applications are logically used and facilitated with telemedicine and telehealth through the clinical IoT. The maker reviews IoT and enormous data in clinical consideration fields. Today, wearables and compact applications maintain health, prosperity preparing, following, and agreeable contamination of the board and care coordination.

As per Shah [26], ongoing upgrades in development and accessibility have incited the ascent of IoT and AI applications in various endeavors. Their chapter thinks about the impacts of progressions, for instance, IoT and AI in clinical consideration through a detailed review of 75 partners explored adroit journal articles.

The assessment reveals outstanding advancement in the number of articles appropriated in the latest decade, a wide variety of dispersion sources, a huge number of essayists, and various applied and plans science chapters, all exhibiting a rising field with phenomenal conveyance potential future years. The creator moreover includes key encounters for the top application classes, which join wearables and accessibility, illness disclosure and treatment, steady thought, and sensor associations, and perceives openings and future investigation headings related to development plan and affirmation, rules for data security and assurance, and structures feasibility and prosperity.

As indicated by Pramanik et al. [27], the advances in intelligent clinical contraptions and unavoidable systems are changing-related clinical considerations into a thriving stage for certain clinical considerations. The IoT, splendid sensors, and wearables have augmented the clinical consideration structure, enabling removed checking and supporting the sickness of the patient every single through focus. This segment plans to fill in as a brief presentation on the progression of insightful and certain clinical consideration systems. The part starts with a chart of IoT, splendid sensors, and unpreventable structures and besides their interrelationships. The role includes the challenges the current clinical administration systems looked at and separates how to overcome these with the help of unpreventable clinical administrations.

As indicated by Wan et al. [28], of late, they have seen electrifying progressions of versatile clinical administration robots, which like various ideal conditions over their human accomplices. Past correspondence networks for clinical consideration robots reliably experience the evil impacts of high response inertness just as repetitive handling demands. Amazing and fast correspondences and speedy dealing with are essential, at times major explicitly under clinical consideration robots, to the clinical consideration recipients. As a good course of action, offloading delay-tricky and passing on simple tasks to the robot depends on improving the organizations and leeway customers. In their chapter, they review a couple of top tier progressions, for instance, the human–robot interface, condition and customer status seeing, course, great correspondence, and mechanized thinking, of a versatile clinical consideration robot and discussion about in nuances the altered demands over offloading the count and correspondence tasks.

As shown by the trademark solicitations of functions over the association use, they request limits of a standard clinical administration robot into elective classes: the edge functionalities and the middle functionalities. For instance, various dormancy delicate tasks, such as customer association, or monotonous endeavors, including prosperity gatherer status affirmation and self-administering moving, can be set up by the robot without progressive correspondences with worker farms.

As indicated by Han [29], the creator examines the main estimates when they plan a clinical consideration robot. Heaps of robots for clinical administration circumstances are being developed; in any case, very few of them have won in the certifiable field. In like manner, they endeavored to acquaint another perspective with the push toward this issue. Their chapter proposes a framework that affirms comfort by interpreting the robot plan from the services cape perspective. Nursing robots' customer testing results were assessed using four services cape elements: equipment, design, decor, space, and ambiance. Stuff was necessary to the robot's comfort, so it was primarily considered, and the GUI plan's limit was Design and Deco. Space was an issue highlighted all over the earth as the robot moved, for example, the width of the passage and the state of the floor.

Fan et al. [30] indicated that the IoT makes all articles interconnected and intelligent, seen as the accompanying innovative upset. As its typical case, IoT-based canny reclamation systems improve to deal with calm issues related to developing peoples and the absence of prosperity specialists. Despite how it has come into this present reality, fundamental problems exist in modernizing the plan and reconfiguring such a structure, enabling it to respond to the patient's requirements rapidly. Their chapter gives a thought to the power-based mechanizing plan approach (Adaptive Delta Modulation) for intelligent rebuilding systems in IoT. Cosmology helps PCs understand the signs and clinical resources, which helps make a recuperation strategy and reconfigure clinical resources according to patients' specific essentials quickly and normally.

As per Bodur et al. [31], the finish of their investigation demonstrates that should lock into IoT advancement with nursing and clinical preparation. Further examinations should be directed to organize mechanical examples into clinical consideration and nursing practices. Of the individuals, 70.8% were female, 81.6% were learning at a state-subsidized school, 61.3% were senior nursing understudies, and 38.7% were senior clinical understudies.

A bigger piece of the understudies communicated that the IoT development would impact future clinical and nursing practices. The nursing understudies got the most raised mean score on the thing fundamental actual assessments, for instance, glucose, heartbeat, and ECGs will be easier using IoT advancement (7.36±2.27), and the most unmean score (5.36±2.82) on the thing "Robot specialists and chaperons made through IoT development will give open-minded clinical administrations later on".

5.3 ROBOTICS IN HEALTHCARE

There has been an extraordinary development in the last few decades, and increased uses of robots in medical science know and simplify many aspects of our wellbeing and health improvement. Robots are a rapidly growing part of the modern healthcare landscape. Robots are defined as machines that can do several tasks with a DoF and higher autonomy than humans, and it is difficult different from other machines. On the other hand, the service and system of healthcare have become a huge campus. With the advent of technology, robots are integrated to reduce such complex nature of healthcare and innovation, and research in the field is still growing.

Medical services present a decent occasion to unravel the utilization of robots in different issues and back patients' soundness. Coordinated obligations are performed utilizing robots for the medical services and clinical business zones of mechanical and hardware, for example, power or development estimations or space, sensor framework innovation, and so forth are the worry expenses brought about by the robot care of patients, recovery, prostheses, clinical mediation if vital, E-wellbeing, checking. By that definition, clinically advanced mechanics is viewed as of extraordinary worth. Medical care regarding wellbeing, social and monetary advantages, and mechanical technology can give answers to a critical extent, particularly for tolerant gatherings needs, such as amputees, stroke victims, or intellectual or mental handicap patients.

With the quick improvement in advanced mechanics, AI, and IoT, they have all the bits of innovation to do this, and it won't be long when these bits of the invention coordinate to change the way they carry on with our lives. Advanced mechanics is worried about customized machines intended to perform work concentrated work. AI is the study of making PCs and machines work without being modified to do as such. Blends of advanced mechanics and machine robots result from discovering that they can chip away at their own.

Progressed condition of AI knowledge is with IoT. Numerous robots can interconnect. IoT stage gives extraordinary office to the interrelationship between items or individuals, moving information cooperation between people without PCs or humans. IoT can be applicable for observing and catching information related to everything without exception media, ecological checking, and framework the executives, for an organization fabricating, energy the board, building and home robotization or transportation, clinical and wellbeing frameworks. Contingent on applications and market examination, there are six regions of clinical mechanical technology:

- Smart clinical containers
- Surgical advanced mechanics
- Prosthetics utilizing careful robots
- Motor co-appointment investigation and treatment by robots
- The robot helped mental and social treatment
- Robotized quiet observing frameworks

Many robots with devoted jobs are composed of an organizer that approaches and an assortment of encompassing sensors. The essential thought isn't just to offer types of assistance inside the condo of a solitary client, yet additionally to traverse the usefulness across structures and a local location to outside zones and maybe even an entire town. Information is traded and incorporated utilizing a typical middleware. Logical data is disengaged from the fixed and robot sensors and the client orders and put away in the setting mindfulness module.

In Figure 5.6, generally speaking, the idea and design of the Robot-Era stage for surrounding helped living and older consideration. The end clients and parental figures collaborate with the framework utilizing a discourse interface or a purposefully basic tablet-based graphical User Interface. The Physically Embedded Intelligent Systems middleware layer incorporates surrounding sensors, client watching sensors, robots, and intelligent devices.

The framework and robots are made easier by the setup organizer.

Robots assume a significant function in medical services for executives. Robot frameworks don't have feelings, can't drain them, and never have any consideration. On the off chance that this seems like the correct specialist, it was additionally the reason behind numerous robots that are now utilized in top clinics around the globe. There is a ton of work in a clinic, and not just specialists can use some assistance. Attendants and medical clinic laborers can profit with the aid of robots. The robot deals with resting, bringing items, and cleaning so that attendants can invest increasingly more energy with patients and give a human touch while pounding the machine. Administration robots can perform human assignments, for example, causing debilitated or old patients to feel forlorn. Conversational and partner robots can help these patients remain positive, remind them to take their prescription, and perform basic routine checks, for example, temperature, pulse, and sugar levels. Operational effectiveness can be increased and can achieve cost reduction in some cases. A job can be played by robots in

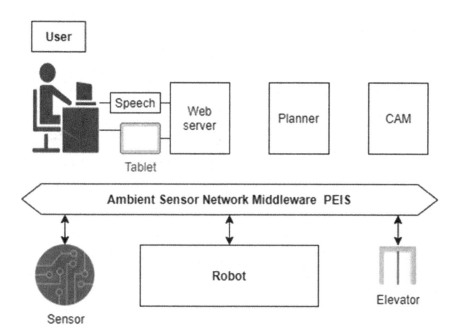

FIGURE 5.6 Healthcare with robotics.

medical care the board in three regions: medical procedure partner jobs (helped during a medical procedure measure), understanding help jobs (supporting patient post-surgical techniques), and administration uphold positions (general activities help). It is essential to improving these jobs, persistent wellbeing, and medical services execution, enhancing patients and speculators. In medical procedures, advanced clinical mechanics demonstrated that it lessens both time and danger. Because of its predominance, prostate and cardiovascular strategies are today played by robots in numerous nations. Robots additionally demonstrated their capacity in recovery and insight. Prosthesis nowadays, social mechanical technology is a thorny branch created to screen and rouse patients. Expanding interest for data innovation in medical services and clinical area prompts advanced mechanics.

Moreover, mechanical technology has progressed applications. Healthcare space advances market development in the coming years. The idea of automated technology frameworks is the connection between true information and the physical world. Advanced mechanics is continually interdisciplinary designing, yet it incorporates biomechanics, computational science, nervous system science, psychological science, sports science, biomedical, etc. The principal challenge is to challenge interface sensors, engines, and human selection with clinical advanced mechanics abilities in various conditions.

The information flow in Figure 5.7 helps people for data information with the actual world to complete the given task. When discussing clinically advanced

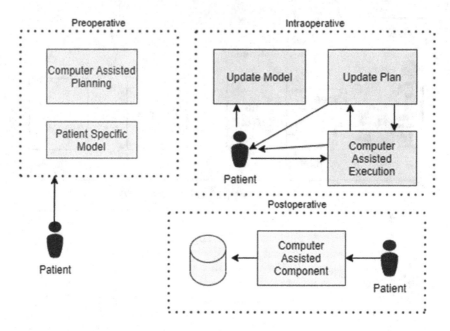

FIGURE 5.7   The information flow for computer-integrated surgery system.

mechanics, a few components movement is initiated remembering direction, self-rule, insight, and so forth, a framework pivoting in more than one hub and inside its current circumstance. Independence reveals the degree of human interest in supervising tasks robot or automated gadgets both in ordinary activity and particularly when issues or deformities in the framework.

5.4   AI IN HEALTHCARE

The use of computations and AI programming to copy human expertise in the search, understanding, and perception of detailed medical information and clinics are referred to as AI in medical services. AI is the computer's ability to calculate for ostensibly information-dependent purposes. Gathering information, measuring it, and offering outstanding performance to the end customer is what AI innovation recognizes from typical improvements in healthcare. AI computations and deep learning are used by simulated intelligence to accomplish this. These computations can detect ongoing undertakings and justify their existence.

It should build an AI model with broad data measures to pick up valuable bits of knowledge and expectations. AI algorithms vary from humans in two ways:

- **Literal Algorithms in AI:** when an objective is set, the calculation gains only from the information and can just comprehend what it has been customized to do.

- **Block Boxes Deep Learning Algorithms**: Calculations can foresee with outrageous accuracy yet offer next to zero fathomable clarification to the rationale behind its choices besides the information and sort of calculation utilized.

Breaking the links between treatment or counter-attack processes and patient outcomes is at the heart of AI wellness applications. AI programs apply to practices, for example, determination measures, treatment convention improvement, drug progression, personalized medication, and patient observation and care.

The condition was diagnosed and prevented by computer-based intelligence computations to examine a significant amount of data from electronic health records. In radiology, simulated intelligence emphases the field of radiology to recognize and examine infections within patients through computerized tomography (CT) and magnetic resonance imaging (MRI). AI applications in psychoanalysis are presently at the proof-of-concept stage. Chat-bots and conversation specialists that imitate human behavior and are assessed for uneasiness and low level are examples of zones where testing quickly spreads.

In primary care, AI has been utilized for supporting dynamic, prescient displaying, and business examination. Regardless of the quick advances in AI advances, general experts' view on the job of AI in essential consideration is extremely restricted, principally centered around managerial and routine documentation assignments.

Through mass Electronic Health Records control, AI can significantly assist professionals in disease diagnosis and patient conclusion. Diseases have become increasingly complex, and with a long history of falsifying computerized healthcare data, the risk of case duplication is significant. Even though a person with a rare illness is less likely to be the only person who has ever had an infection, clinicians face a substantial obstacle when they cannot locate cases from appropriately indicated birthplaces. Using AI to locate similar issues and medicines and factor in boss indications and assist clinicians in posing the most appropriate questions helps patients achieve the most accurate diagnosis and therapy.

The rise of possible AI applications has been demonstrated by the proliferation of telemedicine and patients' care from afar. By observing their data through sensors, simulated intelligence can aid in distant thinking about patients.

5.5 HEALTHCARE WITH IOT BASED ON FUSION OF AI AND ML

As the most recent innovation patterns keep on driving the worldwide medical services industry, we are seeing clinical gadget suppliers offering a scope of creative answers to improve the nature of patient consideration. In driving those gadgets, from actual devices to smart gadgets, new innovative progressions permit specialists and patients to participate recently, communicate important information continuously, and recognize dangerous episodes quicker than at any other time.

It is assisting with relieving. According to the World Health Organization (WHO) [2] report, the clinical administration's IoT market segment is prepared to hit USD 117 billion by 2020. Dynamically, new organizations find new applications inside clinical administrations and use connected sensors to investigate better, screen, and supervise patients and treatment. Many are based on the clinical-grade wearable to even more powerfully track tolerant information, while others see open entryway for sensor networks inside centers and practices to improve clinical consideration movement and screen persistent adherence [32].

Robots filling different capacities and needs in the clinical/wellbeing and social consideration areas past the customary extent of care and recovery robots are set to get one of the main mechanical developments of the 21st century. Robots have been executed from multiple points of view to help the coordination of wellbeing and social consideration. Applications incorporate medical clinic and care home conditions and reach from explicit arrangements tending to generally very much characterized issues. In the current cell phone period, an ever-increasing number of shoppers are getting settled with the possibility of video counsel with their doctor, distant checking through wellbeing applications, and utilizing individual symptomatic gadgets in cell phones as a prepared reckoner. Robots are wherever from sci-fi to your nearby medical clinic, where they are evolving medical services. Robots start to influence medication (utilizing science and innovation to treat and forestall injury and illness treatment) and medical care (accessibility of therapy and an earlier notice of sickness). Robots additionally demonstrated their capacity in recovery and knowledge prosthesis. Another approach to upgrade quiet mind and wellbeing informatics with more prominent availability is through live-in robots that encourage telemedicine to give ceaseless basic consideration to patients. When the robot is joined, a specialist can teach the patient to hit the hay. Utilizing the robot's two-way general media video chatting highlight, specialists and patients can without much stretch and normally offer clinical data. Robots in medication help assuage the clinical workforce from routine errands, redirect their time from all the more squeezing obligations, and make operations more secure and affordable for patients. They can likewise do exact medical procedures in small areas and transport unsafe substances. Mechanical clinical associates screen persistent indispensable insights and ready medical caretakers when a human presence is required in the room, permitting attendants to screen different patients all the while. These mechanical partners likewise naturally enter data into understanding electronic wellbeing records. Robotic trucks can be observed transporting supplies through emergency clinic corridors. Robots are again aiding a medical procedure, permitting specialists to do a medical system through little entry points instead of inch-by-inch cuts. Advanced mechanics is again having a significant effect in different fields of medication.

Distant analysis and automated helped medical procedures are ordinarily utilized worldwide. The fast movement with which Information and Communication Technologies is developing implies that significantly more opportunities for these innovations turn into a reality. A distant conclusion permits a specialist to examine indications distantly. This medium is particularly gainful for provincial regions without close-by clinical assets and patients who can't head out to see a specialist.

For instance, as of now, in any case, pictures got from 3D CAT examines, for example, those delivered by Imaginaries, have a few gigabits, and the present uplink channels are not adequate for far-off live determination. Uniting CAT check pictures and explicit codec advances custom-made to the force and speed of 5G organizations will make complex, distant diagnostics conceivable later on. With the assistance of a machine, specialists would now be able to perform complex techniques with more accuracy and adaptability and diminish the hatred of the activity. This medium altogether decreases the time it takes the patient to do the medical procedure and improves the exactness of the action. Nonetheless, this is just conceivable through advances in programming and consistent transmission of data. The automated medical process offers numerous advantages to patients contrasted with an open medical approach, including:

• Small hospitalization
• Reduce pain and discomfort
• Fast recovery time and return to normal activities
• Small incisions, which reduces the risk of infection
• Anemia and transfusion
• Minimal stain

Four significant sorts of clinical robots are as follows:

5.5.1 CLINIC ROBOTS

Hospital robots can play various assignments to lessen the everyday trouble on specialists, medical attendants, and specialists. This medium incorporates disseminating patient information, such as medications, lab tests, and other delicate materials around the emergency clinic – American mechanical technology organization. Aethon has built up a self-governing portable robot called TUG, which is fit for achieving these undertakings – setting aside cash to zero in on patient consideration and saving time for medical service experts. Mechanical frameworks are additionally being intended to sanitize gadgets and hardware in wellbeing frameworks.

5.5.2 CAREFUL ROBOT

The most well-known employments of advanced mechanics in medical procedure incorporate automatic weapons with a camera or potentially careful instruments, constrained by a specialist. Robot-helped activity implies that it can finish intricate cycles with more remarkable precision and with extra controls. They are likewise regularly insignificantly obtrusive, offering a choice to open a medical procedure, which has a more prominent related danger and requires a more extended recuperation time. Instances of robot-helped methods incorporate biopsy, the expulsion of malignant tumors, fix of heart valves, and gastric detour.

5.5.3 Care Robot

While many of these advances are intended for use in emergency clinics and other medical services places, care robots can help old or impaired patients in their homes. Right now, care robots are essentially used to finish straightforward undertakings, for example, assisting patients with getting up. An illustration of this is Robier – a bear-molded robot created by the Japanese examination organization RIKEN and development organization Sumitomo Rico.

5.5.4 Exoskeletons

Global Data Research has discovered that the exoskeleton market is one of the quickest developing areas in all mechanical technology. The exoskeleton utilizes sensors mounted on the skin to recognize electrical signs in the patient's body and respond with movement in their joints. It intends to give actual restoration to patients recuperating from lower appendage problems, such as stroke and spinal rope wounds.

Figure 5.8 indicates insight concerning the extent of mechanical connection with both the physical and virtual worlds. AI (machine learning) will give moment

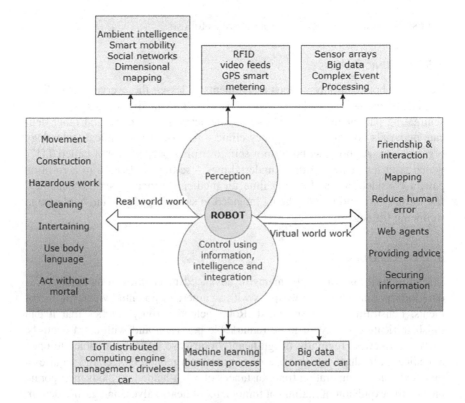

FIGURE 5.8　Flow of AI, IoT with robotics in the real world.

improvement to huge numbers of the weight's medical service frameworks across. As the world faces, others guarantee that AI is minimal relief rather than false and will never replace human-transmitted cures. It isn't easy to imagine how judgment about silent practices, answers, and reactions, distinctions of actual evaluation, especially perception and exploration, can be anything other than human.

It thinks about the scope of information sources (both dynamic control and discernment driven) and shows numerous potential yields, activities, or jobs that can happen. Function of Information Technology (IT) administrations, utilizing such a thoughtful and important piece of the robot association biological system, starts arising.

A robot may have an actual direct articulation that permits it to precisely work and respond in reality. Yet, it can likewise work in virtual the world is at long last utilizing data innovation as a type of arrangement real-world availability (for example, conveying important data to distant spectators). A robot can likewise have discernment. For instance, it can absorb this present reality. Information sources make "applicable signifying" from them and work as indicated by their programming and realized. It presents a gathering of slides that cover the accompanying themes: m-IOT, medical care IT, medication, versatile medical care, Long-Term Evolution, and 4G wellbeing [33].

In the coming days, the interest in the improvement of IoT will be expanding quickly. It will be important to give simple advancement devices that associate the actual world to IoT-based organizations. Robotic studies, IoT, and the expansions in wellbeing informatics are forecast to be the factors for healthcare systems in the future [34–40]. Since IoT is another creating innovation, the apparatuses for different arrangements in the IoT stage are not completely dependable grown at this point. In such a manner, ROS gives appealing occasions to the IoT stage for the foundation network. ROS has qualities like high deliberation level pulls in specialists and logical associations to get to any equipment.

5.6   INTERNET OF HEALTHCARE

The vision of an IoHT world, in which we continuously collect patient data and use it to improve health, is becoming a very real prospect in the near future. Sensors may collect raw data in real time, all the time.

When IoHT data compare with the past data, individualized insights emerge, allowing healthcare practitioners to become "more efficient, economical, and targeted" in their care delivery. Data. There's data everywhere. So, what's next? As previously said, data collected by sensors drive the IoHT, but how that data is used and processed is crucial to translating it into actionable information in real-world contexts.

While healthcare data analysis is pretty well developed, as evidenced by cost-effectiveness and healthcare quality research, clinical or claims databases are used frequently. A most large-scale study built on these datasets, from which analysts are familiar. Due to the enormous number of potential data sources, the type of data obtained, and it is gathered with the frequency, IoHT data is less well clear.

The further data we collect, the more precise our analysis becomes, and the better we comprehend a patient's health. With enough data, it will eventually forecast medical issues that may arise on a population level, with minimal human interaction or research. While costs are still a barrier to widespread adoption of this capacity, rising competition is bringing costs down and developing innovation.

5.6.1 SECURITY

In healthcare, IoT devices can collect data on a patient's physical characteristics and communicate it with doctors, nurses, and family members. The old method of manually recording body characteristics and reporting them to doctors is employed the majority of the time. Nurses gather this information for all patients on a regular basis. Their valuable time is better spent caring for patients than constantly documenting physiological metrics. The IoT-enabled health sector is the answer to this problem.

Those who benefit from IoT technology can share information and connect with smart devices among themselves. IoT delivers additional convenience to doctors, nurses, and patients in the healthcare sector [41,42]. It becomes much more economical for monitoring and diagnosing people with illnesses while also lowering costs. In the healthcare system, there are several security breaches and malicious assaults that are particularly vulnerable, such as forgery and privacy leakage. Figure 5.9 explains the working architecture of Internet of Healthcare.

The IoT collects physical objects and embedded technologies connected to the Internet and includes machine learning, legitimate analytics, embedded devices, and commodity sensors. IoT systems would generate a lot of data as the number of sensors and linked devices grows (big data is the heart of machine learning).

Machine learning and the IoT are so intimately linked. NLP is becoming increasingly significant in IoT as a critical component of machine learning (especially healthcare). These have significant consequences for how businesses grow their agile approach, plan their IT infrastructure, manage their data from the point of origin to the end of consumption, and monitor their security and privacy.

In addition to embedded analytics, cognitive computing is an essential tool for advancing the IoHT's impact. AI, machine learning, and NLP are all used in cognitive computing to ingest and analyze various forms of structured, unstructured, and semi-structured data. Because of the variety of data acquired by sensors and the need to make sense of it all, this is a vital component of the IoHT.

As a result of these obstacles and issues in security based on authentication and communication, the situation has gotten worse. BC technology, which safely enables data exchange, has recently become a crucial advancement in security. Much current research could benefit from the inclusion of BC technology in the health system. The fundamental goal of this technology is to successfully share data between patients and other medical service providers based on features such as authentication, immutability, decentralized storage, scalability, private BC, and trustworthiness.

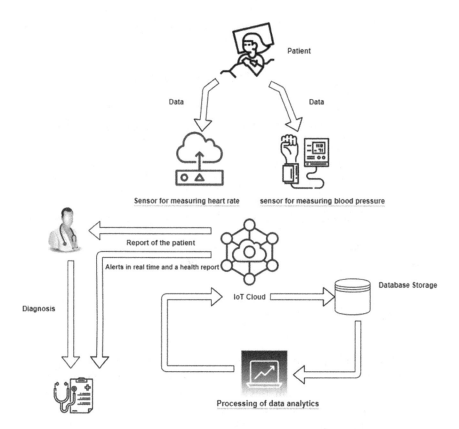

FIGURE 5.9 Working of Internet of Healthcare.

5.6.2 APPLICATION OF IoT IN HEALTHCARE

The IoT has now become identified with technologies being integrated into various businesses, particularly healthcare, which is seeing IoT developments in a variety of domains. IoT is heavily used and invested in by companies that specialize in technology or healthcare. They give important data that helps health practitioners make advances in their respective fields, from Wi-Fi or Bluetooth-enabled X-ray machines to wearables like bio-sensors.

5.6.3 THE ADVANTAGES OF IoT IN HEALTHCARE

The IoT in Healthcare From patients with chronic conditions on one end of the scale to disease prevention on the other, the IoT plays a key role in a wide range of healthcare applications. Here are a few examples of how it's already delivering on its promise: some areas where IoT in Healthcare is used are cancer treatment, diabetes management, treatment of asthma, and IoT in mental healthcare. Figure 5.10 depicts the benefits of Healthcare in IoT.

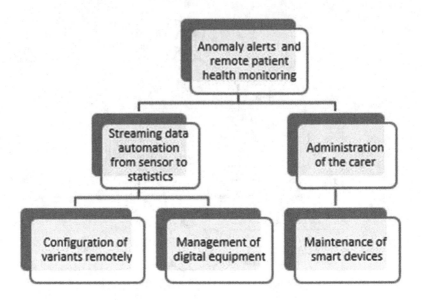

FIGURE 5.10   Benefits of IoT in healthcare.

- **Clinical Care**: IoT-driven, noninvasive monitoring can monitor hospital-ized patients whose physiological status necessitates particular attention continuously. This system uses sensors to collect detailed data, then anal-yses and stores the data using bridges and the cloud before sending the studied digital signals to careers for additional evaluation and discussion.
- **Remote Monitoring**: Many people in the world could be suffering due to the lack of readily available health monitoring. However, compact, powerful wireless solutions connected through the IoT now allow moni-toring to come to the patients rather than the other way around.

Despite being very functional and groundbreaking, the "Internet of Medical Things" faces its own set of obstacles [43,44]. These difficulties include tech-nological concerns as well as adjustment delay issues that must be addressed. Security, functionality, risk, and regulation are the primary issues affecting vari-ous businesses (including healthcare) that overlap through the use of IoT tech-nologies [45–50].

5.7   CONCLUSION AND FUTURE SCOPE

Robots are everywhere, from science writing to the restricted clinic, where they are moving medical care. Mechanical advancements look as though they are in various zones that unswerving touch understanding consideration. They can be cast-off to refine persistent places and working supplements, falling imperils for patients and wellbeing staff. They work in a research lab to make representations and to enter, explore, and collect them. The automated workshop partner can pinpoint that holder and draw the blood with less distress and apprehension for the patient. Robots likewise define and circulate drugs in pharmacological labs. IoT in medical care improves routine; however, huge duties to recuperate quiet outcomes and receipt a portion of the channel off wellbeing experts. Regular positions, for example, far off patient nursing, lead development musings, and the instance of antibodies are on the whole proficiencies of clinical strategies with coordinated IoT. For the past decade, robotics has been one of the emerging, exciting, developing, and imaginative fields of exploration among industrial scientists and universities.

It is exceptionally difficult to recognize robots from different machines; robots can be characterized as machines equipped to perform various tasks with more self-governance and freedom (LoF) than people. Today's healthcare administrations and facilities become extremely unpredictable, incorporating countless building blocks described by shared, dispersed, and heterogeneous devices, devices, and data and communication technology. With the IoT method, robots synchronize as one "thing" and establish links to different things on the Internet.

REFERENCES

1. Miorandi, D., Sicari, S., Pellegrini, F. D., Chlamtac, I. (2012). Internet of Things: vision, applications, and research challenges. *Ad Hoc Netw.* 10 (7), 1497–1516.
2. Gubbi, J., Marusic, S., Palaniswami, M. (2013). Internet of Things (IoT): a vision, architectural elements, and future directions. *Futur. Gener.* 29, 1645–1660.
3. Islam, S. M. R., Kwak, D., Kabir, M. H., Hossain, M., Kwak, K. (2015). The Internet of Things for health care: a comprehensive survey. *IEEE Access.* 3, 678–708. Doi: 10.1109/ACCESS.2015.2437951.
4. Aktas, F., Ceken, C., Erdemli, Y. (2016). Internet of Things technology applications of the biomedical field. *Duzce Univ. J. Sci. Technol.* 4, 37–54.
5. Qi, J. et al., (2017). Advanced Internet of things for personalized healthcare systems: a survey. *Pervasive Mob. Comput.* 41, 132–149.
6. Li, S., Xu, L., Zhao, S. (2018). 5G Internet of Things: a survey. *J. Ind. Inf. Integr.* 10, 1–9. Doi: 10.1016/j.jii.2018.01.005.
7. Xu, L.D., Xu, E.L., Li, L. (2018). Industry 4.0: state of the art and future trends. *Int. J. Prod. Res.* 56 (8), 2941–2962. Doi: 10.1080/00207543.2018.1444806.
8. Yang, P. et al., (2018a). Lifelogging data validation model for Internet of things enabled healthcare system. *IEEE Trans. Syst., Man, Cybernetics: Syst.* 48 (1), 50–64. Doi: 10.1109/TSMC.2016.2586075.
9. Yang, P. et al., (2018b). The Internet of things (IoT): informatics methods for IoT-enabled health care. *J. Biomed. Inform.* 87, 154–156, 2018. Doi: 10.1016/j.jbi.2018. 10.006.
10. Daecher, A., Cotteleer, M., Holdowsky, J. (2018). *The Internet of Things: A Technical Primer.* Deloitte. Available: https://www2.deloitte.com/insights/us/en/focus/internet-of-things/technical-primer.html.
11. Ray, P. P. (2018). A survey on Internet of Things architectures. *J. King Saud Univ.-Comput. Inform. Sci.* 30(3), 291–319.
12. Steve, T. K. J., Vatche, I., Vinod, M. (2020). AI trust in business processes: the need for process-aware explanations. Proceedings of the AAAI Conference on Artificial Intelligence 34(8). https://doi.org/10.1609/aaai.v34i08.7056.

13. Kshetri, N. (2017). Blockchain's roles in strengthening cybersecurity and protecting privacy. *Telecommun. Policy* 41(10), 1027–1038.
14. Lin, J., Yu, W., Zhang, N., Yang, X., Zhang, H., Zhao, W. (2017). A survey on Internet of Things: architecture, enabling technologies, security and privacy, and applications. *IEEE Inter. Things J.* 4(5), 1125–1142.
15. Liu, Y.-l., Chou, Y. J. (2018). Big data, the Internet of Things, and the interconnected society. *Telecommun. Policy* 42(4), 277–281.
16. Zhang, H., Tang, Z., Jayakar, K. (2018). A socio-technical analysis of China's cyber-security policy: towards delivering trusted E-government services. *Telecommun. Policy* 42(5), 409–420.
17. Patel, A. R., Patel, R. S., Singh, N. M., Kazi, F. S. (2017). Vitality of robotics in healthcare industry: An Internet of Things (IoT) perspective. Editors: Bhatt, C., Dey N., Ashour, A. (Eds). *Internet of Things and Big Data Technologies for Next Generation Healthcare, Studies in Big Data*, Springer, Cham, 23, pp. 91–109. https://doi.org/10.1007/978-3-319-49736-5_5.
18. Guntur, S.R., Gorrepati, R.R., Dirisala, V.R. (2019, Jan 1). Robotics in healthcare: An Internet of medical robotic things (IoMRT) perspective. In *Machine Learning in Bio-Signal Analysis and Diagnostic Imaging*, Academic Press, pp. 293–318.
19. Islam, S. R., Kwak, D., Kabir, M. H., Hossain, M., Kwak, K. S. (2015, Jun 1). The Internet of Things for health care: a comprehensive survey. *IEEE Access.* 3, 678–708.
20. Grieco, L. A., et al. (2014, Dec 1). IoT-aided robotics applications: technological implications, target domains and open issues. *Computer Commun.* 54, 32–47.
21. Kumar, M., Shenbagaraman, V. M., Ghosh, A. (2020). Predictive data analysis for energy management of a smart factory leading to sustainability. Editors: Favorskaya, M. N., Mekhilef, S., Pandey, R. K., Singh, N. (Eds.) *Innovations in Electrical and Electronic Engineering*, Springer Book Chapter [ISBN 978-981-15-4691-4], pp. 765–773.
22. Sivaparthipan, C. B., et al. (2019, Dec). Innovative and efficient method of robotics for helping the Parkinson's disease patient using IoT in big data analytics. *Trans. Emerg. Telecommun. Technol.* 11, e3838.
23. Chae, B. K. (2019). The evolution of the Internet of Things (IoT): a computational text analysis. *Telecommun. Policy.* 43(10), 101848.
24. Yoon, S. N., Lee, D. (2018, Jul 16). Artificial intelligence and robots in health-care: What are the success factors for technology-based service encounters? *Int. J. Healthc. Manag,* 1–8. https://doi.org/10.1080/20479700.2018.1498220
25. Tian, S., Yang, W., Le Grange, J. M., Wang, P., Huang, W., Ye, Z. (2019). Smart healthcare: making medical care more intelligent. *Glob. Health J.* 3(3), 62–65.
26. Mandal, S., Balas, V. E., Shaw, R. N., Ghosh, A. (2020, Oct. 2–4). Prediction analy-sis of idiopathic pulmonary fibrosis progression from OSIC dataset. *2020 IEEE International Conference on Computing, Power and Communication Technologies (GUCON)*, pp. 861–865, Doi: 10.1109/GUCON48875.2020.9231239.
27. Dimitrov, D. V. (2016). Medical Internet of Things and big data in healthcare. *Healthc. Inform. Res.* 22(3), 156–163.
28. Shah, R., Chircu, A. (2018, Jul 1). IOT and AI in healthcare: a systematic literature review. *Issues Inf. Syst.* 19(3), 33–41.
29. Pramanik, P. K., Upadhyaya, B. K., Pal, S., Pal, T. (2019, Jan 1). Internet of things, smart sensors, and pervasive systems: enabling connected and pervasive healthcare. In *Healthcare Data Analytics and Management*, Academic Press, pp. 1–58.
30. Wan, S., Gu, Z., Ni, Q. (2020, Jan 1). Cognitive computing and wireless communica-tions on the edge for healthcare service robots. *Computer Commun.* 149: 99–106.

31. Belkhier, Y., Achour, A., Shaw, R. N. (2020). Fuzzy passivity-based voltage controller strategy of grid-connected PMSG-based wind renewable energy system. *2020 IEEE 5th International Conference on Computing Communication and Automation (ICCCA)*, Greater Noida, India, pp. 210–214. Doi: 10.1109/ICCCA49541.2020.9250838.

32. Han, J., Kang, H. J., Kwon, G. H. (2017, Jun 28). Understanding the servicescape of nurse assistive robot: the perspective of healthcare service experience. In *2017 14th International Conference on Ubiquitous Robots and Ambient Intelligence (URAI)*, Graduate School of Technology & Innovation Management, Hanyang University, Seoul, Korea, pp. 644–649. IEEE.

33. Fan, Y. J., Yin, Y. H., Da Xu, L., Zeng, Y., Wu, F. (2014). IoT-based smart rehabilitation system. *IEEE Trans. Ind. Inform.* 10(2), 1568–1577.

34. Shaw, R. N., Walde, P., Ghosh, A. (2020). IOT based MPPT for performance improvement of solar PV arrays operating under partial shade dispersion. *2020 IEEE 9th Power India International Conference (PIICON) held at Deenbandhu Chhotu Ram University of Science and Technology*, Sonepat. India on Feb 28– March 1 2020.

35. Bodur, G., Gumus, S., Gursoy, N. G. (2019, Aug 1). Perceptions of Turkish health professional students toward the effects of the Internet of things (IOT) technology in the future. *Nurse Educ. Today.* 79: 98–104.

36. Mandal, S., Biswas, S., Balas, V. E., Shaw, R. N., Ghosh, A. (2020). Motion prediction for autonomous vehicles from Lyft dataset using deep learning. *2020 IEEE 5th International Conference on Computing Communication and Automation (ICCCA)* 30–31 Oct. 2020, pp. 768–773, Doi: 10.1109/ICCCA49541.2020.9250790.

37. World Health Organization (WHO). (2016). *The World Health Report 2016*, World Malaria Report, WHO Library Catalouguing, Geneva, Switzerland, pp. 8–9.

38. Istepanian, R. S. (2011, Apr 6). The potential of Internet of Things (IoT) for assisted living applications. In *IET Seminar on Assisted Living*, London, pp. 1–40. IET.

39. Feynman, R., Vernon, F. Jr. (1963). The theory of a general quantum system interacting with a linear dissipative system, *Ann. Phys.* 24: 118–173. Doi: 10.1016/0003-4916 (63)90068-X.

40. Dirac, P. (1953). The Lorentz transformation and absolute time, *Physica* 19 (1–12), 888–896. Doi: 10.1016/S0031-8914(53)80099-6.

41. Javaid, M., Khan, I. H. (2021). Internet of Things (IoT) enabled healthcare helps to take the challenges of COVID-19 Pandemic. *J. Oral Biol. Craniofac. Res.* 11 (2), 209–214.

42. Magsi, H., et al. (2021). A novel adaptive battery-aware algorithm for data transmission in IoT-based healthcare applications. *Electronics* 10 (4), 367.

43. de Morais Barroca Filho, I., Aquino, G., Malaquias, R. S., Girão, G. and Melo, S. R. M. (2021). An IoT-based healthcare platform for patients in ICU beds during the COVID-19 outbreak. *IEEE Access* 9: 27262–27277.

44. Bharadwaj, H. K., Agarwal, A., Chamola, V., Lakkaniga, N. R., Hassija, V., Guizani, M., Sikdar, B. (2021). A review on the role of machine learning in enabling IoT based healthcare applications. *IEEE Access* 9: 38859–38890.

45. Jain, G. (2021, Jan. 2). A secure big data layered approach for privacy. *Sambhodi J.* ISSN: 2249–6661, Available at SSRN: https://ssrn.com/abstract=3899380.

46. Jain, G., and Prasad, R. R. (2021). Multi-antenna communication security with deep learning network and internet of things. *Blockchain Technology for Data Privacy Management*, CRC Press, pp. 61–80.

47. Jain, E. G. (2021). A comparative analyzing of SMS spam using topic models. *Innovations in Information and Communication Technologies (IICT-2020)*, Springer, Cham, pp. 91–99.

48. Jain, G. (2021). Application of SNORT and Wireshark in network traffic analysis. *IOP Conference Series: Materials Science and Engineering.* Vol. 1119. No. 1. IOP Publishing, London.

49. Yadav, A., et al. (2021). "Intelligent Moving Machine (IMM) based on battery for an efficient regenerative braking system." *Recent Advances in Mechanical Engineering.* Springer, Singapore, pp. 257–264.

50. Jain, G., Prasad, R. R. (2020). Machine learning, Prophet and XGBoost algorithm: Analysis of Traffic Forecasting in Telecom Networks with time series data. *2020 8th International Conference on Reliability, Infocom Technologies and Optimization (Trends and Future Directions) (ICRITO),* Noida. IEEE.

6 A Machine Learning Approach to Improve the Pharmaceutical Industry Machinery
Case of Zimbabwe

Shadreck N. Tasiyana, Prince
Chitopho, and Tawanda Mushiri
University of Zimbabwe

Abid Yahya
Botswana International University
of Science & Technology

CONTENTS

DOI: 10.1201/9781003224075-6

6.1 INTRODUCTION

The demand for pharmaceuticals is anchored on demand for health itself, and local pharmaceutical production has been a major concern at various international platforms since the 1970s [38,43]. Some studies have also revealed that low production capacity is one of the challenges that result in inadequate access to medicines in East and Southern Africa [29]. According to the 2020 Zimbabwean Heath Budget, capital expenditure allocation doubled between 2019 and 2020, and the health budget constitutes about 32% of the annual budget of Zimbabwe. These facts and the budget trajectory put the nation in a tight corner. The countries (especially developing countries including Zimbabwe) therefore need to employ various strategies to manage this expenditure/demand. Improving the manufacturing process is among many such strategies. According to the Government Gazette (dated 7th May 2021), approval was granted as a pharmaceutical strategy to boost drug production from 30% to 60%. In addition to this, the Pharmaceutical sector has been identified as a priority in National Development Strategy and Zimbabwe National Industrial Development Policy [40–43].

The pharmaceutical industry, among other functions, is responsible for transforming raw materials into a pharmaceutical in an administrable form. Like any other industry, the pharmaceutical industry has also gone through the different stages of the industrial revolution, aiming to increase productivity and profitability while bringing in the aspect of product affordability. The International Society for Pharmaceutical Engineers (ISPE) brought the concept of Industry 4.0 to address the production challenges by proposing the replacement of batch processing by CPM. Unlike the conventional pharmaceutical batch manufacturing system, CPM involves integrating the unit operations into a single continuous production line that is operated through a centralised control platform, with real-time process operational data collection, and subsequently applying the data to control the line to achieve desired product quality efficiently [2].

This research aims to enhance the operational efficiency of local pharmaceutical manufacturing machinery through machine learning (ML) to achieve competitiveness in both the local and regional markets by reducing labour and material wastage and increasing product output quality of machinery. The research touches on local industry background, standards, and manufacturing processes, and the potential impact of artificial intelligence (AI) in manufacturing. The focus is also on comparing the traditional manual and automated manufacturing methods in both time and monetary terms. Potential benefits and some examples are also provided where AI was applied.

6.2 BACKGROUND AND STATUS QUO OF THE ZIMBABWEAN PHARMACEUTICAL INDUSTRY

The Zimbabwean pharmaceutical industry is made up of eight generic pharmaceutical manufacturing companies for finished human medicines. The pharmaceuticals market comprises imported medicines, donated medicines (imported), and locally manufactured medicines. Figure 6.1 shows the statistics of the market distribution for the year 2014 [3].

Zimbabwean export market for pharmaceuticals is insignificant despite the Southern African Development Community providing a US$4.7 billion market

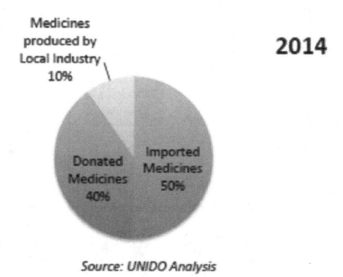

Source: UNIDO Analysis

FIGURE 6.1 Zimbabwean pharmaceutical market distribution for the year 2014. (Reproduced from [3].)

[3]. This is coherent with other reports that show a Zimbabwean economy a trade deficit, whereby imports exceed the exports by at least US$4 billion [4]. The price point indications for selected medicines showed that locally produced products were uncompetitive [3].

In light of the little to no local production in the developing nations, WHO recently launched the Local Production Programme, as a way to promote local production of quality-assured medical products [5]. Some reasons for the low market share of local products in [3] form the basis for this research work (local manufacturers being ineligible and incapacitated to supply the donated drugs and uncompetitive local product prices against imports).

6.2.1 The Manufacturing Process of Pharmaceuticals in Zimbabwe

Since its inception, pharmaceuticals have always been manufactured using a batch process [1]. The manufacturing process starts with weighing the raw materials. The starting materials undergo a series of manufacturing steps until the finished packaged tablet is achieved. Each manufacturing step takes place on an independent machine and in its manufacturing room (cubicle). The process flow in Figure 6.2 shows the manufacturing process of tablets and their packaging into the final consumer pack.

The majority of these machines are manually and individually operated. Consequently, local manufacturers invest heavily in labour resources, high human

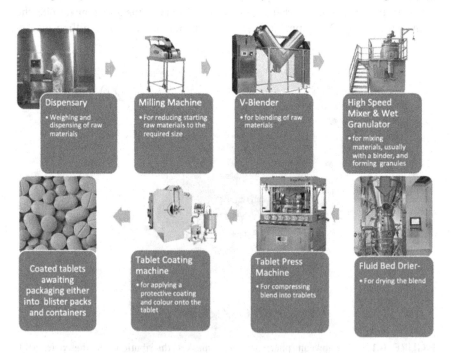

FIGURE 6.2   Process flow for tablets manufacturing in Zimbabwe.

intervention, and labour costs for permanently employed personnel. In manual operations, efficiency also depends on the operator. There are no such challenges in fully automated plants as the traceability and audit trails are inbuilt into the machine's operation software. The other challenge pertains to contamination of the product from particles shed by humans as a natural growth process [1].

Although personnel protective equipment (PPE) is specified and top-level hygiene is advocated for in pharmaceuticals manufacturing, one cannot be confident that an operator will always follow procedure; hence there is some risk of product contamination with manually semi-automated machines. A pharmaceutical plant is also specially designed with a Heating, Ventilation and Air Conditioning (HVAC) system to control the required manufacturing conditions and minimise product cross-contamination.

6.3 PHARMACEUTICAL INDUSTRY EQUIPMENT, PROCESSES, AND STANDARDS

There is more functioning in the pharmaceutical industry, albeit antiquated designed products that require conventional manufacturing processes, hence the prevalence of batch manufacturing process. This section will focus on the traditional equipment/methods and the current technological trends in the manufacturing of pharmaceuticals. Hence, aspects of batch processing, AI, the merits and demerits of each category, and product and process compliance are looked at more closely.

6.3.1 MANUFACTURING OF PHARMACEUTICALS

Figure 6.3 shows a typical conventional batch manufacturing process for tablets and packaging into the final consumer pack.

Conventional manufacturing of pharmaceuticals has relatively low efficiencies and capacity utilisation, high discard and reject levels, and a higher cost of quality [6]. Conventional batch processing requires an offline laboratory analysis of

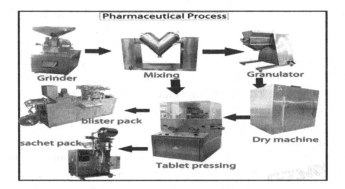

FIGURE 6.3 A typical conventional batch manufacturing process for tablets.

product samples taken at predetermined intervals and different processing steps. The sample collection and testing are mostly in-process and at the end of the batch processing, a concept described as quality by testing (QbT) is also done [7]. The sample's offline test results are then used as feedback in controlling the manufacturing process. The quality system includes process/method/equipment validation, process control through Standard Operating Procedures (SOP) and batch manufacturing instructions or recipes, and offline line testing of product samples at the end of each batch. To support these quality systems, some compliance infrastructures are indispensable, albeit their difficult economic sustenance. As revealed in [6], while the compliance burden has been an enabler for delivering quality medicinal products to the patient, quality has increased to an average of 20% of the total industry cost, which has negatively impacted pharmaceutical manufacturing organisations. The conventional manufacturing paradigm is also functioning sub-optimally as observed from metrics such as capacity utilisation of about 15% or less, discards or reworks of about 5%–10% and an average cycle time of about 95 days [6]. The summarised list of issues with the current paradigm warrants a shift in the pharmaceuticals manufacturing paradigm to one with a smart inline monitoring and intelligent control system with the potential of quality enhancement, reduction in cycle time, and costs, among other benefits [8].

Since the pharmaceutical industry is highly regulated, its approach to manufacturing innovation is usually conservative. The introduction of new manufacturing technologies is believed to delay approvals with the regulatory authorities and present business challenges [9]. Other processing industries have fully embraced the fourth industrial revolution, except for pharmaceutical manufacturing; it is still being established whether this new industry paradigm's ideas and principles are applicable in the pharmaceutical industry. They require some level of customisation (ISPE, 2017). However, there is a need to urgently introduce innovative technological solutions to enable complex drug delivery systems [11]. GEA [12] asserts that organisations should use smart manufacturing, a subset of Industry 4.0, to tap into its numerous and beneficial capabilities, such as agile adaptation to a wide variety of conditions.

An Industry 4.0 (4IR) factory has its machines augmented with wireless connectivity and sensors connected to a system that visualises the entire production line and makes decentralised decisions on its own. Various physical and digital technologies make up the 4IR, summarised as cyber physical systems' connectivity. Henstock [13] regard the industrial transformation purpose as to enhance resource efficiency and productivity to increase the competitive power. The need to control the spiralling costs and the increasing cognisance of the need to drive patient centricity have led to adoption of the 4IR technologies in pharmaceuticals [14]. The ISPE notes that 4IR should be adopted customised to support the industry's current quality and regulatory guidelines. The 4IR acts as an enabler of the pharmaceutical quality requirements. The conventional manufacturing paradigm employs the QbT system, a perspective whereby product quality is verified with the approved specifications at the end of the manufacturing process. However, this has proved to have a negative impact on pharmaceutical manufacturers.

The recent trend in quality for pharmaceuticals is quality by design (QbD) and process analytical technology (PAT). The USA's Food and Drug Association (FDA) has since initiated QbD and PAT to build quality into the product before its inception [15]. Unlike QbT, QbD is a modern approach to pharmaceutical quality that ensures quality into a product by developing a thorough understanding of the compatibility of the product to all the components and processes involved in product manufacturing [16].

A tool kit ensures that quality is built into a product during manufacturing PAT, which subsequently increases the operational efficiencies, capacity utilisation, and process understanding while decreasing operating expenses [6]. PAT is defined as a system to design, analyse, and control pharmaceutical manufacturing processes by measuring and controlling critical process parameters and quality attributes [6]. The FDA notes three main benefits of implementing PAT: an increase in the understanding of process and products, improvement in the control of pharmaceutical manufacturing process, and incorporation of quality into the product at the design stage. Jolliffe et al. [17] asset that online monitoring of the critical process and material parameters is necessary to control the process better and improve its robustness.

Unlike the conventional pharmaceutical batch manufacturing system, CPM integrates unit operations into a single continuous production line. A real-time collection of process operational data such as critical material attribute (CMA) and critical process parameter (CPP) is incorporated through PAT. The data is subsequently applied to control the line with no human input intelligently to achieve a product that meets the desired critical quality attributes (CQAs). Among other benefits, CPM delivers tremendous improvement in process quality and consistency due to unprecedented ability to maintain a state of control, low residence times, and no intermediate hold steps [9].

6.3.2 MACHINE LEARNING

As has been highlighted, CPM calls for machines to relieve humans from intensive physical work, offer intellectual capabilities, and even produce innovations on their own [18]. Limaye et al. [19] assert that real-time process control is highly desired for efficient QbD-based pharmaceutical manufacturing. In their research on the implementation of control systems in the CPM pilot plant (powder to tablet), the authors in [19] carried out a study on advanced model predictive control (MPC) systems, online prediction tools, PAT, and data management tools, among other various tools.

Lin [20] came up with a sketch (Figure 6.4) to show ML's relationship with different disciplines of knowledge. It concluded that "a computer program learns from experience to some class of tasks and performance measure". The performance tasks improve with experience. There are various learning techniques for ML: supervised learning, unsupervised learning, semi-supervised learning, and reinforcement learning [20].

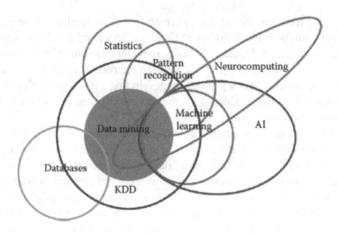

FIGURE 6.4 Relationship between machine learning and other disciplines of knowledge. (Reproduced from Ref. [20].)

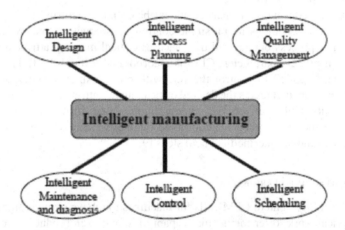

FIGURE 6.5 An intelligent manufacturing system. (Reproduced from Ref. [22].)

6.3.3 Role of AI in Pharmaceuticals Industry

AI contributes to business value drivers such as speed to market, responsiveness, resource productivity, efficiency, customisation, and business model innovation [21].

Figure 6.5 shows the components of an intelligent manufacturing system where Industry 4.0 components such as AI and cloud computing (CC) are utilised to make the system intelligent. Industry 4.0 touches on drug discovery, process control, and quality assurance (QA) in line with the pharmaceutical industry.

6.3.3.1 AI in Drug Discovery

AI has been discovered to be a transformational influence on drug development that can positively impact the system and lead to an annual US$100 billion market. In most cases, what is mostly referred to as AI in the pharmaceutical industry is ML. ML is applied to various drug development areas from disease identification, diagnosis, drug research and manufacturing trials, clinical trials, epidemic outbreak prediction, among other functions [23].

In the preclinical phase, where drug effect and processing are examined, alternate drug formulations are developed to create a drug with the requisite properties. A pharmaceutical drug formulation is determined by the ingredients' type, quantity, and processing conditions. In the past, formulators would use statistical techniques in modelling formulations, and they had to rely on response surfaces to provide an optimisation mechanism. However, this would be misleading at times for complex formulations [24]. AI has since provided a better alternative to formulation generation of pharmaceuticals, such as the use of neural networks, fuzzy logic to assist model formulations.

Clinical development is another critical and potentially lengthy process of drug development. The drug efficacy, as well as the corresponding toxicity and safety levels, is evaluated. Clinical trials are conducted using humans after the drug toxicity has been determined. Patient selection for clinical trials design and optimisation can now be made more efficiently through ML and Natural Language Processing. Internet of things (IoT) and CC enable smart sensors to transmit over the internet and into the pharmaceutical company's cloud as well as provision of real-time data of patients during clinical trials [25]. The large volumes of data generated (big data, BD) are then analysed using ML algorithms to optimise the formulation.

Pharmaceutical companies are also using ML in pharmacovigilance, where adverse event processing or gathering regulatory intelligence is done with real-world data such as claims and electronic health data [23]. The otherwise time-consuming activities are significantly reduced, and a subsequent overall speed reduction to market the developed drug is realised. It is important to note that AI has enhanced operational efficiency in pharmaceutical research and development exercises by developing optimum dose determination, optimum processing, and reducing development costs and, most importantly, time. Speed to market is one of the key business value drivers and using the AI, one can achieve such [21].

6.3.3.2 AI in Process Control and Quality Assurance

Regarding control and QA, issues with intelligent planning, smart scheduling, smart control, and smart quality management are critical components of the Industry 4.0 concept. The concept touches on efficiency, profitability, compliance, quality, and the final product consumer, which is the patient.

Intelligent planning involves determining the optimal configuration of manufacturing resources and execution of resources through intelligent optimisation algorithms, which are the basics of ML. The resulting process plan will be ensuring efficient resource utilisation and, most importantly, minimise possible cross-contamination of products while ensuring compliance to all the applicable regulatory guidelines [5]. Other evolutionary approaches such as genetic algorithms (GA), artificial neural networks (ANN), and particle swarm optimisation (PSO) have been implemented to enhance the AI capabilities of computer-aided process planning systems for delivery of more efficient systems [26].

A large volume of data is generated from customer orders, manufacturing resource status, production capacities, supply chain data, sales data and inventory data, and regulatory guidelines in smart manufacturing. Data analytics (DA) and ML capabilities in enterprise resource planning (ERP) software can thus intelligently produce an optimised production schedule [26]. The smart schedule also considers materials distribution. With actual production progress and various onsite urgency requirements, the suitable material is delivered to the right processing station at the right time.

A smart manufacturing control system has got AI. It includes actuators, process sensors, data processing equipment, equipment connectivity, and algorithms to relate process variables (CPP and CMA) to CQAs. With the advancement in the application of AI in technologies such as PAT, inline measurements are now possible and these enable optimised control of the production process. By integrating the cyber knowledge ontology with the distributed yet collaborative physical equipment, an intelligent manufacturing control system (iMCS) can independently learn from DA and then adapt to the manufacturing system's conditions [27]. PATs, which are process analysers, are the main source of data in an iMCS of a pharmaceutical production line as they continuously measure the CPP, CMA, and product CQA. PAT's various AI approaches are enablers for an iMCS. The approaches provide typical features such as learning, reasoning, and acting. The key technologies to enhance the integration of PAT with the control system include IoT, CC, big data analytics (BDA), and Information and Communication Technologies. The adoption of IoT has enabled the implementation of PAT in the pharmaceutical industry and subsequent continuous manufacturing. Various IoT technologies have made this possible, and today we have smart sensors to communicate [28]. An integral part of the PAT, Near Infrared Spectroscopy (NIR) sensors have been equipped with smart capabilities to communicate the data they generate from CPP process measurement. Thus, IoT enables intelligent running of a manufacturing line, as the ontology and knowledge inference that has replaced the traditional logic controllers in iMacs can autonomously respond to the conditions after receiving the sensed data through IoT mechanisms [27]. CC could enhance the computational services of the data through a virtualised production process; however, challenges such as cyber security, data management, and availability may cripple the production control system [28]. However, this has enabled contamination-free processing of pharmaceuticals as the production line is controlled "off site" without any human being's physical presence. Advanced DA are critical for uncovering hidden patterns and unknown correlations and research in academia and industry showed that one could achieve up to 15%–20% increase on return on investment [28].

BD and ML are indispensable in monitoring, controlling, and optimisation of industrial processes.

BD and ML are used in multivariate statistical process monitoring and soft sensing during manufacturing process' automatic control. In CPM, there is no offline sample testing, and it implies that every CMA and CQA has to be measured in line. Yet, some chemical and physical properties are currently impossible to measure. This has led to an intelligent sensing technology (feature learning soft sensing) where easy-to-measure process variables are used to estimate and predict the hard-to-measure variables. Representation learning is also being used. In this case, probabilistic slow feature analysis is used to induce slowly varying features based on which a simple least squares regression model is built [18]. Unlike the traditional dynamic partial least squares, the slowly varying features represent underlying process variations well, and some tend to be highly correlated to quality indices. Thus, ML's advancement and application to manufacturing process control have significantly enabled real-time monitoring and product release in a more efficient continuous manufacturing paradigm.

In line with quality management, the ICH Q10 document details how a pharmaceutical company can develop and use effective monitoring and control systems for process performance and product quality to assure process capability and continued suitability. Quds and PAT, the main pillars for fourth-generation pharmaceutical QA have been enabled through AI.

6.3.4 THE ADOPTION OF AI, WITH EMPHASIS ON ML IN THE FIRST WORLD TO IMPROVE PHARMACEUTICAL MANUFACTURING

Pharmaceutical manufacturing starts with developing the drug itself, and AI adoption has led to tremendous achievements in the first world. With the availability of big biological and medical data in this present day and advanced ML algorithms, the automated design of drugs is becoming a reality [30]. ML techniques are being used to automate the highly dimensional noisy biological data analysis to success, for example, in drug candidate identification via molecule docking, predicting, and preselect interesting drug–target interactions for further research [30]. Generative Adversarial Networks (GAN) have been used to generate DNA sequences matching specific DNA motifs in protein designs. ML has been applied to Adaptive Clinical Trials (ACT) in terms of drug testing. ML algorithms have been implemented successfully in predicting toxicity, and one good example of such is the DeepTrox algorithm [31]. Several other AI-based computational tools for drug discovery have been developed.

ML and other AI technologies have necessitated CPM implementation as it enables the key concepts of CPM, which are QbD and PAT. QbD and PAT are keys to pharmaceutical manufacturing as they assure the efficacy and overall quality of medicines. QbD ensures quality is built into the product during the design and processing of materials, while PAT introduces the idea of real-time process control and real-time QA [11]. Besides efficiency and quality, CPM is an agile and flexible manufacturing technology that delivers more consistent and reliable tablet production with reduced use and loss of raw materials, less stoppage times, and minimum labour or manual intervention.

6.3.4.1   Drug Development

Supervised, unsupervised, and reinforcement learning have all been applied in drug development. The deepDR approach uses an Auto-Encoder (AE) to generate informative features from heterogeneous drug data. However, the authors in [30] note that careful training and regularisation of neural networks in DL must be taken to ensure the learned features' relevance. This has led to the first world opting for semi-automated drug discovery to reduce the drugs' time and development costs.

Their research [23] observed that 70% of their respondents reported using AI in some way, especially inpatient selection and recruitment for clinical trial studies. It was also noted that some challenges were present in the use of AI such as staff skills which were about 55%, data structure, 52%, and budget constraints which were around 49%. However, several pharmaceutical companies have since invested in AI-based R&D programs and have partnered with AI organisations. Takeda Pharmaceuticals (one of the largest pharmaceutical companies in the world), in collaboration with Recursion Pharmaceuticals (an AI and ML company), recently announced their achievement of identifying novel preclinical compounds for rare diseases [31]. Some other high-profile pharmaceutical companies have partners estimated to be worth USD100 million to reap the competitive advantages of AI [13].

6.3.4.2   Manufacturing Control and QA

Unlike the conventional V-type blenders, in continuous manufacturing, tubular blenders are typically used. Tubular blenders are horizontal cylinders with a bladed shaft that rotates along its central axis (impeller). The formulation components are fed from one end and the impeller-induced axial and radial movements of particles along with the cylinder to the other end determine the blending effectiveness. Limaye et al. [19] developed a framework for implementing the control system in a CPM process. The active pharmaceutical ingredient (API) is effectively controlled during blending, using an advanced predictive model (MPC) and NIR sensor. Figure 6.6 shows a typical GUI for closed-loop operation of CPM.

The API concentration was measured at the end of the blender using a micro-NIR sensor. A partial least squares (PLS) model was developed in UnscramblerX, to predict NIR, and the unscrambler process pulse and a prediction engine (OLUPX) were used for real-time NIR prediction [19]. The blended powder can either be compressed directly or the blend is first granulated and dried in most cases. The coating may be done on the tablets in a continuous coating machine before packing.

The real-time monitoring and advanced computational control pave the way for real-time product QA, namely real-time release (RTR) of pharmaceuticals [33]. In pharmaceuticals packaging, say packing tablets into blisters, image processing and optical defect-recognition have been employed successfully to detect any unfilled or erroneously filled blister pack. Machine algorithms like convolutional

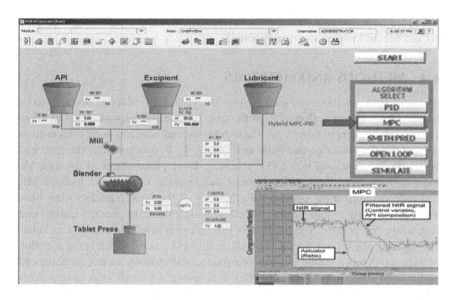

FIGURE 6.6 Graphical user interface for closed-loop operation of CPM. (Adapted from [19].)

neural networks are increasingly used for classification tasks in QA [34]. ML algorithms have offered "validating" mechanisms for real-time monitoring in CPM through soft sensors.

6.3.4.3 GEA (Belgium), a Pharmaceutical Equipment Manufacturer Who has Applied AI and ML to Enable CPM

A leading pharmaceutical equipment manufacturer from Belgium, GEA has done more to pioneer continuous manufacturing for the industry by applying AI and ML in designing its fully integrated powder to tablet CPM solution, the ConsiGma. The ConsiGma consumes less than 50% of the manufacturing facility's space volume than a conventional batch manufacturing line would take. Not only does this benefit the factory's footprint, but it does positively impact the overall operation costs as the HVAC energy consumption are reduced. Adopting AI and ML has seen neuro-fuzzy air quality evaluations yielding energy efficient HVAC designs for intelligent buildings such as a smart factory for pharmaceuticals manufacturing [35].

In their techno-economic feasibility studies of manufacturing Ibuprofen with the AI-enabled CPM, the authors in [35] observed positive cost savings in CapEx and OpEx. The CPM of Ibuprofen and its alternative drug, Artemisinin, showed a great total cost reduction of between 53% and 71%, 27% and 52.6%, respectively. Hence, CPM effectively reduces the costs of producing pharmaceuticals, over and above other benefits such as enhanced quality and response time to supply. Some statistics show that 82% of the companies who have adopted AI in manufacturing technologies have experienced increased efficiency and 45% experienced increased customer satisfaction [37]. Several first-world companies have adopted AI and ML to improve their operations.

6.4 METHODS AND MATERIALS

The case study method was used for this study; it is an inductive research technique. The evidence collected from the case is systematically analysed to allow patterns and concepts to emerge. These patterns and concepts were then used to expand existing theories and build new ones [37]. In this instance, the case was based on PharmaCo (PVT) LTD, a leading local pharmaceutical manufacturing company, and it was the purpose of this research to ascertain whether ML can indeed improve the operational efficiency of the local manufacturing lines and subsequently reduce production costs while enhancing product quality and regulatory compliance. The purpose of this research is to gain concrete and contextual in-depth knowledge on a specific real-world matter, which is the adoption of ML and AI as a whole into the pharmaceutical industry to realise enhanced operational efficiencies. Therefore, this section touches on all associated aspects ranging from data collection and processing methods/tools and programming.

6.4.1 DATA COLLECTION

Both quantitative and qualitative data had to be collected. Quantitative data facilitated the systematic description of ML adoption's impact, and it helped validate the research as it generated reproducible knowledge. The quantitative data collected for the research included the capital expenditure of implementing ML in the local manufacturing industry and its effects on production costs. The local manufacturing industry quantitative data included current status quo; the processing times, product output, product changeover times, and maintenance data. Qualitative data collected facilitated creating a comprehensive technology transfer plan, especially on issues of change management. Quantitative data was mostly through primary sources (structured interviews and questionnaires) to the equipment manufacturers that yielded ML technologies/machinery specifications and cost data.

6.4.2 PROGRAMMING

The data was split into training and testing sets, and the algorithm was validated. Manual validation of the model was done through mathematical calculations, and the model was found to be robust. To simulate the effect of ML, as a way of treating the sample, an algorithm was developed and used to evaluate the impact of ML on a tablet-making machine. Impact simulations of ML capabilities built into a tablet compression machine were evaluated. A ML algorithm was developed using Python language. The selection of python among other languages and packages was based on its higher productivity and its simplified programming syntax, code readability, and English-like commands.

6.4.3 Observations and Interviews

Critical data for programming a ML algorithm was recorded during observation of the production process and interviewing the operators. It was noted that tablet weight was affected mainly by the flow of tablet powder from the hopper down into the turret and the speed at which the tablets were compressed (turret speed). Product manufacturing parameters and costing data were noted through observation (both as a participant and as a non-participant) at the case site (PharmaCo). This was done during the company audit for the selected case. Secondary data sources were explored. During the PharmCo audit, the focus was on manufacturing equipment, processes and facility layout, product manufacturing process details, product costing models, and sales records.

6.4.4 Statistical Tools

It was established a linear relationship between the powder flow rate and machine speed and tablet weight. Hence, the ML algorithm utilised the model, and a linear regression algorithm was used to predict tablet weight [39]. The percentage deviation was then used to predict the adjusted speed, resulting in the achieved target product weight. The R square values of the model (machine algorithm) were obtained through regression analysis.

6.4.5 Data Availability Statement

The data used to support the findings of this study are included within the supplementary information files.

6.5 RESULTS AND DISCUSSION

This section is composed of the results obtained from different respondents and observations and covers the key issues in the manufacturing process of Ibuprofen (taken as a typical drug example). An analysis of the results is also done and represented in various formats for quick analysis. In the manufacturing simulation process, various scenarios were considered and behavioural changes were noted. The results were then discussed accordingly.

6.5.1 Interview with the Managing Director

The interview's main purpose was to understand the top management's perspective and buy in to adopt ML as this is critical in developing a technology transfer plan or roadmap. The MD's responses showed that he is keen on reducing production costs as much as possible. The requirement for strict adherence to product specifications shows the need for optimised manufacturing. This research aims to reduce labour costs by 50%, reducing the total production costs significantly. The drop in costs and product selling costs will enable the organisation to fight

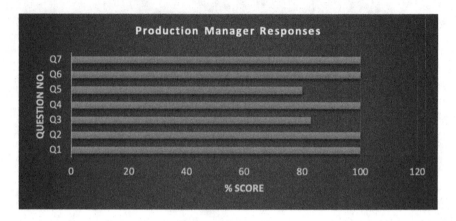

FIGURE 6.7 Production manager responses.

off competition from imported products. That will increase the market share, something that the Managing Director is looking forward to and eager to invest for, as they say, numbers do not lie. The take-home point from the MD's engagement is that he is willing to invest should the ML approach increase his market share and this is a bonus for the ease of adopting the local industry approach, as shown in Figure 6.7.

6.5.2 QUESTIONNAIRE TO THE PRODUCTION MANAGER

The responses by the Production Manager were shown in Figure 6.7.
Key:

Q1: What are you KPIs related to operational efficiency?
Q2: From our initial discussions, what do you understand about ML?
Q3: How would you rate the level of AI adoption in your factory? What about ML? Describe your least and best adoption instances. Describe your least and best adoption instances.
Q4: What benefits are you getting from ML capable machines?
Q5: What challenges are you facing with this level of ML?
Q6: Would you need more ML capable machines? What benefits will you be expecting?
  Discuss areas like labour, product output, material usage, and quality of the product.
Q7: If the tablet manufacturing line were ML-capable, what features do you deem critical to your operations?

The Production Manager responded to the questionnaire as indicated in Figure 6.7. Each question was weighted, and a score was given for each response to quantify the need for the adoption of ML and evaluate the industry's readiness. A high score of 93% (average) shows that ML is a solution to the local pharmaceutical industry's productivity. The discussion shows that the key areas to be addressed in tablet manufacturing are reducing labour cost and improving tablet weight variations and material usage. This is in tandem with the MD's vision of reduced production costs to boost sales and expand market share.

6.5.3 INTERVIEWS WITH OPERATORS

Operators from the tablet manufacturing section were interviewed last. These were oral interviews and were conducted while observing the manufacturing of tablets. During the interview, the operators highlighted three significant challenges: significant tablet weight variation in the acceptable range and the absence of possible settings to adjust the machine to produce tablets with constant weight. Operationally, it was also noted that it takes an average of about 40 minutes in setting the machine before it can be run continuously. Adjusting the machine speed is a challenge since tablet weight will vary depending on the flow rate. Material and product wastage was another concern and drawback that was also highlighted.

Some key issues observed/emanated from the interview with operators touched on issues with having a machine/system capable of keeping a record of the best operating speed for each product to increase efficiency. Therefore, it was vital that the proposed solution of adopting ML was to address these issues. It was also observed that all plant operators showed an appreciation of automation, which made it easier for them to understand AI basics. Eighty percent of the operators welcomed the idea of implementing ML on the machines. About 90% of them are either studying towards an electronics diploma or have already attained one, so introducing ML and AI would enable them to use what they have learned and enhance their careers. In this regard, it was noted that the adoption of ML in pharmaceutical manufacturing would be seamless and as such it is a possibility that an ML approach to improving pharmaceutical machinery can be a success.

6.5.4 MANUFACTURING PROCESS OVERVIEW OF IBUPROFEN 400 MG TABLETS AND REVIEW OF THE BATCH MANUFACTURING RECORD

Ibuprofen is a pain remedy, listed as a critical drug by the WHO. It is also one of the drugs with significantly higher production costs and subsequently costs more than the imported one, hence selecting the case study. The manufacturing process starts with dispensing the starting materials, which is weighing the raw materials. The starting materials undergo a series of manufacturing steps until the finished packaged tablet is achieved. Each manufacturing step takes place on an independent machine located in a manufacturing cubicle (discrete operation units). It can then be deduced from the process description that there are significant inventory build-ups from the process. A slight mistake in production planning may compromise the intermediaries hold times, which negatively affects the final product quality. From the process review, it is apparent that the ML approach will indeed improve operational efficiency.

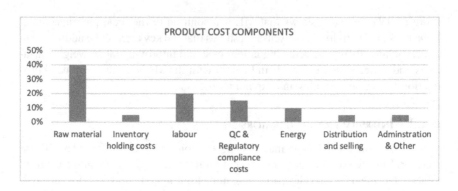

FIGURE 6.8   Product costing at PharmaCo.

6.5.4.1 Product Costing Review

For confidential sake, the product costing was expressed as a percentage rather than actual figures. The organisation uses the absorption costing model, as shown in Figure 6.8. The costing data shows that the top three cost drivers for the production of Ibuprofen 400 mg tablets are raw materials, labour, and quality control/regulatory costs. This is in tandem with the observations from the MD and Production Manager's interviews. It follows that a reduction in product cost will mainly reduce the cost of these three costs.

6.5.4.2 A Machine Learning Algorithm for Tablet Weight
Control on a Tablet Compression Machine

An algorithm was developed using Python programing language. The ML algorithm utilised the linear relationship between product properties, machine parameters, and the product output. Figure 6.10 shows the relationship. The measured product flow rate was the CMA input into the programme. In contrast, the machine speed will be the CPP, and tablet weight the CQA of the product, as shown in Figure 6.9.

In the programme simulation, a product recipe file was created and acted as the training and testing data set for that specific product, in this case, Ibuprofen 400 mg tablets. The machine algorithm was successfully trained and tested. The R squared value for the model was about 0.999, which is satisfactory. Varying the flow rate between the intent and negative and positive deviations yielded the expected adjustment in machine speed and subsequently constant tablet weight. Figure 6.10 shows the set parameters for Ibuprofen 400 mg tablets, with a target weight of 15 g, a target flow rate of 5 m/s, and a target machine speed of 15 m/s.

Scenario 1: When the measured flow rate is equal to the intent.

From the code and output (Figures 6.10 and 6.11), when the measured flow rate (FLOW=5) matched the intent, the program returned the target speed of 60 RPM, and it displayed the details as shown in the output panel (MACHINE SPEED STATUS). The predicted weight, therefore, matched the intent of 15 g. This is the desired control criteria for tablet weight.

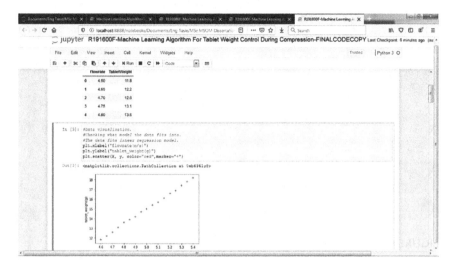

FIGURE 6.9 Linear relationship between the CMA, CCP, and CQA for Ibuprofen 400 mg tablets.

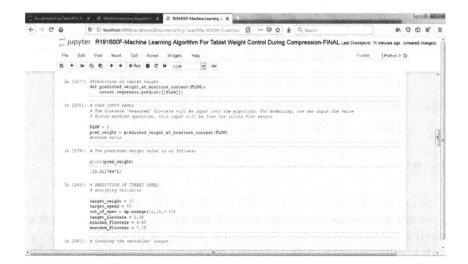

FIGURE 6.10 Learning algorithm for tablet weight control Scenario 1.

Results are shown in Figure 6.11.

FIGURE 6.11 Scenario 1: When the measured flow rate is equal to the intent.

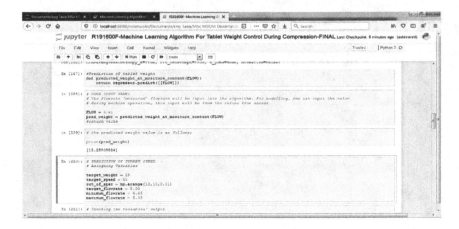

FIGURE 6.12   Learning algorithm using Jupiter Scenario 2.

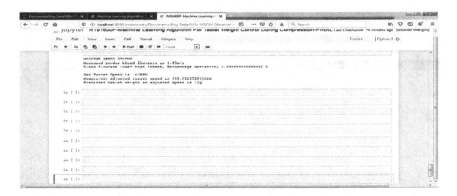

FIGURE 6.13   Scenario 2: When the measured flow rate is less to the intent.

Scenario 2: When the measured flow rate is less to the intent.

From the code and output (Figures 6.12 and 6.13), when the measured flow rate (FLOW = 4.65) is less than the intent, the program predicted weight is 12.2 g. Based on the product's previous training and testing data, the algorithm had to predict an adjusted speed to compensate for the low flow rate, which is lesser than the target speed in this case. The returned speed of 49 RPM led to a final predicted tablet weight of 15 g. This is the desired control criteria for tablet weight.

Scenario 3: When the measured flow rate is higher than the intent.

From the code and output (Figures 6.14 and 6.15), when the measured flow rate (FLOW = 5.35) is greater than the intent, the program predicted a weight of 17.8 g. Based on the product's previous training and testing data, the algorithm had to predict an adjusted speed to compensate for the low flow rate, which is greater than the target speed in this case. The returned speed of 71 RPM led to a final predicted tablet weight of 15 g. This is the desired control criteria for tablet weight.

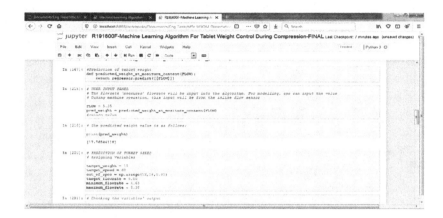

FIGURE 6.14 Scenario 3: Jupiter machine learning.

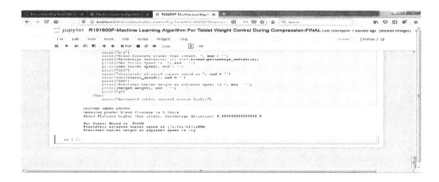

FIGURE 6.15 Scenario 3: When the measured flow rate is higher than the intent.

Results

Scenario 4: When the measured flow rate is out of the acceptable product flow rate.

From the code and output (Figures 6.16 and 6.17), when the measured flow rate (FLOW = 4.1) is out of the acceptable range of 4.65–5.35, the program predicted a weight of 7 g specification.

Such out-of-range flow rate data show a significant deviation in powder CMA or machine failure such as clogging of the powder feed path; hence, operations must be stopped. In this case, the algorithm returned an error code and stopped production for the operator to attend to the problem. This is the desired control criteria for tablet weight as shown in Figure 6.16.

6.5.5 IMPACT OF MACHINE LEARNING ALGORITHM APPLICATION ON A TABLETTING MACHINE

The impact of these benefits on the product price is represented graphically, as in Figure 6.18.

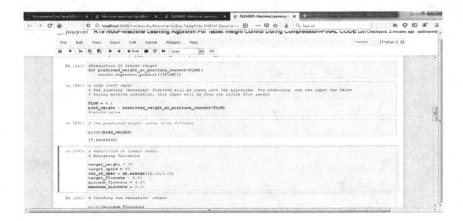

FIGURE 6.16　Jupiter machine learning Scenario 4.

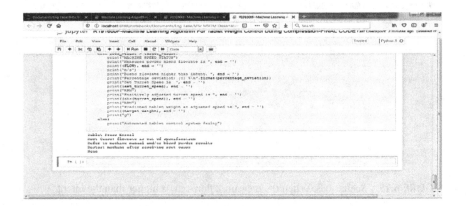

FIGURE 6.17　Scenario 4: When the measured flow rate is out of the acceptable product flow rate.

Adopting a ML capability such as the one discussed in this research would cost about US$735.

6.6　CONCLUSIONS AND RECOMMENDATIONS

6.6.1　CONCLUSIONS

ML algorithm proved to be sufficient in controlling a tablet-making machine. As noted in the results, when varying flow rate, data was introduced for predicting corresponding machine speed to give tablets matching the intent weight, with at least 99.8% confidence, as calculated from the linear model. Other than the enhanced quality benefits, the ML algorithm enabled a remarkable reduction of labour by 50%, material waste by up to 4% (about 80% of initial waste), and set up

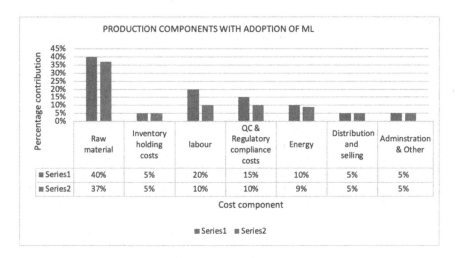

FIGURE 6.18 Effect of ML adoption on product pricing.

time by 13%. Adopting ML thus enables a reduction of total production costs by up to 19%, which translates to a 19% reduction in the price of the locally manufactured tablets. Using the Ibuprofen 400 mg tablets (which were 10% pricier than the imported ones) as an example, it can be concluded that ML can improve pharmaceutical machinery and make the local industry competitive enough to expand their market share locally and regionally. Ordinarily, by varying levels of ML adoption and managing the costs of ML implementation, a break-even point could be achieved, with a minimum level of ML adoption in the local industry that would realise at least a 10% reduction in production cost while at the same time enhancing the quality and regulatory compliance. The positive attitude that representatives from PharmaCo showed on the introduction of ML makes the technology transfer seamless; with little to no resistance from both the operators (who stand to benefit career-wise) and top management (which will eventually realise increased profits for the organisation). Results were processed and analysed using various statistical tools and inductive conclusions made. A technology transfer plan was developed for PharmaCo and can also be adopted by other local pharmaceutical manufacturing companies. Adopting a ML capability such as the one discussed in this research would cost about US$735. It is also worth noting that the research came as a solution for a problem highlighted by the Pharmaceutical Working Group (PWG). The local manufacturing had an operational efficiency issue in their production machines.

6.6.2 Recommendations

It was noted that in-process intermediaries significantly impacted the product throughput negatively. While the solution can be adopted for the tabletting machine only, it is also recommended to adopt ML technology on a whole tablet manufacturing line, from materials weighing up to packing, to realise the full potential of the technology.

REFERENCES

1. ADBG. (2019). *Zimbabwe Infrastructure Report 2019.* Available Online: https://www.afdb.org/en/zimbabwe-infrastructure-report-2019
2. Amaral, G., Bushee, J., Cordani, U. G., KAWASHITA, K., Reynolds, J. H., ALMEIDA, F. F. M. D. E., de Almeida, F. F. M., Hasui, Y., de Brito Neves, B. B., Fuck, R. A., Oldenzaal, Z., Guida, A., Tchalenko, J. S., Peacock, D. C. P., Sanderson, D. J., Rotevatn, A., Nixon, C. W., Rotevatn, A., Sanderson, D. J., … Junho, M. do C. B. (2013). Learning python O'riel. *Journal of Petrology, 369*(1). Doi: 10.1017/CBO 9781107415324.004.
3. Badman, C., Cooney, C. L., Florence, A., Konstantinov, K., Krumme, M., Mascia, S., Nasr, M., & Trout, B. L. (2019). Why we need continuous pharmaceutical manufacturing and how to make it happen. *Journal of Pharmaceutical Sciences, 108*(11), 3521–3523. Doi: 10.1016/j.xphs.2019.07.016.
4. Besharati-Foumani, H., Lohtander, M., & Varis, J. (2019). Intelligent process planning for smart manufacturing systems: a state-of-the-art review. *Procedia Manufacturing, 38,* 156–162. Doi: 10.1016/j.promfg.2020.01.021.
5. Chan, H. C. S., Shan, H., Dahoun, T., Vogel, H., & Yuan, S. (2019). Advancing drug discovery via Artificial Intelligence. *Trends in Pharmacological Sciences, 40*(8), 13. Doi: 10.1016/j.tips.2019.06.004.
6. Cociorva, S., & Iftene, A. (2017). Indoor air quality evaluation in intelligent building. *Energy Procedia, 112*(October 2016), 261–268. Doi: 10.1016/j.egypro.2017.03.1095.
7. Dailey, J. W. (2018). Pharmaceutical industry. In *Encyclopaedia Britannica* (pp. 1–30). https://www.britannica.com/technology/pharmaceutical-industry.
8. de Smith, M. J. (2014). *Statistical Analysis Handbook.* WWW.STATSREF.COM.
9. Dey, R., & Chowdhury, D. R. (2018). Quality by design- a new approach to drug development. *International Journal of Drug Regulatory Affairs, 3*(2), 8–16. Doi: 10.22270/ijdra.v3i2.163.
10. Fedorov, A., Goloschchapov, E., Ipatov, O., Potekhin, V., Shkodyrev, V., & Zobnin, S. (2015). Aspects of smart manufacturing via agent-based approach. *Procedia Engineering, 100*(January), 1572–1581. Doi: 10.1016/j.proeng.2015.01.530.
11. Forum, W. E. (2018). The next economic growth engine: scaling fourth industrial revolution technologies in production. In *World Economic Forum* (Issue January). https://www.weforum.org/whitepapers/the-next-economic-growth-engine-scaling-fourth-industrial-revolution-technologies-in-production%0Ahttp://www3.weforum.org/docs/WEF_Technology_and_Innovation_The_Next_Economic_Growth_Engine.pdf.
12. GEA, B. (2019). *Continuous Processing Solutions for Oral Solid Dosage Forms,* p. 42. Available Online: https://www.gea.com/en/binaries/Pharmaceutical-Continuous-Processing-for-oral-solid-dosage-forms_tcm11-59766.pdf
13. Henstock, P. V. (2019). Trends in pharmacological sciences science and society Artificial Intelligence for pharma : time for internal investment trends in pharmacological sciences. *Trends in Pharmacological Sciences, 40*(8), 543–546. Doi: 10.1016/j.tips.2019.05.003.

14. Ibrić, S., Djurić, Z., Parojčić, J., & Petrović, J. (2009). Artificial Intelligence in pharmaceutical product formulation: neural computing. *Chemical Industry and Chemical Engineering Quarterly, 15*(4), 227–236. Doi: 10.2298/CICEQ0904227I.

15. IPA, T. I. P. A. (2019, January). Pharma times. *Pharma Times, 51*(01), 56.

16. ISPE. (2017). *2017 ISPE Europe Pharma 4.0^TM Conference _ ISPE _ International Society for Pharmaceutical Engineering.*

17. Jolliffe, H. G., & Gerogiorgis, D. I. (2016). Plantwide design and economic evaluation of two Continuous Pharmaceutical Manufacturing (CPM) cases: ibuprofen and artemisinin. *Computers and Chemical Engineering, 91*, 269–288. Doi: 10.1016/j. compchemeng.2016.04.005.

18. Lamberti, M. J., Wilkinson, M., Donzanti, B. A., Wohlhieter, G. E., Parikh, S., Wilkins, R. G., & Getz, K. (2019). A study on the application and use of Artificial Intelligence to support drug development. *Clinical Therapeutics, 41*(8), 1414–1426. Doi: 10.1016/j.clinthera.2019.05.018.

19. Limaye, R., Kumar, L., & Limaye, N. (2018). Fourth generation technologies in pharmaceuticals-revolutionizing healthcare. *Journal of Systems Biology and Proteome Research, 2*(1), 3–7. http://www.alliedacademies.org/systems-biology-proteome-research/.

20. Lin, Y. J., Wei, S. H., & Huang, C. Y. (2019). Intelligent manufacturing control systems: the core of smart factory. *Procedia Manufacturing, 39*(2019), 389–397. Doi: 10.1016/j.promfg.2020.01.382.

21. Lu, Y., & Ju, F. (2017). Smart manufacturing systems based on cyber-physical manufacturing services (CPMS). *IFAC-PapersOnLine, 50*(1), 15883–15889. Doi: 10.1016/j.ifacol.2017.08.2349.

22. Mak, K. K., & Pichika, M. R. (2019). Artificial Intelligence in drug development: present status and future prospects. *Drug Discovery Today, 24*(3), 773–780. Doi: 10.1016/j.drudis.2018.11.014.

23. Mészáros, L. A., Galata, D. L., Madarász, L., Köte, Á., Csorba, K., Dávid, Á. Z., Domokos, A., Szabó, E., Nagy, B., Marosi, G., Farkas, A., & Nagy, Z. K. (2020, December). Digital UV/VIS imaging: a rapid PAT tool for crushing strength, drug content and particle size distribution determination in tablets. *International Journal of Pharmaceutics, 578*, 119174. Doi: 10.1016/j.ijpharm.2020.119174.

24. Meziane, F., Vadera, S., Kobbacy, K., & Proudlove, N. (2000). Intelligent systems in manufacturing: current developments and future prospects. *Integrated Manufacturing Systems, 11*(3), 218–238. Doi: 10.1108/09576060010326221.

25. Mohammed, M., Khan, M. B., & Bashie, E. B. M. (2016). Machine learning: algorithms and applications. In *Machine Learning: Algorithms and Applications* (Issue December). Doi: 10.1201/9781315371658.

26. Peng, T., Huang, Y., Mei, L., Wu, L., Chen, L., Pan, X., & Wu, C. (2015). ScienceDirect Study progression in application of process analytical technologies on film coating. *Asian Journal of Pharmaceutical Sciences, 10*(3), 176–185. Doi: 10.1016/j.ajps.2014.10.002.

27. Rantanen, J., & Khinast, J. (2015). The future of pharmaceutical manufacturing sciences. *Journal of Pharmaceutical Sciences, 104*(11), 3612–3638. Doi: 10.1002/jps.24594.

28. Réda, C., Kaufmann, E., & Delahaye-Duriez, A. (2020). Machine learning applications in drug development. *Computational and Structural Biotechnology Journal, 18*, 241–252. Doi: 10.1016/j.csbj.2019.12.006.

29. Rene, L. (2014). *Regional Network for Equity in Health in East and Southern Africa: Medicines Production and Procurement in East and Southern Africa and the Role of South-South Co-operation.* ISBN: 978-0-7974-6044-7.

30. Saunders, M., Lewis, P. and Thornhill, A. (2007). *Research Methods for Business Students.* 4th Edition, Financial Times Prentice Hall, Edinburgh Gate, Harlow.
31. Schreiber, M., Klöber-Koch, J., Bömelburg-Zacharias, J., Braunreuther, S., & Reinhart, G. (2020). Automated quality assurance as an intelligent cloud service using machine learning. *Procedia CIRP, 86,* 185–191. Doi: 10.1016/j.procir.2020.01.034.
32. Schweidtmann, A. M., Clayton, A. D., Holmes, N., Bradford, E., Bourne, R. A., & Lapkin, A. A. (2018). Machine learning meets continuous flow chemistry: automated optimization towards the Pareto front of multiple objectives. *Chemical Engineering Journal, 352*(April), 277–282. Doi: 10.1016/j.cej.2018.07.031.
33. Scott, B., & Wilcock, A. (2006). Process analytical technology in the pharmaceutical industry: a toolkit for continuous improvement. *PDA Journal of Pharmaceutical Science and Technology, 60*(1), 17–53.
34. Shalev-Shwartz, S., & Ben-David, S. (2013). Understanding machine learning: from theory to algorithms. *Understanding Machine Learning: From Theory to Algorithms,* 9781107057. Doi: 10.1017/CBO9781107298019.
35. Shang, C., & You, F. (2019). Data analytics and machine learning for smart process manufacturing: recent advances and perspectives in the big data era. *Engineering, 5*(6), 1010–1016. Doi: 10.1016/j.eng.2019.01.019.
36. Singh, R. (2018a). Automation of continuous pharmaceutical manufacturing process. *Computer Aided Chemical Engineering, 41,* 431–446. Doi: 10.1016/B978-0-444-63963-9.00017-8.
37. Singh, R. (2018b). Implementation of control system into continuous pharmaceutical manufacturing pilot plant (powder to tablet). *Computer Aided Chemical Engineering , 41,* 447–469). Doi: 10.1016/B978-0-444-63963-9.00018-X.
38. Stuart, O.,Schweitzer, Z., & Lu, J. (2018). Pharmaceutical economics and policy: perspectives, promises, and problems. Doi: 10.1093/oso/9780190623784.001.0001.
39. Su, Q., Ganesh, S., Moreno, M., Bommireddy, Y., Gonzalez, M., Reklaitis, G. V., & Nagy, Z. K. (2019). A perspective on Quality-by-Control (QbC) in pharmaceutical continuous manufacturing. *Computers and Chemical Engineering, 125,* 216–231. Doi: 10.1016/j.compchemeng.2019.03.001.
40. Suresh, S., Roy, S., & Ahuja, B. K. (2015). Quality by design: an overview. *Indian Drugs, 52*(2), 5–11.
41. Tao, F., Qi, Q., Liu, A., & Kusiak, A. (2018). Data-driven smart manufacturing. *Journal of Manufacturing Systems, 48,* 157–169. Doi: 10.1016/j.jmsy.2018.01.006.
42. U.S. Department of Health and Human Services. (2009). Guidance for industry. Q10 pharmaceutical quality system. *Food and Drug Administration, Center for Drug Evaluation and Research, Center for Biologics Evaluation and Research. International Conference on Harmonization of Technical Requirements for Registration of Pharmaceuticals for Human Use (ICH),* April, 1–22. http://www.fda.gov/downloads/Drugs/.../Guidances/ucm073517.pdf.
43. UNIDO. (2017). *Sector Development Strategy for Pharmaceutical Manufacturing in Zimbabwe.* Available Online: https://tii.unido.org/sites/default/files/publications/Zimbabwe%20Pharma%20Strategy%20ebook.pdf
44. Ustundag, Alp & Cevikcan, Emre. (2018). *Industry 4.0: Managing The Digital Transformation.* 10.1007/978-3-319-57870-5.
45. Wang, J., Ma, Y., Zhang, L., Gao, R. X., & Wu, D. (2018). Deep learning for smart manufacturing: methods and applications. *Journal of Manufacturing Systems, 48,* 144–156. Doi: 10.1016/j.jmsy.2018.01.003.
46. Watts, D. C., & Hussain, A. S. (2005, March). Process analytical technology. In *Handbook of Pharmaceutical Granulation Technology,* 2nd Ed., 545–553. Doi: 10.1201/b15426-14.

47. WHO. (2011). *Annex 2 WHO Good Manufacturing Practices for Pharmaceutical* (Issue 961).

48. WHO Expert Committee on Specifications for Pharmaceutical Preparations. Fiftieth report. *World Health Organization Technical Report Series.* 2016;(996): 1-358, back cover. PMID: 27514184.

49. Wong, Y. K., Yang, J., & He, Y. (2020). Caution and clarity required in the use of chloroquine for COVID-19. *The Lancet Rheumatology, 9913*(20), 30093. Doi: 10.1016/S2665-9913(20)30093-X

50. Wood, C., Alwati, A., Halsey, S., Gough, T., Brown, E., Kelly, A., & Paradkar, A. (2016). Journal of pharmaceutical and biomedical analysis near infra red spectroscopy as a multivariate process analytical tool for predicting pharmaceutical co-crystal concentration. *Journal of Pharmaceutical and Biomedical Analysis, 129,* 172–181. Doi: 10.1016/j.jpba.2016.06.010.

51. World Health Organization, A. (2020). *COVID-19: Situation Update for the WHO African Region.* https://apps.who.int/iris/bitstream/handle/10665/331587/SITREP_COVID-19_WHOAFRO_20200325-eng.pdf.

52. Zhong, R. Y., Xu, X., Klotz, E., & Newman, S. T. (2017). Intelligent manufacturing in the context of industry 4.0: a review. *Engineering, 3*(5), 616–630. Doi: 10.1016/J. ENG.2017.05.015.

7 Regression Analysis for Prediction of Blood Pressure from Health Parameter

Biswabandhu Jana
IIT Kharagpur

CONTENTS

7.1 INTRODUCTION

Blood pressure (BP) is a representative parameter of our overall health and one of the best predictors for illness. Over the world, the high BP is a cause of 7.5 million deaths, which are approximately 12.8% of the overall [1]. High BP or hypertension progresses the major hazard for coronary heart diseases, transient ischemic attack (TIA), dementia (brain disease), kidney damage (nephropathy), hemorrhagic stroke as well as several types of chronic diseases [2]. The low BP or hypotension puts a greater risk of serious health conditions such as unsteadiness, dizziness, fainting and others. For adequate control of BP, a continuous health monitoring system is desired for medical professionals. The proposed study aims to estimate systolic blood pressure (SBP) and diastolic blood pressure (DBP) from the biometric parameters, *i.e.*, body mass index (BMI), heart rate (HR) as well as age for early detection and diagnosis. Overall, the developed model facilitates the growth of point-of-care (POC) applications.

DOI: 10.1201/9781003224075-7

The remaining paper is described in a subsequent way. A literature survey is presented in Section 7.2 related to the area of BP studies. In Section 7.3, a model has been developed for estimating SBP and DBP using some biometric factors. The correlations of these parameters with BP are also represented through statistical analysis. Error estimation is computed and the result is validated using t-test in Section 7.4. Finally, a Smartphone application has been developed for predicting SBP and DBP values. The concluding remarks are in Section 7.5.

7.2 LITERATURE REVIEW

Several research articles have shown non-invasive techniques for predicting BP and the effect of high BP. In [3], the authors propose that the overweight can increase the chance of BP and the association between BMI and BP is analyzed using multivariate linear regression analysis. The relationship between BP and BMI is reported for low BMI populations and multivariate regression modeling has been used to examine gender-related differences in the relationship [4]. A comparative study on artificial neural network (ANN) and multiple linear regression (MLR) has been described for continuous estimation of BP using some biometric parameters and pulse transit time (PTT) [5]. The age-related effect on BP is characterized in both normal and untreated high BP subjects [6,7]. Moreover, a continuous and cuffless BP screening method is also presented based on ECG and PPG signals [8,9]. In [10], the authors propose an accelerometer-based method (without using any dedicated external sensors) to display the BP on a tablet touch-screen. A Doppler Ultrasound based BP estimation is also proposed to provide a non-invasive and non-occlusive BP estimation method [11]. Moreover, the deep neural network-based BP estimation model is also proposed based on artificial feature vectors [12]. Some open-source fingerprint-based Android application is also available for monitoring BP. However, the BP application may display an inaccurate reading that can complicate our health or give a false sense of security [13]. To make a difference, this study introduces a Smartphone-based application that can collect health parameters, process and predict BP. Furthermore, the impact of age-adjusted BMI on BP is also extensively reported. The advantages of the proposed approach are lower computational complexity with respect to the small training sample and cuffless estimation of BP can enable the POC system.

7.3 PROPOSED METHOD

The block diagram of the proposed approach is shown in Figure 7.1 to describe the entire process from data collection to prediction of BP.

7.3.1 DATA COLLECTION

To conduct this experiment, BP, HR, age, height and weight are collected from the subjects. Subjects are apparently healthy, have no critical clinical condition at that age and are free from chronic diseases. A trained person has taken the BP

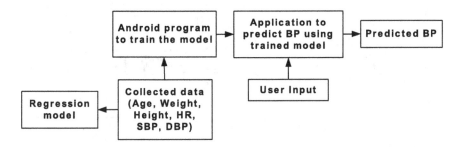

FIGURE 7.1 Block diagram of the proposed method.

while patients are resting supine and it is measured from the auscultation of systolic and diastolic Korotkoff's sound. On the left hand of the Brachial artery, the BP measurement cuff is tried to occlude the artery. BP has been measured using the Rossmax GB102 Aneroid Blood Pressure monitoring device with the help of experienced professionals. BMI is calculated from the ratio of body weight in kg and square value of body height in meters.

The experimental study has been conducted on 156 volunteers aged between 21 and 80 years. The mean and standard deviation (SD) for all obtained parameters are found to be 124.27 ± 13.86 mmHg for SBP, 76.1 ± 8.37 mmHg for DBP, 43.60 ± 18.11 for age, 73.12 ± 7.67 bpm for HR and 24.9 ± 4.35 kg/m^2 for BMI. Patients with BP greater than 140/90 mmHg are considered as hypertensive, prehypertension as 120–140/80–90 mmHg and normal is defined as below 120/80 mmHg.

7.3.2 MODEL

The different Machine Learning-based regression model has been examined based on the training data to obtain the best performance. The linear regression model with 10-fold cross-validation has been selected while the input values are considered as BMI, HR and age. The WEKA Machine Learning toolbox is employed for the proposed model [14]. The model has been trained and saved for predicting BP values for unknown subjects.

In addition, a statistical analysis is performed to determine the input variables as an appropriate predictor [15]. The relationship between all variables is determined using Pearson's correlation while the significance level $P < 0.05$. There is a moderate degree of correlation exists between all these independent variables with BP. The correlation values are found to be as follows (shown in Figure 7.2): SBP and BMI ($r = 0.43$, $P < 0.0001$), DBP and BMI ($r = 0.35$, $P < 0.0001$), SBP and HR ($r = 0.3$, $P < 0.0001$), DBP and HR ($r = 0.44$, $P < 0.001$), SBP and age ($r = 0.47$, $P < 0.0001$) and DBP and age ($r = 0.17$, $P < 0.0001$).

The multivariate linear regression model is used for the evaluation of the independent effect of age, BMI and HR on the output variables of SBP and DBP. The MLR model is chosen as it is the simplest one and the results obtained using this model justify its selection [16]. The residuals (difference between the actual

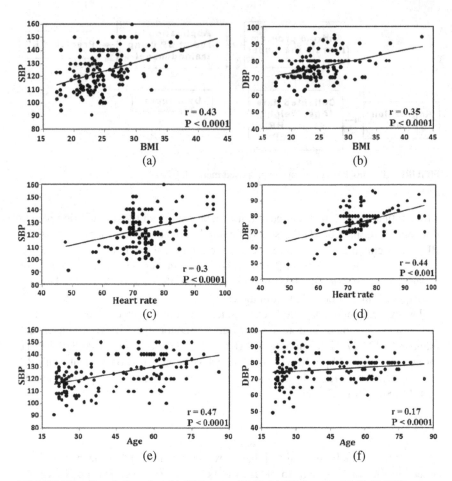

FIGURE 7.2 Correlation plot. (a) SBP versus BMI, (b) DBP versus BMI, (c) SBP versus HR, (d) DBP versus HR, (e) SBP versus age and (f) DBP versus age.

and predicted value) obtained from this model are independent and are not influenced by the previous observations. The residuals are normally distributed and the residual normality plot depicts nearly a straight line. The assumptions prove that the linear regression model can be adapted to describe this data set. The correlation coefficient and probability of relationship between BP and biometric parameters are calculated using the SPSS (statistical package for social science) software. The predicted BP values based on the training data are expressed in equations 7.1 and 7.2.

$$\text{Predicted SBP} = \alpha_0 + \alpha_1 \cdot \text{BMI} + \alpha_2 \cdot \text{HR} + \alpha_3 \cdot \text{Age},$$

$$\text{where } \alpha_0 = 54.77, \alpha_1 = 1.05, \alpha_2 = 0.41, \alpha_3 = 0.31$$

(7.1)

$$\text{Predicted DBP} = \beta_0 + \beta_1 \cdot \text{BMI} + \beta_2 \cdot \text{HR} + \beta_3 \cdot \text{Age},$$

$$\text{where } \beta_0 = 33.06, \beta_1 = 0.43, \beta_2 = 0.40, \beta_3 = 0.059$$

(7.2)

7.3.3 ANDROID APPLICATION

An Android application has been developed using the linear regression-based classifier to predict the SBP and DBP from the user input. The coefficient values are obtained from pretrained model and used for BP estimation. A JAVA platform has been considered for the proposed design and the application is implemented on Moto E (Motorola, Inc.) Smartphone running an Android operating system (KitKat, Google, Inc.) [17].

7.4 RESULT AND DISCUSSIONS

The measurements of 156 subjects are sequentially separated into 106 subjects for training and 50 subjects as an unknown testing set. The BP prediction accuracy of 50 testing subjects is shown in Table 7.1. The performance is observed by measuring mean error (ME), mean absolute error (MAE) and standard deviation of error (SDE) and root mean squared error (RMSE). According to the criteria of Advancement of Medical Instrumentation (AAMI), ME and SDE values of the testing subjects must be below 5 and 8 mmHg, respectively [18]. In Table 7.1, ME values of the proposed approach are lower than the acceptable limit of the AAMI standard. For the SDE criteria, the DBP value is within the margin and SBP is out of acceptable limit based on the acquired dataset.

Table 7.2 also represents an accuracy regarding the criteria of the British Hypertension Society (BHS) standard [19]. The three different thresholds, *i.e.*, error values less than 5, 10 and 15 mmHg, are considered to grade in the BHS standard. Based on the BHS protocol, the proposed methodology for the acquired

TABLE 7.1
Error of Blood Pressure Prediction on Test Data

	ME	MAE	SDE	RMSE
SBP	−1.5	9.36	11.5	11.49
DBP	1.94	4.9	6.48	6.7

TABLE 7.2
Cumulative Error Percentage for SBP and DBP Measurement

	< 5 mmHg	< 10 mmHg	< 15 mmHg
SBP	39.74	69.23	85.25
DBP	57.69	81.4	93.6

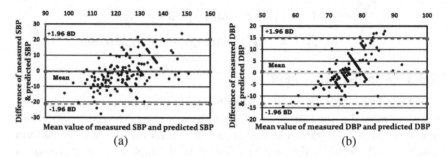

FIGURE 7.3 Bland–Altman plot for error values. (a) SBP differences are shown for the averages of actual and reference values. (b) DBP differences are shown for the averages of actual and reference values.

TABLE 7.3
Odd Ratio Prediction for SBP and DBP

		Hypertension	Prehypertension
Overweight	SBP	7.3	3.82
	DBP	6.3	0.8
Underweight	SBP	0.87	0.38
	DBP	NA	0.25
Normal	Taken as reference		

dataset can be considered as grade B for the estimation of DBP and grade C for the estimation of SBP values.

A scatter diagram of a Bland–Altman plot is shown in Figure 7.3 to examine the difference between the actual and predicted BP values. The y-axis indicates the difference between measured and estimated BP while the x-axis shows the mean value of these two techniques [20,21]. The Bland–Altman plot includes 95% confidence interval for both the upper and lower limits of agreement using a dotted line.

It is evident from the Bland–Altman plot that there is a trend from the bias. The error difference becomes wider with a magnitude of DBP measurement and the proportional error is also increased for predicting high DBP values. In the case of SBP, there is a moderate trend for the standard values and the absolute systematic error is decreasing while predicting high SBP values. Additionally, the correlation between the actual and predicted value is found to be 0.64 and 0.54 for SBP and DBP, respectively.

According to this analysis, a significant positive correlation is found between BMI and BP. An increase or decrease in BMI is significantly associated with the change in both SBP and DBP. However, the exact effect of BMI on BP is still unclear. Table 7.3 shows the odds ratio (OR) for predicting SBP and DBP values [22,23]. As considered from SBP, the overweight people (BMI > 25 kg/m^2) are 7.3 times more likely to have hypertension (SBP > 140 mmHg) and 3.82 times more likely to have prehypertension (SBP 120–140 mmHg) than the normal BMI (18–25 kg/m^2) category people. DBP shows that the overweight persons are 6.3 times more likely to have hypertension and it is less likely than the prehypertension people compared to those of the normal BMI category. The underweight people (BMI<18 kg/m^2) are related to neither hypertension nor prehypertension. In an additional analysis, the BMI has the strongest effect for people who are 60 years and above. OR for SBP is found 11 for hypertension and 1.86 for prehypertension. For DBP measurement, the OR is found to be 8 for the hypertension people. In particular, the aged patients with an unusually high BMI show a progressive tendency towards hypertension.

Moreover, the two-tailed independent samples t-test is performed to observe a statistically significant difference for every pair of BP measurements. In the t-test, a significance level of 0.05 is taken for three parameters (BMI, HR and age). The value of kurtosis and skewness is less than that of the acceptable value to conduct the t-test [24]. Table 7.4 shows the obtained P-values for different pairs of hypertension, prehypertension and normal person. It should be noted that the small value of P defines a better separation among these three cases. The result shows that apart from one instance (P-value of HR for hypertension–prehypertension case), P-value of BMI, HR and age shows a separation of hypertension, prehypertension and normal patients.

Finally, a Smartphone-based Android application has been implemented for predicting the SBP and DBP values using the proposed linear regression model. Figure 7.4 shows the Android application to predict BP based on user input age, HR and BMI. Figure 7.4a and b shows the home screen of Android application and the application predicting SBP and DBP values, respectively.

7.4.1 Limitations and Future Scope

The proposed study has some limitations. The acquired dataset is not following the criteria of the AAMI or BHS standard to observe the performance of the model. In addition, a trend is visible in the Bland–Altman plot while the error values are increasing in high and low BP values. In future, more datasets can be collected according to the international standard protocols to improve the BP estimation values. In addition, the Internet of Things-based system in deep learning framework can extend the work for improving the healthcare system as well as continuous BP monitoring [25,26].

TABLE 7.4
Obtained P-values for Different Pairs of Blood Pressure Cases

	BMI	HR	Age
Hypertension–Prehypertension	0.013	0.36	0.007
Prehypertension–Normal	0.000	0.005	0.000
Normal–Hypertension	0.000	0.005	0.000

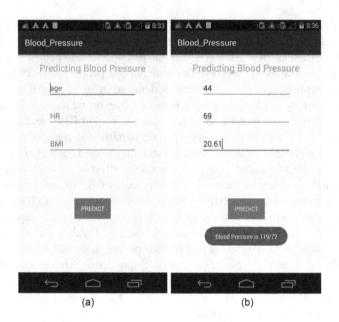

(a)   **(b)**

FIGURE 7.4   Android application. (a) Home screen of Android application and (b) Android application predicting blood pressure.

7.5   CONCLUSIONS

In this study, a non-invasive and non-occlusive BP estimation regression model has been proposed based on the independent effect of biometric parameters. For POC applications, an Android-based platform has also been implemented to monitor the BP continuously in the remote environment. Further, BMI shows a strong predictor for BP measurement and high BMI is the increased risk for hypertension. But the limitation in the existing model is that gender-related differences for predicting BP are not included in this study. For future investigation, it is suggested to include gender differences effect on both BP and BMI for the validation of this model in a larger sample.

ACKNOWLEDGMENT

We are thankful to Dr. Sankar Mitra, EKO Heart Foundation, Kolkata, India and Dr. Kamal Oswal, NCS Diagnostics, Kolkata, India for their help and guidance throughout this work.

REFERENCES

1. WHO, "Global health observatory data," http://web.archive.org/web/www.who.int/gho/ncd/risk factors/blood pressure prevalence text/en/, 2016 [Accessed: 2016-12-8].

2. M. C. Staff, "High blood pressure (hypertension)," http://web.archive.org/web/ http://www.mayoclinic.org/diseases-conditions/high-blood-pressure/in-depth/high-blood-pressure/art-20045868, 2016 [Accessed: 2016-12-22].

3. W. B. Droyvold, K. Midthjell, T. I. L. Nilsen, and J. Holmen, "Change in body mass index and its impact on blood pressure: a prospective population study," *International Journal of Obesity*, vol. 29, no. 6, pp. 650–655, 2005.

4. J. S. Kaufman, M. C. Asuzu, J. Mufunda, T. Forrester, R. Wilks, A. Luke, A. E. Long, and R. S. Cooper, "Relationship between blood pressure and body mass index in lean populations," *Hypertension*, vol. 30, no. 6, 1997.

5. J. Y. Kim, B. H. Cho, S. M. Im, M. J. Jeon, I. Y. Kim, and S. Kim, "Comparative study on artificial neural network with multiple regressions for continuous estimation of blood pressure," in *IEEE International Conference Engineering in Medicine and Biology Society (EMBC)*, 27th Annual Conference, Shanghai, China, 2005, pp. 6942–6945.

6. S. S. Franklin, W. Gustin, N. D. Wong, M. G. Larson, M. A. Weber, W. B. Kannel, and D. Levy, "Hemodynamic patterns of age-related changes in blood pressure," *Circulation*, vol. 96, no. 1, pp. 308–315, July 1997.

7. S. Landahl, C. Bengtsson, J. A. Sigurdsson, A. Svanborg, and K. Sv'ardsudd, "Age-related changes in blood pressure," *Hypertension*, vol. 8, no. 11, pp. 1044–1049, 1986.

8. M. Jain, N. Kumar, and S. Deb, "An affordable cuff-less blood pressure estimation solution," in *International Conference of the IEEE Engineering in Medicine and Biology Society (EMBC)*, Lake Buena Vista, FL, Aug 2016.

9. M. Kachuee, M. M. Kiani, H. Mohammadzade, and M. Shabany, "Cuff-less blood pressure estimation algorithms for continuous health-care monitoring." *IEEE Transactions on Bio-Medical Engineering*, vol. 9294, no. c, pp. 1–11, 2016.

10. R. Murthy and D. Kotz, "Assessing blood-pressure measurement in tablet-based mHealth apps," in *Sixth International Conference on Communication Systems and Networks (COMSNETS)*, Bangalore, India, 2014.

11. B. Jana, K. Oswal, S. Mitra, G. Saha, and S. Banerjee, "Windkessel model-based cuffless blood pressure estimation using continuous wave doppler ultrasound system," *IEEE Sensors Journal*, vol. 20, no. 17, pp. 9989–9999, 2020.

12. S. Lee and J.-H. Chang, "Oscillometric blood pressure estimation based on deep learning," *IEEE Transactions on Industrial Informatics*, vol. 13, no. 2, pp. 461–472, 2017.

13. Harvard Heart Letter, "Don't trust this smartphone app to measure your blood pressure," http://www.health.harvard.edu/heart-health/dont-trust-this-smartphone-app-to-measure-your-blood-pressure, 2016 [Accessed: 2016-12-15].

14. M. Hall, E. Frank, G. Holmes, B. Pfahringer, P. Reutemann, and I. H. Witten, "The WEKA data mining software," *ACM SIGKDD Explorations Newsletter*, vol. 11, no. 1, 2009.

15. E. T. Lee and J. W. Wang, *Statistical Methods for Survival Data Analysis*, 4th ed. Wiley Publishing, New York, 2013.

16. R. O. Duda, P. E. Hart, and D. G. Stork, *Pattern Classification* (2nd Edition). Wiley-Interscience, New York, 2000.

17. G. Developers, "Android developers," https://developer.android.com/index.html, 2016 [Accessed: 2016-10-09].

18. "Non-Invasive Sphygmomanometers—Part 2: Clinical Validation of Automated Measurement Type, ANSI/AAMI/ISO Standard 81060-2," 2009.

19. E. O 'brien, J. Petrie, W. Littler, M. De Swiet, P. L. Padfield, D. G. Altmanu, M. Blandg, A. Coats@, and N. Atkins, "The British Hypertension Society protocol for the evaluation of blood pressure measuring devices," *Journal of Hypertension*, vol. 11, no. 2, pp. 43–62, 1993.

20. S. Puke, T. Suzuki, K. Nakayama, H. Tanaka, and S. Minami, "Blood pressure estimation from pulse wave velocity measured on the chest," in *35th Annual International Conference Engineering in Medicine and Biology Society (EMBC)*, Osaka, Japan, 2013.

21. D. Giavarina, "Understanding Bland Altman analysis," *Biochemia medica*, vol. 25, no. 2, pp. 141–151, 2015.

22. N. K. Mungreiphy, S. Kapoor, and R. Sinha, "Association between BMI, blood pressure, and age: study among Tangkhul Naga tribal males of Northeast India," *Journal of Anthropology*, vol. 2011, pp. 1–6, 2011.

23. M. Szumilas, "Explaining odds ratios," *Journal of the Canadian Academy of Child and Adolescent Psychiatry*, vol. 19, no. 3, pp. 227–229, Aug 2010.

24. H. O. Posten, *Robustness of the Two-Sample T-Test*. Springer Netherlands, Dordrecht, 1984, pp. 92–99.

25. S. Goyal, N. Sharma, B. Bhushan, A. Shankar, and M. Sagayam, *IoT Enabled Technology in Secured Healthcare: Applications, Challenges and Future Directions*. Springer International Publishing, Cham, 2021, pp. 25–48.

26. A. Khamparia, P. K. Singh, P. Rani, D. Samanta, A. Khanna, and B. Bhushan, "An internet of health things-diven deep learning framework for detection and classification of skin cancer using transfer learning," *Transactions on Emerging Telecommunications Technologies*, 2020, vol. 32, pp. 1–11.

8 Revolutionizing Healthcare

Decentralized Data Management of IoT Devices Using Blockchain Technology

Kavitha Rajamohan, Sangeetha Rangasamy, Surekha Nayak, R. Anuradha, and Aarthy Chellasamy
Christ (Deemed to be University)

CONTENTS

DOI: 10.1201/9781003224075-8

8.1   INTRODUCTION

Traditionally, healthcare was restricted to a two-party relationship between doctor and patient, but of late has seen a transformation with a third-party like technology getting involved. Advancements in information technology have strengthened the healthcare industry to an extent where the industry is now ready to offer competent healthcare services with security and interoperability. A few years ago, as the Internet of Things (IoT) made its way into the industry, security breach was a looming challenge. However, with the emergence of blockchain technology (BCT), the security issue is no longer seen as a challenge. Being indispensable, the healthcare industry is gradually embracing

BCT and is evolving rapidly in addition to witnessing an exponential growth. Through the years, the healthcare industry has been quick in experimenting and adopting IoT-enabled devices. Currently, the industry is at a nascent stage and has made technological progress by engaging decentralized management systems to its IoT enabled medical devices. This is evident in the fact that the global figures for the investment in BCT infrastructure in the healthcare market stood at USD 76 million in 2019. The figures are much more promising with the projections for 2026 standing at USD 1,922.9 million [1]. Continuous progress as well as adoption to the evolving technologies has made the medical field move towards precision, leading to reduction in mortality rates and providing timely treatment. The by-product of these technological advancements is the big data, which has brought in the need to manage data that is varied, voluminous and veracious. This big data that is also characterized by velocity needs to be processed through advanced analytics, algorithms, models and tools and it must be transmitted at a lightning speed without compromising on the security and safety of data. This can be ensured through the decentralized management of IoT healthcare devices, which are embedded with consensus algorithms, distributed ledger and smart contracts. The focus of this chapter is to provide the readers with in-depth information on the Internet of Medical Things (IoMT) in the healthcare sector and how decentralized management of IoMT can bring in unprecedented capabilities. It further focuses on the advancements of BCT specific to the healthcare sector and addresses the notable challenges. Further sections give an overview of healthcare, advancements in healthcare, IoT and big data.

8.1.1 HEALTHCARE

The healthcare spectrum is evolving and transforming at a faster pace than ever before. What started as a sickness care sector that put patients at the centre of focus, has now transpired to be a healthcare sector making health as the focal point. Thus, individuals these days will not wait to be sick to take care of their health, but puts health as a priority by adopting a healthy lifestyle. This necessitates a healthcare ecosystem that not only prioritizes diagnosis, treatment and rehabilitation, but also distinctly places importance on the
maintenance of health. This shift has indeed brought in huge stress on the existing healthcare facilities, which is evident in the polarity noticed in the doctor to population ratio. The existing figures show 43% of the World Health Organization (WHO) member countries disclose less than one physician per 1,000 population for the year 2018, which is in stark contrast to the WHO recommended ideal ratio of one doctor for every 1,000 population [2]. This drastic shortage has necessitated the medical fraternity to look into alternatives, which can assist humans in providing medical services. However, the shortcomings in the healthcare verticals are being addressed through the recent advancements in the space, the M, E and U of healthcare widely known as Mobile, Electronic and Ubiquitous healthcare.

8.1.2 ADVANCEMENTS IN HEALTHCARE

Responding to the need to strengthen healthcare facilities across the globe, an interesting concept was set into motion, with the aid of digital revolution that combined digital technology with healthcare and was named Mobile health (M-Health). It is an effective platform through which medical vigilance and medication of a patient is done remotely, if required through the help of family members, using mobile phones and wireless technologies. These devices are used to capture and transmit health data for further actions. M-health just scratched the surface of the vast opportunities available in the technologically driven medical space. Internet triggered health delivery services came into existence recognized as E-healthcare. Diving deeper, the industry also discovered the Clinical Decision Support System and named it as U-healthcare system [3]. It is an advancement in providing medical services through the use of information and telecommunication technologies that manage the prevention, diagnosis, treatment and follow-up of medical actions. Thus, E-health has assured greater improvements, higher precision and accessible healthcare round the clock resulting in specialised individual feedback in real time.

8.1.3 INTERNET OF THINGS

IoT is reckoned as a network of devices, systems and services that are interconnected within the boundaries of the existing internet infrastructure [4]. The complexity of the IoT can be calibrated depending on the required application. It can be as simple as a wearable device or complex one in the form of sensor and ingestible cameras or medical robots that collects and stores person-specific data and allows retrieval of data at any time. This, in turn, has revolutionized the medical field and has made remote health monitoring a reality by diffusing the data gathered by these devices to various health networks. IoT has found a firm foothold in medical circles due to the fact that it not only facilitates critical healthcare but also takes preventive measures by predicting illness.

8.1.4 BIG DATA

Big data is making big waves across the globe literally in every quarter, be it business, politics, economy, legal or the social environment. Big data refers to a voluminous amount of data that is extremely arduous to process using the traditional technology. Thus, big data is defined typically by pointing out its characteristics in terms of the V's, which grew in number gradually over the years. The initial three V's – Volume, Variety and Velocity – was given by Doung Laney [5], an industry analyst in 2001. Further, the author [6] described big data through five V's – Volume, Velocity, Variety, Value and Variability, along with a C for Complexity. Later, SAS (Statistical Analysis System) went ahead to add two additional dimensions, viz Variability and Veracity [7].

Medical services are opted by patients not by choice but forcefully without an option, which naturally accumulates a staggering amount of data every second.

These data are either not captured due to lack of technological advancement in the network or captured but not analyzed due to the constraints in managing data in terms of time and cost. Notwithstanding all the accruing benefits, the healthcare industry has not moved as quickly as expected to embrace the goodness of the big data and the decentralized management of IoT. This sluggishness can be due to the existing gap in connecting big data and IoMT devices. In addition, privacy and security are given utmost priority and cannot be compromised at any cost. Hence, an intervention of BCT with big data and IoMT devices are the prerequisite for a better healthcare system.

8.2   INTERNET OF MEDICAL THINGS

IoMT is a system wherein the connectivity-enabled medical devices are hooked to the healthcare information systems through the internet. These medical devices are not just the ones that are used personally by an individual and linked to his/her computer systems but can also be the ones that are connected to medical experts and health providers. The popularity and usefulness of IoMT is further strengthened as the medical devices are getting ultra-portable with advanced in-built technological features. Globally, the IoT healthcare market is estimated at a whopping USD 446.52 billion in 2028 from USD 89.07 billion in 2021 [8]. The healthcare industry is all set to up its game and make medical facilities affordable, convenient and cost-effective [9]. Notably another concept known as Health Internet of Things (HIoT), which is often used interchangeably with IoMT, started branching out to further explore the use of wireless networks and sensor technologies for tracking medical conditions [10]. Based on the recent technological advancements happening in the healthcare sector that has brought in a sea-change, the authors broadly categorize the IoMT devices as Internet of Informative Medical Things and Internet of Intelligent Medical Things. These are further discussed in the following sections.

8.2.1   INTERNET OF INFORMATIVE MEDICAL THINGS

Medical devices that gather data and transform those data into information to enable further processing are termed informative medical devices. For example, a medical device that monitors and records the blood pressure of a person and compares the reading with the threshold levels that are already fed into the device. When it detects an anomaly, the device sends signals to the wearer to seek immediate medical intervention. Some of the informative medical devices that are used at homes and/or in the healthcare verticals are blood glucose level monitors, blood pressure monitors, fetal monitoring devices, heartbeat and pulse monitoring devices that are designed to monitor the patients round the clock. In similar lines, informative medical devices can also be used by healthy individuals to keep a check of their body mass index, to monitor the intake of calories, to nudge them to take a walk if seated for a long time or to drink water at frequent intervals. When these devices are enabled to connect automatically to a mesh of networks through the internet, they are called Internet of Informative Medical Things.

8.2.2 INTERNET OF INTELLIGENT MEDICAL THINGS

An instrument, an equipment or a machine which has in-built computing capabilities is known as an intelligent device. Intelligent medical devices, therefore, not only gather data and transform the data into information, but also processes it further to help provide intelligent output instantly without human intervention. To this effect, these devices can be pre-programmed to be just reactive machines or can be intelligently programmed. When it is pre-programmed to be reactive, these intelligent medical devices have the capability to make self-adjustments by processing the gathered data. For example, a medical device that spontaneously administers medications or a medical equipment that automatically takes over the breathing process when the patient's vitals hit a certain reading can be considered reactive devices. On the other hand, when intelligently programmed with cutting-edge technologies such as machine learning and artificial intelligence (AI), these medical devices can decipher the commands and perform tasks accurately with or without human intervention. For example, the use of robots in telesurgery which is infused with voice-activated robotic arms and haptic feedback can be considered intelligently programmed medical devices.

Thus, IoMT can be described as a system wherein medical devices automatically configure and instantly connect to a mesh of networks. This interconnected network adopts the distributed ledger system and dispenses services through intelligent interfaces either involving human intelligence or through AI. When the distributed ledger system, smart contract, and BCT gets involved in this loop of IoMT, the entire process becomes secured and safe, thereby mitigating the biggest challenges of the medical industry, viz privacy, safety and security of data.

8.3 ARCHITECTURE OF DECENTRALIZED IOMT USING BCT

The architecture of the Blockchain-based decentralized IoMT system consists of physical, network and application layers. The physical layer being the first stage of human–machine interface comprises wearables, hospital and clinical devices, which collect healthcare data of patients. The network layer is bifurcated into communication layer and blockchain layer. The communication layer comprises Wi-Fi, IoT gateway and routers of various devices that will communicate and connect with the blockchain layer [11]. The collected data will enter the blockchain layer, through the communication protocols. This layer will save the transactions, authenticate the same using smart contracts, validate them by certification or matched keys or encryption and facilitate payment gateway. Every time a transaction is validated using consensus algorithm, a new block is generated. This block is immutable, traceable and secured, to store data that is owned by the patient and accessible only when it is permitted.

The validated data enters the application layer, which has two divisions of data analytics and user clients. The validated data is stored in the cloud for wider access and for further interpretative, diagnostic and predictive analysis using deep

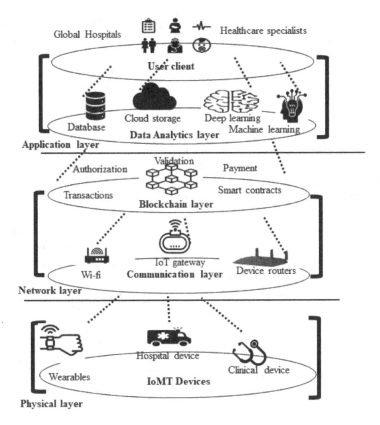

FIGURE 8.1 Decentralized IoMT architecture based on BCT.

learning or machine learning techniques. The user client layer comprises health-care providers and hospitals that will access the stored, authenticated and updated patient data for treatment or medical research and many more. The data collected from various decentralized IoMT devices, across clinics and hospitals around the globe, validated and authenticated by blockchain consensus algorithm, stored in the cloud with enhanced functional values, can serve various research require-ments of vaccination development, identifying the pattern of spread of diseases, geographic and demographic ailment analysis, paediatric issues, organ availabil-ity and many more use cases. The decentralized IoMT architecture based on BCT is given in Figure 8.1.

8.4   HEALTHCARE DATA MANAGEMENT

The authors [12] mentioned that a minimum of 44,000 people to a maximum of 98,000 people die in hospitals due to medical errors. Medical errors are possible due to wrongly placed information on diagnostic, treatment and pre-ventive care. There comes the requirement for an effective healthcare database management system connecting the emerging technologies. Healthcare data is the one which is collected from the healthcare sector. Nowadays, the emerging technologies play a major role in gathering the data. The advent of the internet paved the way to the new world where devices can interact, create, store and exchange the data. Gone are the days in which decisions are based on structured data. IoT and big data are the magical terms through which people, products and producers are having better access to a wealth of data. This data also facilitates a well-informed decision by the stakeholders. Blockchain is another disruptive technology, which has joined hands with IoT and big data to support the data management in various sectors such as finance, education, governance and recently healthcare [13]. One cannot deny the advantages these three technologies have brought into the healthcare sector like reduction in waiting time during emergencies, easy tracking of all the stakeholders (Hospitals, Doctors, Nurses, Druggist, Clinical Lab, Ambulance and Insurance agency), improved drug management and reservation of diagnostic medical services. Perhaps the successful introduction of numerous wearables brought in confidence in the minds of patients that they are monitored 24 hours a day [14]. These devices are user friendly and capable of performing wireless data transmission, real-time feedback and alert mechanism. They facilitate healthcare providers by transferring live data of the patients like blood pressure, blood glucose and breathing pattern [15]. Hence, they have immense potential in the healthcare sector with the help of IoT, Big data and BCT for data management. The following subsections discuss the data management mechanism linking healthcare with IoT, big data and BCT.

8.4.1 PATIENT

Patients are monitored by the service providers through sensors fixed in wearables or embedded in stationary monitoring devices called Remote Patient Monitoring (RPM). These devices can be connected effectively to generate, collect, transfer and store data with the help of IoT (to generate/collect/store), Blockchain (to transfer with privacy and security) and cloud (to store). One cannot deny the grave privacy risks associated with Big Data management. However, to overcome security and privacy issues, blockchain provides a cryptographic mechanism. This will ensure an efficient data management system, which saves the life of patients without delay in treatment.

8.4.2 MEDICAL PROFESSIONALS

Electronic Health Record (EHR) is defined [16] as

> Computerized medical records relating to patients' physical and mental health. The data in the record can be of past, present and future data stored in an electronic system which captures, transmits, receives, stores, retrieves, links and manipulates multimedia data for the purpose of providing effective healthcare and health related services.

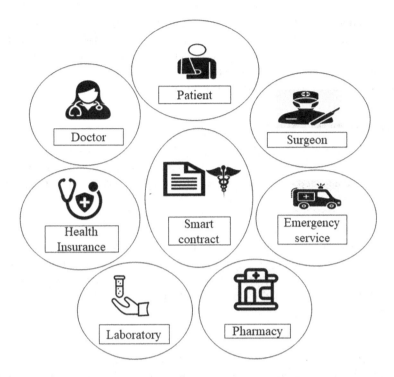

FIGURE 8.2   Various medical professionals connected with smart contracts.

The authors [17] mentioned that there are three parties involved in database man-agement, namely patients, medical institutions and third-party agencies such as insurance companies. Medical institutions create and keep the data, which is owned by patients. These processes are controlled and monitored through BCT with the support of IoMT and big data. So, the third-party agencies require permission from the patients and medical institutions, which has to be handled through smart contract using Ethereum [18]. Figure 8.2 depicts the various medi-cal professionals connected with smart contracts.

8.4.3   MEDICAL INSURANCE

The health insurance sector consists of stakeholders like insurance companies, beneficiaries, service providers, third-party administrators, intermediaries, rein-surers, Insure Techs, start-ups, diagnostics, pharmacies, government regulatory agencies and government. Interaction among these stakeholders may take place in a network and related information can be stored in servers, in the form of EHR or scanned copy of the handwritten prescriptions. Initiatives have been taken to convert the manual processes into digital mode, which facilitated underwrit-ing records, claim records and medical records to be managed in cloud systems with the involvement of third parties. However, to ensure the smooth flow of information to avoid delay in treatment and further processes, there is a requirement for a decentralized distributed ledger to establish transparent and participatory workflows. Smart contract implementation will facilitate self-enforced mechanisms to automatically execute an order to claim the insurance based on the execution of a predefined health framework [19].

8.4.4 AMBULANCE SERVICES

In a medical emergency, on-time delivery of services in the healthcare industry might solve the problem of life-or-death scenarios. In case of emergencies, since patients are connected through smart contracts, they can send a request to hospitals for required services. Since it is connected through smart contracts, the request of the patients can be sent to nearby hospitals and based on the queue the hospital can accept or reject the request. Once the hospital accepts the request, the patient has to provide the public key through the hospital to access the patient's EHR and instruct the smart ambulance to start the treatment. Various check mechanisms can be ensured through smart contracts, which will bind the smart ambulance and hospitals morally and ethically to maintain their integrity and trust.

8.4.5 TRACKING OF MEDICINES

Counterfeit drugs are a serious threat to the industry, society and economy. The authors [20] expressed that developing countries' exposure to spurious drugs is approximately 30%, leading to the loss of life of patients. Considering the huge loss to all spheres of the economy, there is a requirement to build a system to overcome this huge loss. The stakeholders involved in healthcare products especially medicine-based supply chain are manufacturer, Food and Drug Administration (FDA), distributor, pharmacy and patient. To make the distribution very effective with the enhanced traceability, smart contracts and Interplanetary File system (IFPS) can be added [20]. It also has the mechanism to upload the specifications and images of the medicine to facilitate the authenticity and identity of the medicine along with its manufacturers.

8.4.6 CLINICAL LABORATORY

Clinical lab results of patients form the major source of raw data that routes the medical practitioners to identify and diagnose their health conditions. Security and privacy of these data is the primary concern. At the same time, the data should be available as and when required by different stakeholders. Considering these requirements, the amalgam of IoMT, big data and blockchain might facilitate the creation and management of data from laboratories. There are different kinds of blockchain platforms like Ethereum, Ripple and Hyperledger already in use. Each of them is unique in terms of consensus mechanism and protocol [21]. Table 8.1 summarizes the discussions presented in this section. Based on the earlier discussion, the steps involved in developing a blockchain-based database management system are listed below:

TABLE 8.1

Stakeholders in Healthcare Data Management of IoT Devices using Blockchain

Stakeholders	Applications
Patient	RPM embedded with IoT and Blockchain will facilitate better connectivity among the medical devices, medical practitioners and patients.
Medical professionals	IoT along with Blockchain will not only enhance the accessibility but also retains privacy aspects of the medical records by allowing only the medical institutions and related third parties such as insurance companies to be privy to the EHR.
Medical insurance	Insurance companies, beneficiaries, service providers, third-party administrators, intermediaries, reinsurers, Insure Techs, diagnostics, pharmacies, government and its regulatory wing can be connected through smart contract to facilitate self-enforced mechanisms. This will automatically initiate an order to claim the insurance based on the execution of a predefined healthcare framework.
Ambulance services	Smart contract can be established between patients with IoMT devices and smart ambulance in case of emergency.
Tracking of medicines	Smart contracts and IFPS can be put into place to have control among manufacturers, FDA, distributor, pharmacy and patient to overcome counterfeit drugs.
Clinical laboratory	Security and privacy of clinical lab results can be retained with the amalgam of IoMT, big data and blockchain.

Step 1: Initiate the interaction between a patient, medical practitioners and service providers through the creation of data, namely medical history, present status and other health-related updates.

Step 2: Create a patient's EHR. It consists of lab records, scan details (medical images), nursing details, drugs prescribed and medical history.

Step 3: Assign the ownership of EHR to the patients since it involves highly sensitive content.

Step 4: Provide authenticated access to medical service providers.

Step 5: Link the patients' EHR with blockchain and store the same in the cloud.

Step 6: Facilitate additional access to the users via electronic gadgets with the distributed ledger mechanism.

8.5 DECENTRALIZED MANAGEMENT OF IOT DEVICES

The IoMT is nothing but medical devices that are connected through the internet globally. It helps to manage the stakeholders in the decentralized environment in the form of preventive healthcare, care from home, intensive healthcare, diagnostic healthcare, rehabilitation healthcare, therapeutic healthcare, chronicle healthcare and clinical trials.

8.5.1 PREVENTIVE HEALTHCARE

Preventive healthcare facilitates healthier practices like nutritional diet and mental and physical fitness leading to a better lifestyle for wellbeing. The advent of wearable devices and implantable devices has a great role in preventive healthcare. As per the study conducted by WHO (2003), there were 75% adult patients who were not adhering to the prescriptions and not following the doctor's suggestions properly in terms of medicines, diet and exercise. Blockchain combined with IoT will not only help patients to be on track but also the healthy patients to track their performance.

8.5.2 CARE FROM HOME

Traditional healthcare systems have undergone massive transformation with the help of IoT by providing nursing and caretaker services at home. Monitoring patients' health behaviour is made simple at the doorstep with the introduction of IoMT devices. However, privacy, safety and security of personal data on patient's improvement are a matter of concern, which can be resolved with the introduction of the blockchain mechanism. Various sensor devices are connected to smartphones which in turn store the data in a distributed ledger that can be connected to various stakeholders with patient authorization [22].

8.5.3 INTENSIVE CARE

Recently, a variety of IoMT healthcare monitoring systems are proposed to increase the performance of intensive care units with less human support. Wearable or environmental embedded IoMT interconnected devices gather an ICU patient's electrophysiological parameters. Gathered parameters can be sent to the monitoring system, which consists of a ubiquitous environment that initiates proactive and immediate treatment. Since it is decentralized, after identifying an emergency situation, it alerts the doctors, pharmacist, ambulance, etc. It also avoids human errors, provides fast communication and helps doctors to make the right decision with error-free information.

8.5.4 DIAGNOSTIC HEALTHCARE

Recent technologies of IoMT are a wearable diagnostic digestive system that finds glucose, salt and alcohol levels from the intake diets. Also, it assesses heartbeat rate and measures the stress level to make it available through the diagnostic information without any persistent tests in clinical settings. These technologies monitor the patient regularly and warn/alerts by forecasting the health issue.

Tracking the drug effectiveness, monitoring the quality of sleep and reminding the refill of medicine are examples of diagnostic healthcare.

8.5.5 REHABILITATION HEALTHCARE

Rehabilitation procedure requires that the doctor and patient work out a detailed course of therapeutic plan that spans over a considerable period of time and is divided into three phases, namely evaluation, intervention and results. Evaluation is a detailed assessment of the patient's case, current health condition and his/her profile. In the intervention stage, the therapist/doctor works alongside the patient in the rehabilitation centre. Assessing the progress made by the patient and deciding whether to further the treatment or end the treatment is done in the result stage. In all these phases, IoMT now plays a decisive role. In the evaluation phase, IoMT is used for diagnosis, and in the intervention phase, it is applied to monitor the bodily changes of the patient while exercising or doing the required activities. In the results stage, IoMT aids in tracking the achievement of the patient in the previously laid therapeutic plan. By adopting IoMT, the complete rehabilitation process can be carried out remotely in the comforts of the patient's home in addition to speeding up the whole process.

8.5.6 CHRONICLE HEALTHCARE

Chronic diseases are not curable and patients have to live with them throughout their life. Chronicle healthcare patients require continuous monitoring, mental and dietary counselling, to avoid escalation of the disease, which may prove fatal. IoMT devices such as blood sugar level monitoring, body weight, bone strength monitoring and electrolyte concentration helps diabetic and arthritis patients to continuously monitor for any anomaly. Ingestible pills help in monitoring medicinal intake by Alzheimer or bipolar disorder patients. Wearable and app-based devices with diet counselling for various chronic illnesses linked with vital parameters will prevent several critical situations. Support group help, counselling, success stories through shared apps, community-based links with medical and pharma support available for chronic conditions are possible through decentralized IoMT.

8.5.7 CLINICAL TRIALS

Clinical trials involve the testing of drugs/vaccines, medical devices, medical and surgical procedures primarily on small voluntary groups, followed by larger groups. The main aim is to test the scientific validity and ability to reproduce the results. This involves huge costs and longer time periods. IoMT will remove both the disabilities, by expediting the time and better monitoring as large data can be collected through IoMT for quality analysis. The use of AI and machine learning/deep learning will reduce the analysis time of huge data collected. Sharing of data on severe after-effects of drugs, effects with co-morbidities can be done more effectively through the IoMT network. Cloud storage will reduce data storage issues and blockchain technology will make the data stored and secured.

8.6 PERFORMANCE EVALUATION

In recent years, there are many notable technologies proposed by researchers and developers. There is a big challenge to benchmark the performance of technologies with suitable metrics. Specifically, in multilayered computing paradigms like Cloud, Fog and Edge, IoMT architectures are not having standard metrics to evaluate. The author [23] has given the summary of computing characteristics with performance metrics of Cloud, Fog and Edge computing. The comparison says that edge computing has a better result than cloud computing and fog computing. The authors [24] identified a set of common metrics for multi-layered architecture and elaborated on the measurable metrics with respect to each computing layer and common metrics for all layers. Based on the computing characteristics and requirements, healthcare system developers can choose any combination of computing paradigms to provide better security, smart analysis, and interdevice communication.

8.7 RECENT BLOCKCHAIN TECHNOLOGIES IN HEALTHCARE

In recent years, many applications have been developed in the healthcare industry. RPM is one such application where the IoT devices are deployed in the patient body or in the form of wearable devices. The sensed data is sent to the remote server via network, stored in the cloud and accessible only by the respective healthcare providers. The advancement in information technology and BCT made a great transformation in healthcare research and industry. The blockchain-based healthcare applications allow the stakeholders like patients, doctors, hospitals and diagnostic centres, to share and access patient information as an EHR in a safe and secure way. As mentioned in Section 8.3, the decentralized IoMT architecture that is based on BCT consists of three layers. This section discusses the recent technologies with respect to layers, namely Perception layer (Healthcare IoT devices), Network layer (Edge Computing, Fog Computing and Cloud Computing) and Blockchain layer (Data encryption). Figure 8.3 shows the hierarchical view of recent blockchain technologies in healthcare.

8.7.1 HEALTHCARE IoMT DEVICES

Different types of IoT sensors are used in RPM, especially the portable healthcare IoT devices that upgraded the quality of healthcare systems by providing data to analyse the patient's health condition. Generally, smartphones, wearable sensors and health monitors at hospitals are used as IoMT devices. Earlier, temperature sensors, ECG sensors and blood pressure sensors were used commonly to monitor the condition of healthy patients. Nowadays, advanced sensors such

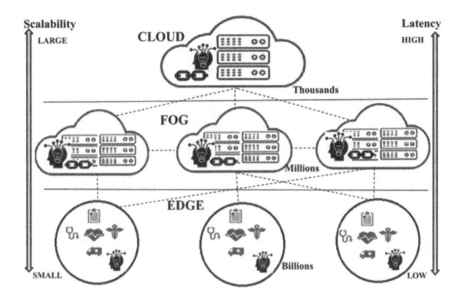

FIGURE 8.3   Hierarchical view of recent blockchain technologies in healthcare.

as spirometer, glucometer, pulse meter and airflow are used to monitor critical bedridden patients [25]. The sensed information is transmitted to data stores through network communication devices such as Wi-Fi, wireless sensor network and Bluetooth. These devices are responsible for the routing mechanism and network gateway.

8.7.2   CLOUD COMPUTING

Cloud computing is one of the key technologies in the healthcare industry that has configurable computing resources such as servers, applications, networks, storage and services. It provides cost-effective and efficient services all around the world. Healthcare systems are introduced to collect, transmit, store and analyse data retrieved from the patients' IoT healthcare devices [26]. Cloud computing allows stakeholders to access the patients' health records from various sources and process the details in real time via the Internet. An increase in the number of devices leads the entire system to suffer from issues like latency, computing power, shortage of bandwidth and slow response.

8.7.3   FOG COMPUTING

Fog computing extends the cloud computing services to the IoMT network and provides mobility support, low latency and location awareness features, which are more important in most of the healthcare systems. It provides a greater user experience with low latency and improved quality of services since it hosts most of the cloud services at the network edge [27]. It is a greater gift for real-time big data analytics.

8.7.4 EDGE COMPUTING

There is a big challenge in collecting different patient health data using heterogeneous IoMT devices from various networks and transmitting the sensed data to the server without any fault like missing and corruption of data. Edge computing collects the data from IoMT devices and processes the data in a distributive way in real time at the edge of the network which leads the system to respond more faster. In edge computing, each device acts as a server; this benefits most of the computing process being taken care of by the edge itself. Perhaps, it challenges the hackers to access thousands of distributive devices, which are not practically possible [28]. Edge computing made it possible to serve the urgent medical request since most of the computing happens at the edge level.

8.7.5 ARTIFICIAL INTELLIGENCE

AI empowers the implementation of the healthcare system to solve complex real-time problems. Both IoMT and AI need each other to enhance the solution from millions of sensed data and to understand patterns like humans. The deployment of AI software embedded in IoMT with edge and fog computing solutions brings intelligence to the entire healthcare system. AI can be deployed in different levels as edge, fog and cloud layers in the healthcare system. HealthFog uses an ensemble of deep learning in the fog layer to diagnose heart diseases [29].

8.7.6 DATA ENCRYPTION

In recent days, there is a tremendous increase in usage of devices and technologies in the IoMT healthcare system. So, there is a need to emphasize on security and privacy of the data and network. In order to secure data, in blockchain-based IoMT healthcare systems, the encryption happens in two layers, namely network layer for data transmission and blockchain layer for data security [30,31]. The healthcare system architecture follows different security mechanisms in each layer to prevent the attack on EHR. To provide privacy and security [15] proposed a novel structure for distributed IoT devices using sophisticated cryptographic primitives like symmetric and asymmetric encryption.

8.8 CHALLENGES IN DECENTRALIZED MANAGEMENT OF IOMT DEVICES IN HEALTHCARE

The healthcare sector is struggling to embrace and tap the unlimited potential offered by decentralized management of IoMT due to a lot of inherent and practical challenges. These challenges are divided into two categories, namely challenges in IoMT and challenges in decentralized management in IoMT, which are discussed below.

8.8.1 CHALLENGES IN IoMT

Challenges in IoMT are significantly related to the security aspects of the medical devices involved.

8.8.1.1 Device Vulnerability

IoMT includes radio frequency identification (RFID) tags, implantable medical devices (IMDs) and wearable devices that are prone to security risks. Security challenges in RFID tags can be by way of electromagnetic interference and wireless attacks. IMDs are exposed to security risks such as radio attack, power denial attack, authentication issues, prohibited traffic monitoring, device cloning issue, problems in firmware updates and tampering issues. Wearable external devices face the risk of hijacking and third-party intrusion. All these can lead to a serious security issue that causes sufferings to patients and healthcare providers since privacy is breached and also paves way for trust concerns. Thus, there is a serious challenge to find a solid protection against such active and passive attacks.

8.8.1.2 Energy Challenges

IoMT includes small medical gadgets that run on restricted battery power. These gadgets get on to the power saving mode when there is no need for sensor observations and execute their function at low speed of CPU when the function to be performed is not crucial. These features pose a challenge of finding an energy aware protection solution.

8.8.1.3 Security Update Challenge

Security protocols need to be regularly updated to mitigate the high-risk vulnerabilities and this can be achieved by maintaining the devices' protection patches up-to-date. In this regard, the underlying major challenge is to develop a method that aids speedy updating of protection systems.

8.8.1.4 Heterogeneity of Devices

The devices used in healthcare are of different varieties with different networks, computing capabilities, inbuilt memory, embedded software and energy consumption. Hence, there exists a challenge of structuring a customized protection of these devices.

8.8.1.5 Challenge of Scalability

With the advancement in technology, the number of new medical devices flooding the healthcare space is huge. When these devices get connected to the internet, it becomes a humongous task resulting in scalability challenges.

8.8.1.6 Limited In-built Memory

Most of the medical devices are with limited in-built memory, which requires these devices to be enabled through system software. This memory limitation may hinder the device from taking the load of complex protocols. These devices have limited computational abilities and usually operate as a sensor as well as actuator. Finding a solution to limit the usage of memory turns out to be a daunting task.

8.8.1.7 Challenges of Accuracy

Accuracy concerns arise due to the malfunctioning of the device. Inaccuracy and lack of precision may be due to the malfunctioning of the medical robots, false diagnosis and incorrect medical prescriptions. Such malfunctions in medical devices turn out to be very costly since they might result in partial or permanent injury to the patients and in extreme cases might end up in loss of life.

8.8.1.8 Challenge of Standardization

Medical devices need to adhere to standardization since these devices need to operate in sync with the IoT technology. As such, if the devices are not standardized, it will be difficult to standardize the security measures that will prevent the devices from getting hacked.

8.8.2 Challenges in Decentralized Management of IoMT

Some of the challenges that arise due to the implementation of a decentralized management system using IoMT are given below.

8.8.2.1 Challenges in Cyber Security

Open wireless networks always pose a threat to security of data and this threat gets transmitted to IoMT devices that rely heavily on these networks. However, healthcare data needs to be vehemently protected since it is a sensitive matter that relates to life and death of the patient. Thus, protection from cybercrimes such as data theft, hacking and tampering turns out to be a serious challenge, which is eased out through the decentralized management system. However, a decentralized management system is not fool proof. The involvement of many IoMT devices and their spread might breach the protocol and expose the identity of the patients, thus threatening privacy and security.

8.8.2.2 Challenge of Scalability

The data storage capabilities at the healthcare facilities will be fiercely challenged in the case of decentralized management systems since it stores a complete ledger in each of the network's nodes. The number of information blocks generated will be huge in addition to the increased number of nodes. There is a lower latency which is an advantage, but there is a compromise on throughput rate.

8.8.2.3   Challenge of Investment

Currently available facilities in IoMT lack computational power to handle the encryption algorithms with the necessary capacity, time and speed. As such, huge investment is required by the healthcare providers for installing the computational facilities in decentralized mechanisms. Nevertheless, there are major costs involved in terms of deployment and maintenance when the healthcare provider shifts his existing system to the decentralized-based system.

8.8.2.4   Regulatory Challenges

Decentralized mechanisms such as blockchain lack legal or compliance code as they are designed to be compliance with laws such as Health Information Technology for Economic and Clinical Health Act (HITECH) (HHS.gov U.S. Department of Health & Human Services, 2009), General Data Protection Regulation (GDPR) [32] and Personal Data Protection (PDP) Bill [33] depending upon the region to which the healthcare provider belongs. Since different types of connections are established with the blockchain (decentralized) application and economic, social and healthcare systems, it turns out to be a challenge when there is a void in terms of legal or compliance code to be followed, especially in the healthcare domain.

8.8.2.5   Challenge of Infrastructure

The healthcare infrastructure needs to be robust in terms of socio-technical alignments to withstand the complexities of adapting decentralized mechanisms (blockchain) across the country.

8.8.2.6   User Challenges

The lack of expertise in using and operating the IoMT devices is yet another challenge since the healthcare sector faces a lack of trust among the patients and other communities.

8.8.2.7   Challenge of Immutability

Audit trail records of the decentralized system are immutable and as such provide the much-needed data protection and trust. But this immutability stands challenged and destroys the trust factor in case false information is fed into the blockchain system that has a malicious intent.

8.9   CONCLUSION

Quality health facility is a top-notch factor for determining the standard of human life in a country. Advanced remote monitoring of a patient was made feasible with the help of IoMT, which has increased satisfaction of the patient and practitioner. There is a big leap in augmenting BCT in IoMT devices, which aims for safe, secure, transparent and guided medical assistance. This chapter discussed a decentralized IoMT architecture along with the BCT, which consists of three layers such as physical, communication and application layers. Different use cases on data management regarding patient, medical professional, medical insurance claims, ambulance service, tracking of medicines and clinical laboratory were deliberated. This study can be further directed by implementing a safe and secure healthcare system using advanced IoMT devices, blockchain technologies and SDN (Software Defined Networking) embedded strong computational layers aiming at better performance.

REFERENCES

1. Blockchain Technology in Healthcare Market share and industry growth revenue 2021: Regional overview latest technology, business status, top growing factors and market dynamics forecast to 2027 with impact of covid-19," MarketWatch, 06-May-2021. [Online]. Available: https://www.marketwatch.com/press-release/blockchain-technology-in-healthcare-market-share-and-industry-growth-revenue-2021-regional-overview-latest-technology-business-status-top-growing-factors-and-market-dynamics-forecast-to-2027-with-impact-of-covid-19-2021-05-06. (Accessed: 10-Jun-2021).

2. World Development Indicators, Worldbank.org. [Online]. Available: https://databank.worldbank.org/reports.aspx?source=2&series=SH.MED.PHYS.ZS&country=. (Accessed: 10-Jun–2021).

3. Touati, F., and R. Tabish. 2013. "U-healthcare system: state-of-the-art review and challenges." *Journal of Medical Systems* 37 (3). doi:10.1007/s10916-013-9949-0.

4. Cremer, D.d., B. Nguyen, and L. Simkin. 2017. "The integrity challenge of the Internet-of-Things (IoT): on understanding its dark side." *Journal of Marketing Management*. Routledge. doi:10.1080/0267257X.2016.1247517.

5. Explanation of 3V's Model of Big data Given by Doug Laney, *Cosoit.com*, 2021. [Online]. Available: https://www.cosoit.com/explanation-of-3v-model-of-big-data. (Accessed: 10- Jun-2021).

6. Oguntimilehin, A. 2014. "A Review of Big Data Management, Benefits and Challenges IT Governance View Project Students' Enrolment into Tertiary Institutions in Nigeria: the Influence of the Founder's Reputation-a Case Study View Project Ojo Ademola Institute of Enterprise Management and Analytic Journal of Emerging Trends in Computing and Information Sciences A Review of Big Data Management, Benefits and Challenges" 5 (6). http://www.cisjournal.org.

7. "Big Data: What it is and why it matters," What it is and why it matters I SAS India. [Online]. Available: https://www.sas.com/en_in/insights/big-data/what-is-big-data.html. (Accessed: 10-Jun-2021).

8. "Internet of Things [IoT] in healthcare Market Size & Trends, 2028." Fortune businessinsights.com, 2021. [Online]. Available: https://www.fortunebusinessinsights.com/internet-of-things-iot-in-healthcare-market-102188. (Accessed: 10- Jun-2021).

9. Van Oranje-Nassau. C., H.R. Schindler, A.M. Vilamovska, and M. Botterman. 2012. "Policy options for radio frequency identification (RFID) application in healthcare; a prospective view: final report (D5)." *Rand Health Quarterly* 1(4):5.

10. Jara, A.J., M.A. Zamora-Izquierdo, and A.F. Skarmeta. 2013. "Interconnection framework for MHealth and remote monitoring based on the Internet of Things." *IEEE Journal on Selected Areas in Communications* 31 (9). Institute of Electrical and Electronics Engineers Inc.: 47–65. doi:10.1109/JSAC.2013.SUP.0513005.

11. Dai, H.-N., M. Imran, and N. Haider. 2020. "Blockchain-enabled Internet of Medical Things to combat COVID-19." August. http://arxiv.org/abs/2008.09933.

12. Rao, M v, D. Thota, and P. Srinivas. 2014. "A study to assess patient safety culture amongst a category of hospital staff of a teaching hospital." *IOSR Journal of Dental and Medical Sciences (IOSR-JDMS) e-ISSN* 13. www.iosrjournals.orgwww.iosrjournals.org.

13. Saxena, S., B. Bhushan, and M.A. Ahad, 2021, "Blockchain based solutions to secure IoT: Background, integration trends and a way forward." *Journal of Network and Computer Applications*, doi: 10.1016/j.jnca.2021.103050.

14. Lee, J., D. Kim, H.Y. Ryoo, and B.S. Shin. 2016. "Sustainable wearables: wearable technology for enhancing the quality of human life." *Sustainability (Switzerland)* 8 (5). MDPI AG. doi:10.3390/su8050466.

15. Dwivedi, A.D., G. Srivastava, S. Dhar, and R. Singh. 2019. "A decentralized privacy-preserving healthcare blockchain for IoT." *Sensors (Switzerland)* 19 (2). MDPI AG. doi:10.3390/s19020326.

16. Murphy, G. F., and Waters, K. A., 1999. EHR vision, definition, and characteristics, in *Electronic Health Records: Changing the Vision*, eds. Murphy, G. F., Hanken, M.A., and Waters, K. A., W.B. Saunders Company, Philadelphia, PA.

17. Chen, Y., S. Ding, Z. Xu, H. Zheng, and S. Yang. 2018. "Blockchain-based medical records secure storage and medical service framework." *Journal of Medical Systems* 43 (1). Springer New York LLC. doi:10.1007/s10916-018-1121-4.

18. A. Kumar, K. Abhishek, B. Bhushan, and C. Chakraborty, 2021, "Secure access control for manufacturing sector with application of ethereum blockchain." *Peer Peer Network*. Application. doi: 10.1007/s12083-021-01108-3.

19. PWC and FICCI, Federation of Indian Chambers of Commerce and Industry, 2021. "Revamping India's health insurance sector with blockchain and smart contracts." 2021. Pricewater house Coopers Pvt Ltd, New Delhi, India.

20. Musamih, A., K. Salah, R. Jayaraman, J. Arshad, M. Debe, Y. Al-Hammadi, and S. Ellahham. 2021. "A blockchain-based approach for drug traceability in healthcare supply chain." *IEEE Access* 9. Institute of Electrical and Electronics Engineers Inc.: 9728–43. doi:10.1109/ACCESS.2021.3049920.

21. Khezr, S., M. Moniruzzaman, A. Yassine, and R. Benlamri. 2019. "Blockchain technology in healthcare: a comprehensive review and directions for future research." *Applied Sciences (Switzerland)* 9 (9). MDPI AG. doi:10.3390/app9091736.

22. Jeong, S., J.H. Shen, and B. Ahn. 2021. "A study on smart healthcare monitoring using IoT based on blockchain." *Wireless Communications and Mobile Computing* 2021. Hindawi Limited. doi:10.1155/2021/9932091.

23. El-Sayed, H., S. Sankar, M. Prasad, D. Puthal, A. Gupta, M. Mohanty, and C.T. Lin. 2017. "Edge of things: the big picture on the integration of edge, IoT and the cloud in a distributed computing environment." *IEEE Access* 6 (December). Institute of Electrical and Electronics Engineers Inc.: 1706–17. doi:10.1109/ACCESS.2017.2780087.

24. Aslanpour, S. S. Gill, and A. N. Toosi, 2020, "Performance evaluation metrics for cloud, fog and edge computing: a review, taxonomy, benchmarks and standards for future research." *Internet of Things* 12. doi:10.1016/j.iot.2020.100273.

25. Jamil, F., S. Ahmad, N. Iqbal, and D.H. Kim. 2020. "Towards a remote monitoring of patient vital signs based on IoT-based blockchain integrity management platforms in smart hospitals." *Sensors (Switzerland)* 20 (8). MDPI AG. doi:10.3390/s20082195.

26. Dimitrov, D.v. 2019. "Blockchain applications for healthcare data management." *Healthcare Informatics Research* 25 (1). Korean Society of Medical Informatics: 51–56. doi:10.4258/hir.2019.25.1.51.

27. Sun, L., L. Sun, X. Jiang, H. Ren, H. Ren, and Y. Guo. 2020. "Edge-cloud computing and Artificial Intelligence in internet of medical things: architecture, technology and application." *IEEE Access* 8. Institute of Electrical and Electronics Engineers Inc.: 101079–92. doi:10.1109/ACCESS.2020.2997831.

28. Hartmann, M., U.S. Hashmi, and A. Imran. 2019. "Edge computing in smart health care systems: review, challenges, and research directions." *Transactions on Emerging Telecommunications Technologies*. Wiley Blackwell. doi:10.1002/ett.3710.

29. Tuli, S., N. Basumatary, S.S. Gill, M. Kahani, R.C. Arya, G.S. Wander, and R. Buyya. n.d. "HealthFog: an ensemble deep learning based smart healthcare system for automatic diagnosis of heart diseases in integrated IoT and fog computing environments." 104: 187–200. doi:10.1016/j.future.2019.10.043.

30. Bhushan, B. C. Sahoo, P. Sinha, and A. Khamparia, 2021, "Unification of blockchain and Internet of Things (BIoT): requirements, working model, challenges and future directions," *Wireless Network*, doi:10.1007/s11276-020-02445-6.

31. Bushan, B. P. Sinha, K.M. Sagayam, and J. Andrew, 2020, "Untangling blockchain technology: a survey on state of the art, security threats, privacy services, applications and future research directions," *Computer and Electrical Engineering*, doi: 10.1016/j.compeleceng.2020.106897.

32. Tikkinen-Piri, C., A. Rohunen, and J. Markkula. 2018. "EU general data protection regulation: changes and implications for personal data collecting companies." *Computer Law and Security Review* 34 (1). Elsevier Ltd: 134–53. doi:10.1016/j.clsr.2017.05.015.

33. Prasad, D.M., and S.C. Menon. 2020. "The personal data protection bill, 2018: India's regulatory journey towards a comprehensive data protection law." *International Journal of Law and Information Technology* 28 (1). Oxford University Press: 1–19. doi:10.1093/ijlit/eaaa003.

9 Introduction to Blockchain and Smart Contract – Principles, Applications, and Security

Adarsh Singh, Ananya Smirti, and Raghav Gupta
Manipal University Jaipur

Chamitha de Alwis
University of Sri Jayewardenepura

Anshuman Kalla
University of Oulu

CONTENTS

DOI: 10.1201/9781003224075-9

9.1   INTRODUCTION

The last couple of years have witnessed a tremendous increase in the popularity of blockchain technology. The first most popular use case of blockchain technology is *Bitcoin* (cryptocurrency), which came into existence in the year 2008. Since then, researchers, developers, and practitioners have realized the potential of blockchain technology and have leveraged it for numerous other applications in various sectors such as healthcare, supply chain management, e-voting, energy management, education, and telecommunications. Blockchain has emerged as a decentralized, distributed, and secure technology to store records of transactions and digital assets of values. Blockchain is created by connecting computing and storing machines called nodes in a Peer-to-Peer (P2P) fashion, making exhaustive use of cryptographic mechanisms and running consensus algorithm(s) at all the nodes. Indeed, blockchain is a type of Distributed Ledger Technology (DLT) that essentially replicates the database at all the nodes in the underlying P2P network. Moreover, the use of cryptographic techniques and decentralized decision-making make the blockchain a very promising technology.

A brief history of blockchain technology is as follows. Bitcoin, the most famous use case of blockchain, was introduced by a group or individual under the pseudonym Satoshi Nakamoto in 2008. The pseudonym published a white paper focusing on a peer-to-peer electronic cash system [1]. The main aim of the paper was to provide a solution to the double-spending problem in a decentralized trustless environment. This electronic cash system gave birth to bitcoin cryptocurrency. However, the underlying technologies and concepts such as Merkel tree, hashing, digital signature, P2P networking, and distributed storage existed much before the advent of bitcoin (and the blockchain as underlying technology). For instance, Ralph Merkle introduced the idea of a Merkle tree or hash tree in the year 1979 [2]. Stornetta and Haber introduced a system that aims to digitally timestamp electronic documents in the year 1991 [3]. The concept of a smart contract was proposed by Nick Szabo in the year 1994 [4]. Thus, Satoshi profitably combined these existing technologies and concepts to reiterate the meaning of blockchain technology.

The rest of the chapter is organized as follows. Section 9.2 presents the fundamentals of blockchain, generic block structure, the process flow of transactions, salient features of blockchain, and types of blockchain. Smart contract, its features, and different platforms that support smart contracts are discussed in Section 9.3. A wide range of applications of blockchain and smart contracts are discussed in a nutshell in Section 9.4. Various security attacks on blockchain and smart contracts are briefly presented in Section 9.5. Finally, Section 9.6 concludes the chapter.

9.2   BLOCKCHAIN

To begin with, let us try to understand what blockchain is, how it operates, and what are its salient features. In simple words, blockchain is the most popular type of DLT where all the records of transactions and data (of value) are stored, shared, and synchronized across all the nodes of a P2P network [5]. This collection of records or database is called a *digital ledger*. The nodes in the P2P network are the participating machines that dedicate their computing and storage capacities to establish and maintain blockchain facility. Moreover, since the digital ledger in the blockchain is shared; thus, it is replicated at all the nodes resulting in a distributed ledger. This implies that all the nodes in the P2P blockchain network have the exact copies of the entire database (i.e., digital ledger) stored locally. Any legitimate update in the ledger, performed by any node, is broadcasted so that each node is synchronized in terms of the current state of the distributed digital ledger.

What distinguishes blockchain from other types of DLTs is the data structure that it uses for the distributed ledger. From the data structure point-of-view, blockchain is a linked list of records (aka blocks) connected in chronological order [6]. Every record or block bundles together (using cryptographic techniques) a set of valid transactions that occur in a time window. Moreover, every block stores a pointer (i.e., hash value) of the previous block. After expiration of a given time window, a new block is created and is logically connected with the previous block using a cryptographic hash-based chain. Thus, the technology is called "*blockchain*". As time goes, more blocks are created, timestamped, and appended to the existing blockchain. Thus, the size of blockchain grows with time, and new blocks are added in exclusively append mode. It is worth noting that blockchain exhaustively uses cryptographic techniques to keep the ledger (i.e., database) secure since it is kept at various (untrusted) nodes in the P2P network. Furthermore, a consensus algorithm is required to establish agreement among the nodes for every update to be performed in a blockchain.

9.2.1 BLOCK STRUCTURE

Now, it is time to learn what is the structure of a block in a blockchain. A block is simply a container that is used to store a set of valid transactions and data. Although a typical structure of a block can vary depending on the needs, platforms, and applications, to understand the basic ideas, we discuss the structure of a block in the bitcoin blockchain. Conceptually, a block is divided into two parts; block header and block body. The structure of the bitcoin block header has six fields with a total size of 80 bytes [1]. The body of the block is of variable size and stores a set of transactions along with the transaction counter. Moreover, on average, a bitcoin transaction has a size of at least 250 bytes with an average transaction size of 500 bytes [7,8]. Furthermore, the number of bitcoin transactions per block is usually more than 500, with an average of 2,000 transactions per block [7,8]. The first block of any blockchain is named genesis block, and it has no previous/parent block to point. Figure 9.1 shows the structure of a block.

9.2.1.1 Block Header

A brief description of the six fields in the bitcoin block header is given in Table 9.1. The version field is basically to track the blockchain (software) upgrades. The timestamp field registers the Unix epoch time when a miner starts mining a new block. To connect each block with its previous block, the *"previous block hash"*

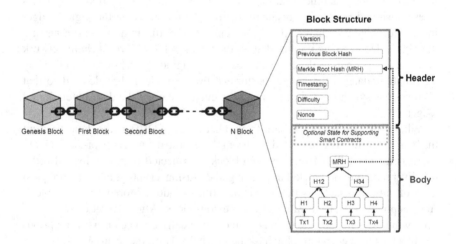

FIGURE 9.1   Block structure.

TABLE 9.1
Fields of Block Header in Blockchain [12]

Field	Size of the Field	Data Type	Brief Description
Version	4 bytes	Int32	Indicates the set of validation rules to be followed for the current block.
Timestamp	4 bytes	Unit32	Stores the Unix epoch (number of seconds passed since 1970-01-01 00:00:00 UTC [13]) at the start of the mining process by a miner.
Previous block hash	32 bytes	Char	Stores double SHA-256 hash of previous block such that all the blocks are logically chained together.
Difficulty/nBits	4 bytes	Unit32	Encoded version of target threshold.
Nonce	4 bytes	Unit32	An arbitrary number added by a miner to block header so that when the block hash is computed, the obtained value is less than or equal to the target threshold.
Merkle Root	32 bytes	Char	Contains the final (root) hash value that is obtained by using Merkle tree hashing. In this tree, all the leaf nodes are basically the hash values of all the transactions in the current block.

field is used. This field is of 32 bytes and stores the cryptographic hash (usually SHA256 hash [9]) of the previous block.

The field nbits is simply an encoded and compact representation of the target hash value (a 256-bit number) to mine a new block [10]. The nonce is a field that the mining nodes keep changing to compute the hash value of the current block header such that the obtained value is less than equal to the target value. In other words, a miner keeps hashing the block header by trying random numbers for the nonce field and stops when the block hash value is less than equal to the target value. The target hash value is set according to the current difficulty level [10].

The *difficulty* is basically a relative level of computation (work) required to find an acceptable block hash value for mining a new block. The difficulty for genesis block is considered to be 1. If the current level of difficulty is 2, then this implies that the computational effort required to mine a new block is twice the computation required for mining the genesis block.

After mining a set of 2016 blocks, the difficulty is recomputed, which then sets the target value, and accordingly, the value of nbits field is decided. The reason behind varying the difficulty level is to ensure the inter-block mining time stays approximately constant, i.e., 10 minutes in bitcoin [11]. It is worth pointing out that the above explanation assumes the use of the Proof-of-Work (PoW) consensus algorithm.

To compute the value of the Merkle Root field, cryptographic hashes of all the transactions in the current block are taken as the leaf nodes of the Merkle tree. The non-leaf nodes are then computed by hashing the concatenated (hash) values of the child nodes. In the case of the binary Merkle tree, every non-leaf node has two child nodes. The process of computing the value of non-leaf nodes is continued till the root hash value is obtained. Thus, the Merkle root hash field provides a way to compactly represent (i.e., fixed-size bits) all the transactions in the current block. This field allows any entity to verify the legitimacy of the transactions bundled in a given block [14].

9.2.1.2 Block Body

The block body contains a finite set of valid transactions, which need to be confirmed on the blockchain. The body of a bitcoin block consists of transactions and the transaction counter. However, for other blockchains, the content of the body differs. For instance, in the Ethereum blockchain, the block body contains an additional part named state to enable the storage and execution of smart contracts [15]. The number of transactions in a block depends on the maximum allowed block size (e.g., 1 MB for bitcoin blockchain [7]) and the size of each transaction to be included in a block. Therefore, miners tend to select transactions with small sizes and high transaction fees from the transaction pool. In other words, miners aim to maximize their profits by accommodating as many transactions as possible in the new block. Here, the transaction fee is the amount promised by the transacting user to be paid to the miner who confirms his/her transaction on the blockchain by successfully mining a new block. In summary, the block body can contain transactions and smart contracts. Also, the size of the block body is variable in size because the number of transactions included in a block is not fixed.

9.2.2 Process Flow in Block Mining

The complete process of block creation is divided into several steps, as depicted in Figure 9.2. These steps require the involvement of multiple entities and mechanisms that are necessary for creating a new block. These are discussed below.

The first step is to initiate a transaction between two digital accounts belonging to Bob and Alice. A simple example of a transaction can be sending cryptocurrency (e.g., bitcoin) from one account to another account. Every account in blockchain has an associated pair of public and private keys. An account is identified using its address, which is simply an encrypted public key associated with that account. The users can access these addresses through their wallets, which are software applications used for creating and managing multiple addresses to perform transactions [16].

As shown in figure 9.2, Bob sends some cryptocurrency to Alice and uses his private key to digitally sign the transaction. Once the transaction is signed, it is broadcast to the directly connected nodes in the blockchain P2P network. Each node in the P2P network validates the transaction and forwards it to its peers (i.e., direct neighbours). Thus, the new transaction propagates throughout the P2P network [17]. Each mining node, a node empowered to create new blocks on the blockchain, maintains a temporary collection (Mem-pool [18]) of unconfirmed transactions. Subsequently, participating miners select the set of unconfirmed

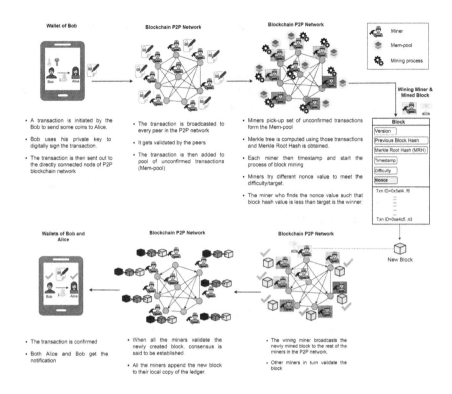

FIGURE 9.2   Flow of transaction and block mining.

transactions from their mem-pool. It is worth pointing out that some blockchains allow users to specify a transaction fee s/he is willing to pay to the miner who successfully processes the transaction. In such a case, miners often select unconfirmed transactions based on the transaction fee to maximize the profit. Next, every participating miner forms a Merkle tree of the selected transactions and eventually obtains a Merkle Root Hash [1]. Following this step, a new block can be mined. In order to mine a new block, a miner timestamps the block, fills the different fields in the block header, and adds the transactions to the block body. The miner then proceeds to compute the hash value of the block within the predefined difficulty target (as discussed in Section 9.2.1). Block mining requires the miner to keep changing the nonce value in the block header until a block hash value is obtained, which satisfies the difficulty level and is less than or equal to the target (see Section 9.2.1). Such computation requires a lot of energy as the hashing block header is carried out in a brute force manner.

All the miners then compete with each other to calculate the block hash value before others. The miner who successfully finds the hash value at the earliest is the winning miner [19]. This winning miner then broadcasts the newly created block to the blockchain P2P network [17]. Each miner validates the newly created block by first verifying the transactions in the received block and then, using the nonce value in the header, recomputes the block hash to ensure compliance. If a majority of the miners approve the newly created block, a consensus is established, and the nodes then add the new block to their local copy of the blockchain. Likewise, the new block is appended to the blockchain while all the transactions in the new block are confirmed. Moreover, the winning miner then receives a reward for mining a new block to the blockchain.

9.2.3 FEATURES OF BLOCKCHAIN

Blockchain offers a multitude of features, as illustrated in Figure 9.3. These features include transparency, non-repudiation, decentralization, pseudonymity, immutability, availability, provenance, automation, auditability, fast processing, trust-building, and lower-OPEX.

9.2.3.1 Immutability

As discussed earlier, blockchain is an append-only database, wherein only new information (i.e., a new block containing transaction data and optionally smart contracts) can be added. However, altering or deleting any existing information is computationally infeasible, making blockchain immutable or tamperproof. Fundamentally, immutability results from the way blocks are created using

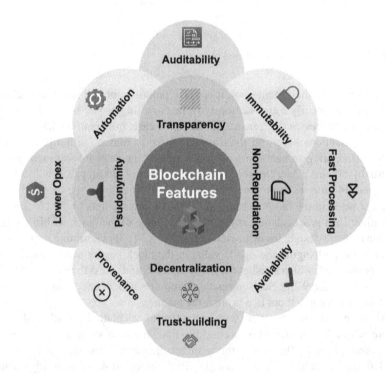

FIGURE 9.3 Blockchain features.

cryptographic techniques, chained together logically using a hash-based chain, and replicated at all the nodes in the P2P blockchain network using a consensus algorithm. Any slightest change in the data produces a different hash value. Thus, any change in a confirmed transaction within a block changes the hash value of that block. As the blockchain grows and the size of the P2P blockchain network increases, the data stored on the blocks become more difficult to alter. For example, if any data corresponding to the block number 100 is modified, then the hash of that block will change. Since the hash of a previous block connects the next block, any change in the block hash of the block number 100 will affect the hash of the subsequent blocks, i.e., 101, 102, so on till the most recent block. Such a cascading effect becomes evident in the blockchain network, making blockchain immutable [20].

9.2.3.2 Decentralization

The property implies that blockchain is not governed by a central authority. This is because every node in a P2P blockchain network has an equal right to participate in all operations, and thus, any node can add a new block to the existing distributed ledger [21]. As compared to traditional systems, decentralized architecture prevents any system from single point of failure. Centralized systems are prone to single point of failure, implying that any vulnerability can bring down a system completely or partially. Such a failure may lead to compromised data and compromised Identity and Access Management (IAM) functions [22]. Thanks to the decentralized and distributed P2P network (that collectively manages blockchain), even if one of the nodes is compromised, the other nodes in the network continue to operate and ensure the smooth working of the system. Decentralization also leads to disintermediation, i.e., all the intermediaries, which are usually present in a centralized system, are not required anymore in a blockchain-based system.

9.2.3.3 Transparency

Transparency has been one of the major issues of centralized systems wherein the details such as who is accessing the user's data and how the data is being processed are not available to the users. Moreover, the issue of transparency becomes even more important when there are multiple third parties in such centralized systems. Blockchain provides a solution to this problem by allowing the members of the P2P network to read the transactions, data, and other activities happening in the blockchainized system. Furthermore, depending on the type of blockchain (e.g., public or private) and the domain of application, the level of transparency can differ. For instance, in the case of a public permissionless blockchain, such as the bitcoin, the data is transparent and open to be read or queried by any user (i.e., no restriction at all). However, in the case of a permissioned blockchain, the data remains confidential and available only to the authenticated authority [23]. Nonetheless, once an entity is a member of the blockchainized system, everything present in the blockchain is transparent.

9.2.3.4 Pseudonymity

Blockchain allows its users to participate and play different roles without the need to disclose their real-life identities. This is made possible by assigning unique digital identity (ID) to every entity in the blockchainized system. Usually, a public–private key pair is uniquely generated for each entity, and the ID is somehow derived from public keys. In simple words, the ID is an encrypted public key where hashing is one of the processes involved in the encryption. Using such IDs does not reveal the real-life identities of the participating entities [21]. Nevertheless, it is worth noting that it is possible to trace the users back to their real identities if the system is not well designed or the users are not careful enough [24]. Thus, user's privacy is preserved as long as the transactions cannot be traced back to the users.

9.2.3.5 Non-repudiation

Non-repudiation implies that any entity cannot deny/refute any activity once performed and committed on the blockchain [25]. The goal of non-repudiation service is to generate, gather, and preserve the evidence of the performed digital activities so that later the false denials can be proved [26]. In the blockchain, cryptographic techniques such as asymmetric encryption and digital signature enable the realization of non-repudiation [27,28]. Every transaction is digitally signed by the sender before it is pushed to the blockchain platform. Thanks to the non-repudiation property of blockchain technology, neither a sender can deny what it has sent nor a receiver can deny what it has received [27].

9.2.3.6 Fast Processing

Usually, a traditional system comprises a centralized authority that may employ one or more third parties to run and manage all the operations and relevant data. This is basically required to build trust in the traditional system [29]. At times, there are multiple third parties that together make the system. For instance, a financial transaction may face several trusted intermediaries in the form of clearinghouses, depositories, and payment gateways [30]. The existence of such intermediaries inflates the operational/processing delay. Another example to illustrate the fast processing capability of blockchain is when it is used to enable 5G-IoT ecosystem [31]. In particular, empowering the edge and core network with blockchain can eliminate the need for the IoT messages to travel all the way to centralized systems like the cloud. Thus, blockchain, being decentralized and distributed technology, allows disintermediation of such third parties, which leads to fast processing.

9.2.3.7 Low Cost

Any transaction in a blockchain-based system can be carried out at the peer level without the need for trusted third parties. Usually, the trusted party charge some amount of fee for the services they provide. For instance, an international banking transaction using Society of Worldwide Interbank Financial Telecommunication (SWIFT) system may have to pass through many intermediary banks. Each of these banks charges some fee in addition to the SWIFT fee and exchange rate fee [32]. In a blockchain-based system, the third-party intermediaries are not present; thus, the overall cost is lower than traditional systems.

9.2.3.8 Provenance

Provenance is a way to provide the entire history of the data lifecycle, i.e., one can track back the various state changes or alterations that have happened from the current point to the inception [33]. In other words, data provenance, therefore, provides complete information on how the data were obtained, where they were kept, how it was utilized, and more. The provenance property well characterizes blockchain since the ledger is distributed over the P2P network, which is accessible to every node in the network. Provenance turns out to be a useful property of blockchain technology for areas such as supply chain management, land record registration, and jewellery trading [34].

9.2.3.9 Auditability

Every transaction on the blockchain is time-stamped and digitally signed using the private key of the user. This enables the network to validate each transaction [21]. Timestamp allows the nodes to trace previous records and document specific details about a transaction. This improves the transparency and security of the transactions [35].

9.2.3.10 Availability

Availability ideally means a given system should always be up and provide the required services to its users irrespective of any fault, issue, or ongoing attacks. This feature is available in blockchain due to its decentralization and distributed nature. Unlike a centralized system, any node in the decentralized blockchain system is equally capable of providing access to the distributed ledger. Moreover, availability applies to both system and transaction availability [36]. Here, the data of the block must be available to legitimate users on demand so they can view transaction data at any time and from any location without it being corrupted, inaccessible, or inconsistent [25,36].

9.2.3.11 Automation

Blockchain facilitates automation by using smart contracts, which are self-executing computer programs emulating the terms and conditions of an agreement. Automation forms the basis for developing decentralized applications (dApps) and increases the efficiency and the speed of transactions [37]. Moreover, automation in blockchain reduces human intervention, eliminates the need for third parties, and improves the operational efficiency of each sector dependent on blockchain [38].

9.2.4 Types of Blockchain

Three different types of blockchain are discussed in this section.

9.2.4.1   Public Blockchain

A public blockchain is an open, unrestricted, and permissionless distributed ledger system. In such an open network, the nodes have the authority to access all the records, add data on the blockchain, ability to verify transactions, and even be a part of the mining process [39]. Public blockchain utilizes the property of decentralization and accessibility to the fullest (though not completely [40], without any restrictions. The most common examples of public blockchain are Bitcoin and Ethereum.

The advantages of using public blockchain are highly transparent, trustless, open, and optimally decentralized [41]. Since everything is recorded and visible to everyone, public blockchain forms a trustless environment by eliminating the need for trusted third parties. Each entity in the network contributes to grow the blockchain and prevent the need for intermediaries. The extent of decentralization in a system implies the level of fault resiliency of the system. A fully decentralized system provides better security and fault resiliency as compared to centralized systems [42]. However, the downsides of public blockchains are energy inefficiency, less privacy due to high transparency, slow convergence, more prone to attacks, and highly unregulated, so not suitable for some applications [41].

9.2.4.2   Private Blockchain

A private blockchain is a closed, restricted, and permissioned blockchain, where the accessibility of the network is different for each node [43]. Most of the nodes in such a network have access to only specific rights, while some nodes can have full access to the network. Therefore, this type of blockchain is not entirely decentralized, as a part of the allowances is restricted to a central authority [44]. Examples of private blockchain are Corda and Hyperledger [45].

The advantages of the private blockchain (compared with public blockchain) are higher throughput, low latency, better privacy, and more scalable. Since the authoritative nodes in the network are less in number, it takes less time to reach a consensus. Thus, private blockchain can cater to the requirement of high transaction throughput (i.e., speed of the transactions in transactions per unit time). With private blockchain, thousands of transactions can be processed in a second [46]. As compared to a public blockchain, private blockchains are more scalable. This is possible due to the less number of authorized nodes managing and validating transactions and related data. A private blockchain is aimed at businesses and enterprise organizations that require maximum privacy and stability in the processes [47]. The private ecosystem enables such organizations to operate with better efficiency, speed, and less downtime. On the other hand, the drawbacks of private blockchain are the need for trusted nodes, regulatory authority, and the tendency to be centralized in nature since it is managed by a single organization [41].

9.2.4.3   Consortium Blockchain

A consortium is defined as the alliance of two or more individuals, organizations, or governments to achieve a common goal. In a consortium blockchain, all the members in the consortium have the right to write and verify data on the blockchain. It is also a permissioned blockchain like the private blockchain [48]. Therefore, only selected nodes from each member of the consortium can participate in operations related to the blockchain. This makes consortium blockchains a semi-decentralized network, where, although the authority is distributed amongst the members of the consortium, only authorized nodes from each member are allowed to participate in the mining and validation process. The nodes cannot add information to the blockchain on their own without the confirmation of each node. Each member participates equally in reaching a consensus, which, unlike public blockchain, requires significantly lower computational power and uses less energy [49].

The advantages of consortium blockchain are as follows. Transactions do not require any fee since all the infrastructure is provided by the members themselves, eliminating the need of incentivizing transactions [50]. The distribution of power in consortium blockchain protects it from a monopoly. Operations such as blockchain rollback, the rectification of erroneous transactions, and other operations related to the blockchain are brought about by the agreement of all the members [51]. The less number of participating nodes facilitates the faster accomplishment of consensus and synchronization. The transaction throughput is higher as compared to a public blockchain, resulting in better scalability.

9.3   SMART CONTRACTS

9.3.1   INTRODUCTION

The concept of smart contracts was introduced in the 1990s by Nick Szabo, a computer scientist and a cryptographer [4]. The concept was introduced as a set of promises in a digital form together with protocols that should be followed to fulfil what is promised. This concept was analogized to the operation of a vending machine. Furthermore, the concept of the smart contract is expected to follow simple and clear logic and verification through cryptographic methods to be more useful and functional compared to traditional paper-based contracts. In recent years, the concept of smart contracts has been identified to be more useful in conjunction with the growth in the blockchain and DLTs [52].

Blockchains enable smart contracts through the decentralized decision-making banking on consensus mechanisms to facilitate many emerging blockchain-based applications such as data markets, Energy Internet (EI), and micro transactions [53,54]. Smart contracts convert the contractual clauses in traditional contracts into logical and executable computer programs with well-defined conditions [37]. Once the predefined requirements are satisfied, contract statements are executed. Furthermore, as smart contracts follow an object-oriented approach, each instance of a smart contract can be accessed through its unique address, whereas all the smart contract instances can reside on the blockchain. Smart contracts are stored as immutable records in blockchain and ensure strict access control.

9.3.2 FEATURES OF SMART CONTRACTS

Smart contracts, when deployed on the blockchain, offer an assortment of features and advantages. Below are some of the important features of smart contracts (running on top of blockchain) based on [37,38,55,56].

9.3.2.1 Decentralized Operation

Smart contracts are operated as decentralized programs in a blockchain network. This enables smart contracts to overcome various issues faced by centralized applications. For instance, the decentralized operation ensures resilience against single-point failures to operate autonomously even if one or more nodes of the network are compromised. Furthermore, smart contract services are immune to Denial of Service (DoS) attacks and provide guaranteed service availability. In addition, the decentralized operation minimizes data transmission cost and latency.

9.3.2.2 Immutability

The execution of a smart contract is securely stored in the form of a transaction on the blockchain. The blockchain network validates these cryptographically sealed transactions while being added to the blockchain. Once a smart contract is recorded in the blockchain, it cannot be altered. Moreover, the immutability of the smart contract increases as the blockchain grows because the time to alter a blockchain (under attack) increases with a longer chain of blocks.

9.3.2.3 Elimination of a Third Party

Trusted third parties are required for the operation of centralized applications. However, the decentralized property of smart contracts on blockchains enables functioning without requiring any third-party service. This will enable a large number of connected devices to make decisions and perform transactions in a decentralized fashion.

9.3.2.4 Autonomous Execution

dApps on blockchain operate according to the terms and conditions defined in smart contracts. These applications continue to operate until it reaches terminating conditions, while the execution of smart contracts cannot be intervened by any authority or third party.

9.3.2.5 Transparency

Operating in a decentralized peer-to-peer network enables the nodes to access the transactions on the blockchain. Each clause operated by a smart contract is visible and available for inspection to the entire network. This gives smart contracts an advantage over centralized applications as the execution process is visible to the network. It provides transparency to the execution process and enables the participating users as well as the other nodes to inspect the process flow of smart contract execution.

9.3.2.6 Accuracy

Traditional applications involve human intervention for database management, which may result in erroneous data being stored in the database. This will raise concerns related to the accuracy of the data being stored. However, smart contracts verify the prescribed conditions prior to execution, and any human intervention is eliminated while improving accuracy. Furthermore, smart contracts are unbiased and establish a trustworthy execution environment by providing a transparent, immutable, and accurate execution.

9.3.2.7 Speed

Process execution in centralized applications requires documentation and authorizations on different levels for each process. It also requires the involvement of third parties and other intermediaries, which increases the complexity and the overall execution time of a process. In contrast, smart contracts execute the predefined conditions agreed upon by the stakeholders while eliminating the involvement of different authorizations and intermediaries. Hence, the entire processing time depends on the time required for contract execution and verification. This increases the processing speed.

9.3.3 DIFFERENT BLOCKCHAIN PLATFORMS SUPPORTING SMART CONTRACTS

Several blockchain platforms have already adopted smart contracts as an integral feature. Brief descriptions of such platforms are provided below:

9.3.3.1 Ethereum

Vitalik Buterin developed Ethereum in 2015 with the intention of providing a platform that is capable of supporting dApps [57]. Ethereum also supports the use of smart contracts to create and deploy dApps on the network. Each smart contract on Ethereum has its own Ethereum address that resides on the Ethereum Blockchain. The Ethereum address refers to a unique value assigned to users and smart contracts for identification. This address allows smart contracts to retain assets while performing transactions over the Ethereum network. Furthermore, Ethereum uses "Gas Fee", which is the fee that is required to perform a transaction [58]. This fee includes the computational cost of executing a contract. Each function or operation requires a gas fee based on the complexity of the operations performed. In addition, Ethereum supports the use of programming languages such as Solidity, Serpent, LLL, and Muran [37]. These programs are compiled into machine codes and loaded on the EVM (Ethereum Virtual Machine) for execution.

9.3.3.2 Hyperledger Fabric

Similar to Ethereum, Hyperledger Fabric is also a distributed ledger platform capable of running smart contracts and dApps [59]. Hyperledger Fabric is designed to support enterprise applications using a permissioned blockchain environment. Smart contracts, also known as Chaincode in Hyperledger, operate in a permissioned environment and do not require any transaction fee. Unlike Ethereum (which uses virtual machines to run smart contracts), Fabric uses a Docker container. Docker is an open-source platform using OS-level virtualization to facilitate the operation of applications independently [60]. This results in lower overhead, resulting in enabling the platform and applications to function in a faster and energy-efficient manner. Furthermore, Fabric supports high-level programming languages such as Java and Golang [37].

9.3.3.3 Corda

It is an open-source distributed ledger platform designed for businesses, allowing them to transact, ensuring strict privacy [61]. Corda supports the use of high-level programming languages operating on the Java Virtual Machine (JVM), such as Java and Kotlin [62]. Smart contracts in Corda are not neatly encapsulated into packages, as is the case with Ethereum and Hyperledger Fabric. Instead, contracts are split into different parts to increase flexibility while fulfilling the needs of regulated financial and industrial institutions. The data of a smart contract is stored in the state objects known as ContractStates. These ContractStates contain opaque data that are used to perform the functions and operations as defined in the contract. The participating parties can rely on these contracts in case of legal disputes [37].

9.3.3.4 Stellar

Stellar is an open-source blockchain-based platform, which facilitates trading currencies and payments [63]. Stellar allows users to perform operations such as creating, sending, and trading digital representation of multiple forms of money. Furthermore, Stellar supports languages such as Python, JavaScript, Golang, and PHP [37]. Similar to Fabric, Stellar also requires Docker containers to execute programs [60]. In addition, the transaction processing time of Stellar is much faster as compared to other platforms. This is due to the usage of Anchors. Anchors issue credits to the Stellar networks by holding user deposits. Stellar transaction occurs based on the issued anchors. This results in reducing the transaction time to less than even 5 seconds [37].

9.3.3.5 EOS

EOS is a decentralized and scalable platform designed for enterprise-grade applications that can also run dApps. This platform supports both public and private blockchain deployment [64]. The contracts are Turing complete and are developed in C/C++. Furthermore, smart contracts used in EOS are similar to Ethereum, where a new instance of the contract is created every time the contract is executed. In addition, contracts in EOS do not require any transaction fee [37]. Furthermore, the nodes in EOS cooperate in producing blocks without competing, which also increases the security [65].

9.4 APPLICATIONS OF BLOCKCHAIN AND SMART CONTRACTS

Blockchain, along with smart contracts, brings tremendous opportunities due to its salient features such as decentralization, immutability, transparency, non-repudiation, pseudonymity, and fast processing. Healthcare [66], finance [67], real estate, music industry [68], insurance [69], and media [70], to name a few, are some of the sectors that have already realized the potential benefits of blockchain and smart contracts and thus have started using them. For instance, in the healthcare sector, blockchain can enable digital maintenance of records of patients and medical equipment, pharmaceutical supply chain management, remote patient monitoring, and health data analytics [71]. Some of the companies that ventured into this space are Medicalchain [72], IRYO [73], and Burstiq [74]. Many such companies aim to provide patients total control and ownership of their electronic medical records and allow the patients to decide with whom to share their medical records. Insurance is another sector that can be uplifted using blockchain and smart contracts. Some of the functionalities that can be enabled by blockchain and smart contracts in the insurance sector are eliminating the need for intermediaries, detecting fraud more efficiently, assisting in the development of a dynamic insurer/client relationship, and making the application process in a more client-centric manner [75].

Yet another sector that has embraced blockchain is real estate. Customers may rent, purchase, invest, and lend in a safe and efficient environment due to smart contracts and decentralized ledgers. For instance, Propertyclub, a company based on blockchain, allows users to utilize blockchain to browse, sell, rent, purchase, and invest in properties using their portal [76]. Thus, blockchain is emerging as a promising future technology that can support and enhance many sectors and domains of businesses.

9.5 SECURITY ASPECTS OF BLOCKCHAIN AND SMART CONTRACTS

Blockchain and smart contracts have immense potential and are considered secure due to the underlying features such as cryptographic techniques, decentralization, and distributed database, making it extremely difficult for attackers to hack or manipulate. In particular, the blockchain-based system does not suffer from issues related to a centralized system such as single point of failure, the necessity of third party or intermediaries, authorities keeping full control, and most importantly, the privacy of the user.

Nevertheless, blockchain itself has its security and privacy issues. Many security attacks in the past, such as the DAO attack, selfish mining attack, Parity Multi-sig attack, and the 51% attack [77–79], show that the technology is still in its development stage. Some of the security attacks pertaining to blockchain and smart contracts are briefly discussed in Table 9.2. Nevertheless, the blockchain

TABLE 9.2

Various Attacks on Blockchain and Smart Contracts

Focus of Attack	Attack	Brief Description
Blockchain	Majority attack	When an attacker has accumulated more mining power than others, it is able to control the entire blockchain and alter the view of the honest nodes on the network [79,80]
	Eclipse attack	The attacker populates the data structures of an honest node in order to isolate it and manipulate its view of the blockchain (i.e., the ledger in a P2P network). The attack is a building block to other attacks such as majority attack and DDoS attack [81].
	DoS attack	An attacker floods the network with an abnormally large number of requests, crippling the network's capacity to handle genuine traffic [82]. Attackers aim to disconnect a network's mining pools, e-wallets, crypto exchanges, and other financial services [80].
	Sybil attack	Multiple nodes that are controlled by a single user. By utilizing them, it may outcast honest nodes. This attack is generally used to take control over the network, and it can also pave the path for bigger attacks such as DDoS attack or the majority attack [83].
	Selfish mining attack	A malicious miner (or group of miners) mines new blocks privately and do not publish them to the rest of the network. Such a miner keeps mining new blocks until its local copy of (private) blockchain becomes longer than the current publically available blockchain. On achieving sufficient lead, the selfish miner publishes (broadcasts) a longer blockchain, which gets accepted by the network. One obvious intention of selfish miner is to maximize the earned rewards [28,80].
	Race around attack	A race attack is a sort of double-spend attempt. It necessitates that the receiver accepts unconfirmed transactions as payment. This is accomplished by sending the fraudulent transaction to the target and the legitimate transaction to the mining pool [83,84].
Smart contract	The DAO attack	The DAO hack took place in June 2016, and the attacker was able to steal over 3.6 million Ethers (worth 60 million USD, then). A vulnerability called re-entrancy in the smart contract was the source of the DAO attack [77,85].
	Parity Multi-Sig wallet attack	The developers of the wallet created a public library that was deployed over Ethereum to save the gas cost incurred for every transaction. The attacker exploited this public library and stole over 150,000 ETH (30M USD) [77,86].
	Integer underflow/ overflow attack	The vulnerabilities in Ethereum and solidity create a way for the attacker to pass some parameters that can be exploited to fetch more balance in his/her account than available originally [77].

community and alliances are continuously working towards the mitigation of these attacks.

9.6 CONCLUSION

This chapter presents a detailed discussion on blockchain and smart contracts. The blockchain concept is introduced, explaining the block structure, process flow in block mining, blockchain features, and types of blockchain. Subsequently, the concept of smart contracts is introduced while elaborating its features and the blockchain platforms supporting smart contracts. Then, the applications of blockchain and smart contracts are presented. In addition, security and privacy concerns of blockchain and smart contracts are presented, highlighting the possible attacks. The unique features of blockchain qualify it as promising technology towards developing novel and innovative applications and services. However, blockchain and smart contracts require further research and development work, especially in the areas of scalability, transaction speed, and security, to establish as a robust and agile platform enabling future applications and services.

REFERENCES

1. Nakamoto S, Bitcoin A. A peer-to-peer electronic cash system. *Bitcoin*; https://bitcoin.org/bitcoin.pdf. 2008;4.
2. Merkle RC. *Secrecy, Authentication, and Public Key Systems*. Ph.D. Thesis. Stanford University; http://www.merkle.com/papers/Thesis1979.pdf. 1979.
3. Haber S, Stornetta WS. How to time-stamp a digital document. In: *Conference on the Theory and Application of Cryptography*, Springer, Berlin, Heidelberg, 1990:437–455.
4. Szabo N. Formalizing and securing relationships on public networks. *First Monday*. Published online, https://firstmonday.org/ojs/index.php/fm/article/download/548/469. 1997.
5. Natarajan H, Krause SK, Gradstein HL. *Distributed Ledger Technology (DLT) and Blockchain*. World Bank, https://openknowledge.worldbank.org/handle/10986/29053. 2017.
6. Crosby M, Pattanayak P, Verma S, Kalyanaraman V, others. Blockchain technology: beyond bitcoin. *Appl Innov*. 2016;2(6–10):71.
7. Saad M, Spaulding J, Njilla L, et al. Exploring the attack surface of blockchain: a comprehensive survey. *IEEE Commun Surv & Tutorials*. 2020;22(3):1977–2008.
8. Antonopoulos AM. *Mastering Bitcoin: Unlocking Digital Cryptocurrencies*. O'Reilly Media, Inc., 2014.
9. Martino R, Cilardo A. Designing a SHA-256 processor for blockchain-based IoT applications. *Internet of Things*. 2020;11:100254.
10. Majeed U, Hong CS. On the proof-of-work puzzle hardness in bitcoin blockchain. *Proc Korean Inf Sci Soc*. Published online 2018:1348–1350.
11. Vranken H. Sustainability of bitcoin and blockchains. *Curr Opin Environ Sustain*. 2017;28:1–9.
12. Ma Y, Sun Y, Lei Y, Qin N, Lu J. A survey of blockchain technology on security, privacy, and trust in crowdsourcing services. *World Wide Web*. 2020;23(1):393–419.

13. Singh B, Gupta G. Analyzing windows subsystem for linux metadata to detect timestamp forgery. In: *IFIP International Conference on Digital Forensics*, Springer, Cham, 2019:159–182.
14. Chen P-W, Jiang B-S, Wang C-H. Blockchain-based payment collection supervision system using pervasive Bitcoin digital wallet. In: *2017 IEEE 13th International Conference on Wireless and Mobile Computing, Networking and Communications (WiMob)*; IEEE, 2017:139–146.
15. Khan MA, Salah K. IoT security: review, blockchain solutions, and open challenges. *Futur Gener Comput Syst*. 2018;82:395–411.
16. ur Rehman MH, Salah K, Damiani E, Svetinovic D. Trust in blockchain cryptocurrency ecosystem. *IEEE Trans Eng Manag*. 2019;67(4):1196–1212.
17. Li X, Jiang P, Chen T, Luo X, Wen Q. A survey on the security of blockchain systems. *Futur Gener Comput Syst*. 2020;107:841–853.
18. Coinguides. What is Bitcoin Mempool? Memory pool size, fees, transactions explained. Retrieved on June 30, 2021. Published 2018. Accessed June 30, 2021. https://coinguides.org/bitcoin-mempool/
19. Kasthala V. Blockchain nodes and mining, explained. Retrieved on June 30, 2021. Published 2019. https://medium.com/@venkat.kasthala/how-does-mining-work-in-blockchain-b4fc5f7f3209.
20. Politou E, Casino F, Alepis E, Patsakis C. Blockchain mutability: challenges and proposed solutions. *IEEE Trans Emerg Top Comput*. Published online 2019;9(4):1972–1986.
21. Zheng Z, Xie S, Dai H-N, Chen X, Wang H. Blockchain challenges and opportunities: a survey. *Int J Web Grid Serv*. 2018;14(4):352–375.
22. Nuss M, Puchta A, Kunz M. Towards blockchain-based identity and access management for internet of things in enterprises. In: *International Conference on Trust and Privacy in Digital Business*, Springer, Cham, 2018:167–181.
23. Kritikos M. What if blockchain offered a way to reconcile privacy with transparency? Retrieved on May 30, 2021. https://policycommons.net/artifacts/1335700/what-if-blockchain-offered-a-way-to-reconcile-privacy-with-transparency/.
24. De Filippi P. The interplay between decentralization and privacy: the case of blockchain technologies. *J Peer Prod Issue*. 2016;7:1–19.
25. Hammi MT, Hammi B, Bellot P, Serhrouchni A. Bubbles of trust: a decentralized blockchain-based authentication system for IoT. *Comput & Secur*. 2018;78:126–142.
26. Zhou J, Gollmann D. Towards verification of non-repudiation protocols. In: *Proceedings of 1998 International Refinement Workshop and Formal Methods Pacific*, Springer-Verlag, 1998:370–380.
27. Fang W, Chen W, Zhang W, Pei J, Gao W, Wang G. Digital signature scheme for information non-repudiation in blockchain: a state of the art review. *EURASIP J Wirel Commun Netw*. 2020;2020(1):1–15.
28. CryptoCompare. How do digital signatures in Bitcoin work? Retrieved on June 23, 2021. Published 2015. https://www.cryptocompare.com/wallets/guides/how-do-digital-signatures-in-bitcoin-work/
29. Georgescu A, Cirnu CE. Blockchain and critical infrastructures--challenges and opportunities. *Rom Cyber Secur J*. Published online 2019;1(1):1730–2668.
30. Dhar V, Stein RM. FinTech platforms and strategy. *Commun ACM*. 2017;60(10):32–35.
31. Hewa TM, Kalla A, Nag A, Ylianttila ME, Liyanage M. Blockchain for 5G and IoT: opportunities and challenges. In: *2020 IEEE Eighth International Conference on Communications and Networking (ComNet)*, 2020:1–8.
32. Qiu T, Zhang R, Gao Y. Ripple vs. SWIFT: transforming cross border remittance using blockchain technology. *Procedia Comput Sci*. 2019;147:428–434.

33. Salman T, Zolanvari M, Erbad A, Jain R, Samaka M. Security services using block-chains: a state of the art survey. *IEEE Commun Surv & Tutorials*. 2018;21(1):858–880.
34. Montecchi M, Plangger K, Etter M. It's real, trust me! Establishing supply chain provenance using blockchain. *Bus Horiz*. 2019;62(3):283–293.
35. Ali MS, Vecchio M, Pincheira M, Dolui K, Antonelli F, Rehmani MH. Applications of blockchains in the Internet of Things: a comprehensive survey. *IEEE Commun Surv & Tutorials*. 2018;21(2):1676–1717.
36. Zhang R, Xue R, Liu L. Security and privacy on blockchain. *ACM Comput Surv*. 2019;52(3):1–34.
37. Zheng Z, Xie S, Dai H-N, et al. An overview on smart contracts: challenges, advances and platforms. *Futur Gener Comput Syst*. 2020;105:475–491.
38. Hewa T, Ylianttila M, Liyanage M. Survey on blockchain based smart contracts: applications, opportunities and challenges. *J Netw Comput Appl*. Published online 2020:177:102857.
39. Taskinsoy J. Blockchain: a misunderstood digital revolution. Things you need to know about blockchain. *Things You Need to Know about Blockchain* (October 8, 2019). Published online 2019.
40. Mohan C. State of public and private blockchains: myths and reality. In: *Proceedings of the 2019 International Conference on Management of Data*, https://dl.acm.org/doi/abs/10.1145/3299869.3314116. 2019:404–411.
41. Nitchoun D. Easily understand the difference between private blockchain and public blockchain! Retrieved on July 7, 2021. https://medium.com/@Equisafe/easily-understand-the-difference-between-private-blockchain-and-public-blockchain-2c4f9b2111b.
42. Capponi A, Olafsson S, Alsabah H. Proof-of-work cryptocurrencies: does mining technology undermine decentralization? *Available SSRN*. Published online 2021.
43. Pongnumkul S, Siripanpornchana C, Thajchayapong S. Performance analysis of private blockchain platforms in varying workloads. In: *2017 26th International Conference on Computer Communication and Networks (ICCCN)*, IEEE, 2017:1–6.
44. Cash M, Bassiouni M. Two-tier permission-ed and permission-less blockchain for secure data sharing. *In: 2018 IEEE International Conference on Smart Cloud (SmartCloud)*, IEEE, 2018:138–144.
45. Lin I-C, Liao T-C. A survey of blockchain security issues and challenges. *IJ Netw Secur*. 2017;19(5):653–659.
46. Yang R, Wakefield R, Lyu S, et al. Public and private blockchain in construction business process and information integration. *Autom Constr*. 2020;118:103276.
47. Carson B, Romanelli G, Walsh P, Zhumaev A. *Blockchain Beyond the Hype: What is the Strategic Business Value*. McKinsey & Co. https://www.mckinsey.com/-business-functions/mckinsey-digital/our-insights/blockchain-beyond-the-hype-what-is-the-strategic-business-value. Published online 2018:1–13.
48. Chana M, Luoa H, Mab EZ, Chiub DM. *From Use Case to Benchmark: Comparing Consortium and Private Blockchains*. https://www.parallelchain.io/.
49. Dib O, Brousmiche K-L, Durand A, Thea E, Hamida EB. Consortium blockchains: overview, applications and challenges. *Int J Adv Telecommun*. 2018;11(1&2):51–64.
50. Al-Shaibani H, Lasla N, Abdallah M. Consortium blockchain-based decentralized stock exchange platform. *IEEE Access*. 2020;8:123711–123725.
51. Li K, Li H, Hou H, Li K, Chen Y. Proof of vote: a high-performance consensus protocol based on vote mechanism & consortium blockchain. In: *2017 IEEE 19th International Conference on High Performance Computing and Communications; IEEE 15th International Conference on Smart City; IEEE 3rd International Conference on Data Science and Systems (HPCC/SmartCity/DSS)*, IEEE 2017:466–473.

52. Wang S, Ouyang L, Yuan Y, Ni X, Han X, Wang F-Y. Blockchain-enabled smart contracts: architecture, applications, and future trends. *IEEE Trans Syst Man, Cybern Syst.* 2019;49(11):2266–2277.
53. Saputhanthri A, De Alwis C, Liyanage M. Emergence of Blockchain based IoT Marketplaces In: Joint European Conference on Networks and Communications (EuCNC) & 6G Summit, Grenoble, France, 2021.
54. Andoni M, Robu V, Flynn D, et al. Blockchain technology in the energy sector: a systematic review of challenges and opportunities. *Renew Sustain Energy Rev.* 2019;100:143–174.
55. Peng K, Li M, Huang H, Wang C, Wan S, Choo K-KR. Security challenges and opportunities for smart contracts in internet of things: a survey. *IEEE Internet Things J.* Published online 2021.
56. Alharby M, Van Moorsel A. Blockchain-based smart contracts: a systematic mapping study. *arXiv Prepr arXiv171006372.* Published online 2017.
57. Buterin V, others. A next-generation smart contract and decentralized application platform. *White Pap.* Ethereum Found., Zug, Switzerland, 2014.
58. Kasireddy P. How does Ethereum work anyway. *Publ Mediu* (https//medium com/@ preethikasireddy/how-does-ethereum-work-anyway-22d1df506369).   Published online 2017.
59. Androulaki E, Barger A, Bortnikov V, et al. Hyperledger fabric: a distributed operating system for permissioned blockchains. In: *Proceedings of the Thirteenth EuroSys Conference*, 2018:1–15. doi:10.1145/3190508.3190538.
60. Docker. No Title. Retrieved on July 7, 2021. Published June 2021. https://docs. docker.com/.
61. Brown RG, Carlyle J, Grigg I, Hearn M. Corda: an introduction. *R3 CEV*, August. 2016;1:15.
62. Valenta M, Sandner P. Comparison of ethereum, hyperledger fabric and corda. *Frankfurt Sch Blockchain Cent.* http://explore-ip.com/2017_Comparison-of-Ethereum-Hyperledger-Corda.pdf. 2017.
63. Mazieres D. The stellar consensus protocol: a federated model for internet-level consensus. *Stellar Dev Found.* https://www.stellar.org/papers/stellar-consensus-protocol.pdf. 2015;1–32.
64. EOS. Eosio developer portal - Eosio development documentation. Retrieved July 7, 2021. https://developers.eos.io/welcome/latest/index.
65. Valdeolmillos D, Mezquita Y, González-Briones A, Prieto J, Corchado JM. Blockchain technology: a review of the current challenges of cryptocurrency. In: *International Congress on Blockchain and Applications*, Springer, Cham, 2019:153–160.
66. Al-Megren S, Alsalamah S, Altoaimy L, Alsalamah H, Soltanisehat L, Pentland A. *Blockchain Use Cases in Digital Sectors: A Review of the Literature.* 2018. doi:10.1109/Cybermatics_2018.2018.00242.
67. Zile K, Strazdina R. Blockchain use cases and their feasibility. *Appl Comput Syst.* 2018;23:12–20. doi:10.2478/acss-2018-0002.
68. Sitonio C, Nucciarelli A. *The Impact of Blockchain on the Music Industry.* 2018.
69. Kalsgonda V, Kulkarni R. Applications of blockchain in insurance industry: a review. Published online, *PIMT Journal of Res.* 2020:12(4):1–3 doi:10.13140 /RG.2.2.23708.72322.
70. Voinea DV, others. Blockchain for journalism-potential use cases. *Soc Sci Educ Res Rev.* 2019;6(2):244–256.
71. Agbo CC, Mahmoud QH, Eklund JM. Blockchain technology in healthcare: a systematic review. *Healthcare.* 7;2019:56.

72. Medicalchain. Medicalchain Whitepaper 2.1. Retrieved on May 17, 2021. Published 2018. https://medicalchain.com/Medicalchain-Whitepaper-EN.pdf.
73. IRYO Network. IRYO Global participatory healthcare ecosystem. Retrieved on May 17, 2021, 2021. Published 2017. https://iryo.network/iryo_whitepaper.pdf.
74. Burstiq. Burstiq. Retrieved on May 17, 2021. https://www.burstiq.com/technology/.
75. Deloitte. Analysis blockchain in health and life insurance. Retrieved on June 24, 2021. https://www2.deloitte.com/us/en/pages/life-sciences-and-health-care/articles/blockchain-in-insurance.html.
76. Propertyclub. Propertyclub. Retrieved on May 26, 2021. https://propertyclub.nyc/article/real-estate-tokenization.
77. Praitheeshan P, Pan L, Yu J, Liu J, Doss R. Security analysis methods on Ethereum smart contract vulnerabilities: a survey. *arXiv Prepr arXiv190808605*. Published online 2019.
78. Ye C, Li G, Cai H, Gu Y, Fukuda A. Analysis of security in blockchain: case study in 51%-attack detecting. In: *2018 5th International Conference on Dependable Systems and Their Applications (DSA)*, IEEE, 2018:15–24.
79. Averin A, Averina O. Review of blockchain technology vulnerabilities and block-chain-system attacks. In: *2019 International Multi-Conference on Industrial Engineering and Modern Technologies (FarEastCon)*, IEEE, 2019:1–6.
80. Anna Katrenko MS. Blockchain attack vectors: vulnerabilities of the most secure technology. Retrieved on July 7, 2021. Published 2020. https://www.apriorit.com/dev-blog/578-blockchain-attack-vectors.
81. Heilman E, Kendler A, Zohar A, Goldberg S. Eclipse attacks on bitcoin's peer-to-peer network. In: *24th {USENIX} Security Symposium ({USENIX} Security 15)*, 2015:129–144.
82. DoS vs DDoS. DoS vs DDoS. Retrieved on May 27, https://www.usenix.org/system/files/conference/usenixsecurity15/sec15-paper-heilman.pdf. 2021. https://www.fortinet.com/resources/cyberglossary/dos-vs-ddos.
83. Dasgupta D, Shrein JM, Gupta KD. A survey of blockchain from security perspective. *J Bank Financ Technol*. 2019;3(1):1–17.
84. Race Attack. Race attack vs. double-spending attack: are they same? Retrieved on June 28, 2021. https://bitcoin.stackexchange.com/questions/60164/race-attack-vs-double-spending-attack-are-they-same.
85. Siegel D. Understanding the DAO attack. Retrieved on June 01, 2021. Published 2020. https://www.coindesk.com/understanding-dao-hack-journalists.
86. Palladino S. The parity wallet hack explained. Retrieved on May 17, 2021. Published 2017. https://blog.openzeppelin.com/on-the-parity-wallet-multisig-hack-405a8c12e8f7/.

10 Blockchain Technology in Healthcare

A Systematic Review

Halima Mhamdi
University of Gabes

Ben Othman Soufiene
Prince Laboratory Research

Ahmed Zouinkhi
University of Gabes

Faris. A. Almalki
Taif University

Hedi Sakli
University of Gabes
EITA Consulting

CONTENTS

DOI: 10.1201/9781003224075-10

10.1 INTRODUCTION

The Internet of Things (IoT) is defined as a network of identifiable and unique elements that communicate without human interaction using IP connectivity [1]. This new concept covers several domains: energy [2], smart home [3], agriculture [4], healthcare [5–7], and industry [8]. The integration of IoT in the healthcare sector is giving rise to a new paradigm called the Internet of Medical Things (IoMT). This term refers to a connected infrastructure of devices and software applications that can communicate with various IT systems to provide health-related services [9]. Figure 10.1 shows the different IoMT participants.

Some examples of IoMT include remote patient monitoring for people with chronic or long-term illnesses. This type of treatment saves patients from visiting the hospital or doctor's office every time they have a medical question or a change in their condition as well as inpatient wearable mHealth devices that can send information to caregivers. Another example, in the pharmaceutical sector, is drug tracking. However, it is important to note that the healthcare sector faces many challenges. The major challenge is the processing and analysis of patient records due to the large amount of data collected. The security of this data is another

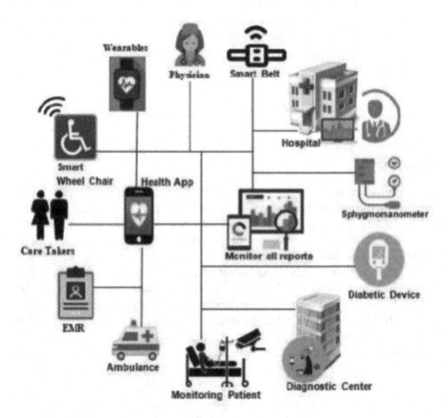

FIGURE 10.1 IoMT system entities.

challenge to consider. Due to the high connectivity, these systems are prone to malicious attacks. In addition, it is difficult to ensure confidentiality due to the exchange of sensitive data. In summary, the main challenges are as follows:

- **Patient Records Management**: Currently, information is not shared between doctors, and the patient must carry over the reports of his previous consultations to each new specialist. This mission is more difficult for an uninformed patient who does not master the medical discussion and does not have a precise idea of the content of his file. With the rise of telemedicine, visits to the doctor are made through multiple channels, making it more difficult for healthcare professionals to update patients' medical records. Therefore, it will be vital for this industry to create a way to record and update medical records for both in-person and virtual visits. This means digitizing these records and sharing them, after patient consent, with healthcare professionals to be updated in real time.
  - **Clinical Trial Certification**: Clinical trials involving drugs are intended to establish or verify a certain amount of data. The sharing of this data including confidentiality, integrity, record keeping, and patient enrollment is often used by researchers in a secure manner. Sharing research between different scientists and organizations could lead to better and more rapid progress on specific topics.
  - **Drug Traceability**: The lack of drug traceability is another issue to which a distributed and public database could provide a start.
  - **Securing Access to Health Data:** This is a major issue in network-to-network data transmission. The dependence of IoMT applications and platforms on a centralized cloud puts security at risk.

Blockchain is an emerging technology that is spreading in various sectors and presents many advantages and opportunities. Blockchain technology is characterized by the immutability of stored data, decentralization, and privacy. Integrated into the health sector, it helps to overcome the problems encountered in the latter.

This chapter is organized as follows. In the second section, we discuss the blockchain technology, its function mode, its characteristics, as well as smart contracts. Section 10.3 presents the application of this technology in the field of health and the solutions proposed by the researchers in this axis. We end with a conclusion.

10.2 THE BLOCKCHAIN TECHNOLOGY BASIC CONCEPTS

In the peer-to-peer network, machines and devices communicate with each other without intermediate entities forming a decentralized network called Blockchain. It is, in fact, a set of connected nodes that share and record transactions. Each node in the network keeps a copy to avoid having a single point of failure. The data shared through the blockchain is structured in blocks that are linked together forming a distributed ledger technology (DLT). The security and immutability of this data is ensured through cryptographic functions. The concept of blockchain is introduced by Satoshi Nakamoto in 2008 [10]. It attracts the interest of several researchers in different fields. Bhushan et al. [11, 12] and Saxena et al. [13] presented an in-depth study on the combination of blockchain technology and IoT. They focused on IoT applications by ensuring security, confidentiality, and privacy in IoT systems. They also investigated the future challenges in this sector. The authors in their article [14], with the same aim to guarantee security and confidentiality, have exposed the contribution of this technology in the design and development of the smart city. Other researchers have exploited the use of blockchain in the supply chain [15, 16]. This use aims to solve the problem of reliability and access to manufacturer information. The proposed solution is based on the use of the Ethereum blockchain and the ERC20 interface. It guarantees data security and traceability as well as interoperability by reducing the cost and making exchanges automatic in the supply chain and manufacturing [17]. They addressed the security and privacy issue in Internet of vehicle using blockchain. In addition, Halima et al. [18] exploited the decentralized feature to ensure communication between vehicles and service providers.

Blockchain technology is mainly characterized by major elements: decentralized, transparent, autonomous, secure, and immutable. As described above [19]:

- **Decentralized**: Blockchain technology is a distributed database where data is stored in all nodes of the network. All nodes can manipulate, access, and update transactions simultaneously and without intermediary via a well-defined protocol. This data is not all held on a central intermediary's server, but instead is "distributed", i.e., hosted by each participant.
- **Transparent**: Since their creation, the transactions in the blockchain are accessible by all users. But they are extended by cryptographic functions so that they cannot be modified. That is to say that the addition of transactions is allowed and not their modification or deletion. As in the Bitcoin network, all transactions are public and verifiable by everyone through a consensus mechanism, which will allow everyone to ensure that each participant owns the Bitcoins they are spending and that they are spending them only once. The transparent nature of blockchains could certainly prevent the modification or theft of this data.
- **Consensus**: The blockchain corresponds to a history of transactions on which everyone agrees. This consensus on the sequencing of transactions solves the so-called "double spending" problem: A Bitcoin spent in one transaction cannot be spent a second time in a transaction that would later be broadcast on the network. The second transaction would be rejected by the network.
- **Secure:** Once recorded in the blockchain, it is impossible to delete or modify a transaction since there are several copies in different nodes of

the network. Therefore, the blocks can be extended and not modified. This gives the blockchain a high level of security and makes it more complicated to attack the blocks of information.

- **Autonomous:** In the blockchain network, the handling of transactions is no longer concentrated in a central organization but is spread over all participants of the network. Transactions can be consulted and stored by each node and even transferred and updated. In this way, the blockchain functions autonomously without the intervention of a trusted third party and keeps the identity of the node anonymous and secure.

10.2.1 BLOCKCHAIN PROCESS AND CATEGORIES

Before starting the process of blockchain operation, we must define a transaction. This is the act of exchanging and sharing information between blockchain nodes. Transactions are in fact data exchanged between network participants and stored in files called blocks. These data are encrypted and then chained to the previous block, forming a chain. Following the addition of transactions, the blockchain evolves each time. The transactions must be verified and validated in advance.

Figure 10.2 illustrates the function process of blockchain transactions. This process begins when someone B requests a transaction from A. The data requested by the other party B will form a new block and will be distributed on the different nodes of the blockchain network. In order to be transferred, the new block is verified and validated by the network nodes using cryptographic techniques. After being validated, it is added to the previous blocks in chronological order. The added block is chained in such a way that it cannot be modified or deleted. At the final stage, user B receives the transaction from A which ends successfully.

According to its characteristics and functionalities, the blockchain is classified into three categories [20]:

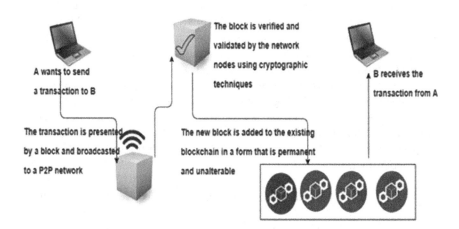

FIGURE 10.2 Blockchain transaction process.

- **Public Blockchain**: In the public blockchain network, transactions are managed by all participants without central control organs. They have the right to consult and even modify the exchanged data. The use of the consensus mechanism guarantees the security and immutability of this type of network. The most famous example of the public blockchain is Ethereum and Bitcoin.
- **Private Blockchain**: In the private blockchain network, only authorized participants can access it. The access is done by invitation from the entities controlling the network. Therefore, to carry out transactions, participants must request permission from third parties. This type of network is usually applied between companies of the same type. Hyperledger Fabric is an example of a private blockchain.
- **Consortium Blockchain:** The consortium blockchain is the fusion between the public and private blockchains. The reading and writing of transactions in this type is both allowed for some nodes and restricted for others. The most notable difference from each system can be seen in the consensus. Instead of an open system where anyone can validate blocks or a closed system where only one entity appoints block producers, a consortium chain has a handful of equally powerful parties that function simultaneously as validators. BigchainDB is an example of a consortium blockchain [20].

10.2.2 SMART CONTRACTS AND ETHEREUM PLATFORM

One of the major assets of blockchain is the utilization of smart contracts and decentralized applications (DApp). Their main role is the exchange of assets and services as well as monetary transactions, without recourse to a third-party authority. In 1994, the smart contracts concept is defined, by Nick Szabo, as "a computerized transaction protocol that executes the terms of a contract" [21]. The smart contract executes transactions automatically, without the need for human intervention. The information handled by the smart contract is received from connected objects and other measuring devices. Miners in the blockchain check the transactions [22, 23] and update them to be saved in the blockchain.

Smart contracts are developed using blockchain platforms like Ethereum. This platform is the most promising blockchain. It can support advanced custom smart contracts using the Turing-complete programming language. Solidity, as a high-level programming language, is used to write smart contracts code which is then converted into Ethereum Virtual Machine (EVM) bytecode. In the EVM, the quantity of gas is the cost or execution fee for each transaction. This fee is calculated as follows:

$$Fee = gasPrice \times min(gasLimit, gasUsed) \qquad (10.1)$$

where gasPrice is the amount of Gwei, as a form of remuneration, received by the miners, gasLimit is the maximum gas amount to complete a transaction, and gasUsed is defined depending on the storage and processing quantity for each transaction [25].

A decentralized application is an application deployed on blockchains and is generally based on smart contracts. It aims to improve the transparency and traceability of the collected information. Given the number of researchers and developers who are attracted to DApp, various sites gather statistics on the different DApp applications [26].

10.3 THE BLOCKCHAIN FOR HEALTHCARE

Thanks to the potential and characteristics of blockchain, this technology is considered a key solution to the problems encountered in the healthcare field. It attracts the interest of many professionals' healthcare. Seven out of 10 of them expect the main benefits of blockchain to apply to clinical trials and medical records, and 6 out of 10 believe that blockchain will help them access new markets and new reliable and secure information [24]. The implication of blockchain in the healthcare sector can be divided into four main categories: patient data management, which includes electronic health record sharing; drug supply chain management, which covers both counterfeit drugs and pharmaceutical Supply Chain; clinical trial; and security in healthcare. Table 10.1 outlines several solutions proposed by the researcher to overcome these problems.

10.3.1 PATIENT DATA MANAGEMENT

When managing medical records, the patient, the doctors, the hospital, the pharmacists, or the medical analysis laboratories are all sources of data, it is difficult to visualize and share all these data in a clear way. This problem is frequently encountered when a patient is admitted to the hospital. Health professionals do not always have access to the patient's history and do not have complete visibility on the treatments he/she is taking on the history of his/her illness or on his/her family history. The ideal would be to have a list of all the places where a patient's medical data is located so that it can be quickly retrieved. This list would be accessible, with the patient's consent, to any health professional who requests it. Thus, instead of having access only to the database of the establishment where one is, one could have access to all the sources of information dispersed in all the databases of the network. Blockchain technology provides just such a solution in the form of a distributed and secure registry that allows patients not only to have visibility over their data, but also to control access to it. So, via blockchain technology, we ensure the interoperability of the platform used by the various health actors. Similarly, for the emergency service, it can access patient data without the need to request it from the patient.

Several researchers have studied this issue. In [25], the authors proposed a platform named BiiMed. This solution aims at sharing the patient's electronic health record between different stakeholders. It ensures data integrity and interoperability, thanks to the blockchain. The proposed architecture is composed of

TABLE 10.1

Summarized Literature Review

Problem Addressed Uses Cases	Paper	Year	Framework	Smart Contracts	Contribution
Patient data management	[25]	2020	NM		• Share the patient's electronic health record between different stakeholders.
	[27]	2016	Ethereum	Yes	
	[30]	2020	Ethereum		
	[26]	2019	NM	No	• Ensures integrity, confidentiality, and interoperability of the data shared.
	[28]	2018	NM		
	[29]	2028	Proprietary		
	[31]	2020	NM		• Resolved the problem of large-scale data management and sharing in an EHR system.
					• Remote monitoring system guarantees the security and privacy of the patient.
Security and privacy in blockchain healthcare	[33]	2018	NM	NM	• Allows the sharing of patient data by controlling the access to these sensitive data.
	[34,35]	2017	NM	NM	
	[36]	2018	NM	NM	
	[37]	2018	NM	NM	• Ensure the security of private data.
	[38]	2017	NM	Yes	• Ensure the confidentiality of messages on the blockchain.
	[39]	2016	NM	NM	
					• Provides access at different levels of granularity without the need for a PKI.
					• Ensures the integrity, security, and confidentiality of private patient data.
Drug/pharmaceutical supply chain management	[41]	2020	NM	NM	• Product identification and tracking in pharmaceutical supply chains.
	[42]	2016	NM		• Maintain security, traceability, and visibility in the pharmaceutical supply chain.
	[43]	2019	NM		
	[44]	2019	NM		
	[45]	2019	NM	Yes	
					• Tracking of pharmaceutical products during distribution.
Clinical trial certification	[46, 47]	2017 2018	Bitcoin NM	NM NM	• Avoid undesirable consequences of drug use.
	[48]	2017	NM	NM	• Development of platforms and systems for collecting and sharing patient data in clinical trials.
	[49]	2018	NM	NM	
	[50]	2016	Ethereum	Yes	
	[51]	2017	Ethereum	Yes	• Support the transparency of the data and documents retrieved during clinical research.
	[52]	2019	NM	NM	
	[53]	2021	NM	NM	
	[54]				• Ensure traceability of clinical data.

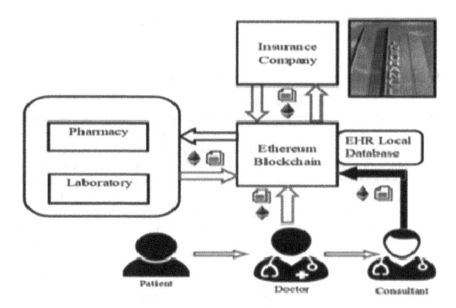

FIGURE 10.3 Management of patient medical records.

two parts: Health Information System and BiiMed blockchain. HIS consists of gathering, saving, and sharing medical data while the BiiMed platform manages the shared data. It is based on the Ethereum blockchain and the smart contract. MedChain [26] is another platform that works on the same principle of sharing data by storing them immutably in the blockchain. The MedRec scheme, proposed [27] by Azaria et al, allows both the integrity and confidentiality of the data shared through a decentralized system that guarantees easy access to this data by the patient, doctors, and any other person included in the process of medical record treatment, as shown in Figure 10.3. The authors of [28] have proposed a system called MeDShare. This system allows the exchange of medical data and keeps electronic medical records secure. The participants in this system are hospitals, service providers, and health research. They use medical data shared by MeDShare. Data confidentiality is ensured by a customized audit control. In the same sense of sharing medical information, the authors have developed the Medblock prototype [29] based on the blockchain. This prototype allows secure access to electronic medical records.

Kazmi et al. [30] have exploited smart contracts to design a system for remote patient monitoring and alerting health specialists in case of emergency. This remote monitoring system guarantees the security and privacy of the patient through blockchain. To solve the interoperability problem, the authors [31] implemented a blockchain-based system. It allows patients to share their clinical data with healthcare providers. The patient has the right to choose the person with whom he shares his data. Access to the data in a secure way is ensured by the identification and authentication of the user. Once identified, they can access and update the patients' data.

10.3.2 Security and Privacy in Blockchain-Healthcare

Healthcare is not a sector like any other and must comply with particularly strict confidentiality rules. To function in the healthcare sector, a blockchain must first and foremost guarantee data protection and the anonymity of patient data. In Europe, the MyHealthMyData project designs a health blockchain model that is compatible with medical privacy, because no information is stored directly on the blockchain: it only stores links to its information. A partner of the giant Siemens, MyHealthMyData aims to facilitate access to and sharing of health data in clinical trials. If a person wishes to delete his or her data from the blockchain, he or she will be able to break the links to his or her information, without having to break the chain. The different blocks will remain in place in the chain but will be permanently deactivated [32].

The authors of [33] tackled the problem of security and patient privacy. They proposed a system based on the immutability and autonomy of the blockchain. This system allows the sharing of patient data by controlling the access to these sensitive data. Discrete wavelets transform and genetic algorithm are the basis of the proposed scheme. To ensure the security of private data, the authors of [34,35] proposed a key management scheme to ensure the confidentiality of messages on the blockchain. In the same context, Zhang and Poslad [36] suggest an access authorization model and scheme called Granular Access Authorization supporting Flexible Queries (GAA-FQ) using encryption and decryption algorithms. This scheme provides access at different levels of granularity without the need for a public key infrastructure (PKI). The signature scheme proposed in [37] is a solution ensuring security and trust. Thanks to the attribute with multiple authorities, which is the backbone of this solution, the patient's public/private keys are not generated and shared. MediBchain is a platform proposed by Abdullah et al. [38]. It ensures the integrity, security, and confidentiality of private patient data. The authors have also exploited cryptographic functions to solve the problem of anonymity faced in other systems. Healthcare Data Gateway (HGD) is another solution based on blockchain technology and presented in [39]. Patient data is shared while keeping privacy.

10.3.3 Drug/Pharmaceutical Supply Chain Management

The traceability of drugs and the fight against counterfeiting is another concrete case of blockchain and IoMT. According to the World Health Organization, 1 in 10 pharmaceutical products is counterfeit. This figure reaches 30% of medicines in developing countries, which represents a market of 200 billion dollars. Moreover, 25 million counterfeit drugs are distributed on the Internet with a value of 43 million euros [40].

Drug traceability is a very sensitive area that needs an urgent solution as it affects the lives of individuals. The use of blockchain technology brings

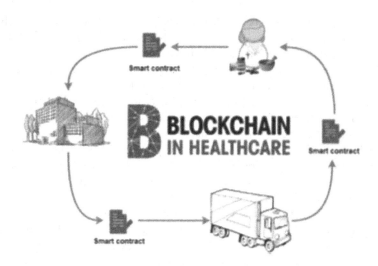

FIGURE 10.4 Pharmaceutical logistics sector based on smart contract [43].

advantages in this context especially in the tracking of pharmaceutical products during distribution. For this use case, the different supply chain actors are identified in the blockchain network. Pharmaceutical companies register their products with a unique identifier. Stores reselling the drugs or pharmacists could check upon receipt of stocks of drugs that they come from valid laboratories; the information related to each drug is updated in the blockchain each time.

Clauson et al. [41] present a detailed study on the application of blockchain technology in pharmaceutical supply chains. This study includes product identification and tracking as well as validity verification. Hyperledger's Counterfeit Medicines Project [42] also helps to fight counterfeit medicines. In their paper [43] as shown in Figure 10.4, the authors exploit the notion of smart contracts and multi-agents' system. They propose a platform allowing the storage of transactions between the different actors of the system in the blockchain. The smart contracts ensure the management of these transactions.

To maintain security, traceability, and visibility in the pharmaceutical supply chain, the authors [44] designed a private blockchain platform to fight drug counterfeiting. Similarly, a proof-of-concept application has been developed by Jamil et al. [45]. This platform consists of a web application whose role is to monitor drug files between doctors, patients, pharmacists, etc. in a decentralized manner. The smart contracts guarantee the confidentiality, security, and transparency of the management process and the sharing of the drug life cycle.

10.3.4 CLINICAL TRIAL CERTIFICATION

In order to develop medical and biological insights, a biomedical research called a clinical trial is done on humans. The objective of these clinical trials is to develop and verify a series of data. They allow, but are not limited to, demonstrating the efficacy, relevance, and safety of a drug in relation to a disease. Indeed, the objective of these studies is to demonstrate a causality between the favorable evolution of a disease and the taking of a specific treatment.

The characteristics of blockchain technology allow it to play a prominent role in the certification of clinical trials. Indeed, blockchain could be used to ensure that data is collected and exchanged, when necessary, while respecting patient privacy or proprietary information. The use of this technology allows one to save the results found as well as the data and reports from the clinical research in an immutable way. This property overcomes the problems of changing results, thus reducing the incidence of fraud and error in clinical trial records. Blockchain brings transparency to clinical trials. Also, the pharmaceutical industry could use blockchain to authenticate clinical trial results.

Several studies have exploited blockchain in clinical research to avoid undesirable consequences of drug use [46–48]. The characteristics of blockchain, notably its immutability, transparency, and decentralization, encourage the development of platforms and systems for collecting and sharing patient data in clinical trials [49,50].

The authors of [51, 52] use the Ethereum blockchain platform and smart contracts. The results found to support the transparency of the data and documents retrieved during clinical research. In the same context, the use of smart contracts and blockchain, Zhuang et al. [53,54] presented an automatic and secure validation system for unmediated clinical trials via distributed databases. The traceability of these data is ensured via the proof of concept and blockchain protocol [47].

In summary, blockchain technology is applied in various sectors of healthcare as shown in Table 10.1. Its adoption allows the advancement of biomedical/health research. For the management of patient medical records, it stores these records on a distributed registry of an authorized blockchain. For the management of patient medical records, it stores these records on a distributed registry of an authorized blockchain, thereby ensuring the integrity of data in the various stages of processing, without human intervention. The DLT conducts a decentralized database containing all the information needed during the research. Researchers can access and manipulate medical data in complete security. The Blockchain, having the particularity of being immutable, facilitates the detection of fraud by prohibiting any duplication or modification in the transaction, and finally allows a transparent and secure transaction. To prevent drug counterfeiting, the Blockchain, thanks to its detailed tracing power, monitors every step of the pharmaceutical supply chain. It controls the origin of the drug, its components, and its owner.

10.4 CONCLUSION

This chapter presents a state of the art on the impact of blockchain technology in the healthcare sector. The most relevant applications in this area are electronic patient record sharing, and pharmaceutical tracking, clinical trial, and security in healthcare. Blockchain brings security, integrity, and transparency to the healthcare field. Despite the promising offers of blockchain in terms of confidentiality and efficiency, there is a lack of realization of solutions proposed by researchers. It is, therefore, necessary to carry out an important upstream work of data digitization, process automation, staff education, and regulatory supervision.

REFERENCES

1. C. Bahhar, C. Baccouche, S. Ben Othman and H. Sakli, "Real-time intelligent monitoring system based on IoT", In: 2021 18th International Multi-Conference on Systems, Signals & Devices (SSD), 2021, pp. 93–96, Doi: 10.1109/SSD52085.2021.9429358.
2. A. Zouinkhi, H. Ayadi, T. Val, B. Boussaid and M.N. Abdelkrim, "Auto-management of energy in IoT networks", *Int J Commun Syst*, Vol. 33, p. e4168, 2020. Doi: 10.1002/dac.4168.
3. T. Malcheand P. Maheshwary, "Internet of Things (IoT) for building smart home system", In: Proceedings of the 2017 International Conference on I-SMAC (IoT in Social, Mobile, Analytics and Cloud) (I-SMAC), Palladam, India, 10–11 February 2017, pp. 65–70. New York: IEEE.
4. L. Minbo, Z. Zhu and C. Guangyu, "Information service system of agriculture IoT", *Automatika*, Vol. 54, No. 4, pp. 415–426, 2013.
5. G. George and S.M. Thampi, "Securing smart healthcare systems from vulnerability exploitation", In: Wang G., El Saddik A., Lai X., Mart inez Perez G. and Choo KK. (eds) *Smart City and Informatization.iSCI 2019. Communications in Computer and Information Science*, vol 1122. Springer, Singapore. https://doi.org/10.1007/978-981-15-1301-5_24
6. F.A. Almalki, S.B. Othman, F.A. Almalki and H. Sakli, "EERP-DPM: energy efficient routing protocol using dual prediction model for healthcare using IoT", *Journal of Healthcare Engineering*, vol. 2021, Article ID 9988038, 15 p, 2021.
7. Faris A. Almalki, Ben Othman Soufiene, "EPPDA: An Efficient and Privacy-Preserving Data Aggregation Scheme with Authentication and Authorization for IoT-Based Healthcare Applications", *Wireless Communications and Mobile Computing*, vol. 2021, Article ID 5594159, 18 pages, 2021. https://doi.org/10.1155/2021/5594159.
8. S. Trab, E. Bajic, A. Zouinkhi, Abdelkrim, M.N. and H. Chekir, "RFID IoT-enabled warehouse for safety management using product class-based storage and potential fields methods", *International Journal of Embedded Systems*, Vol. 10, No. 1, pp. 71–88, 2018.
9. A.H. Mohd Aman, et al, "IoMT amid COVID-19 pandemic: application, architecture, technology, and security", *Journal of Network and Computer Applications*, Vol. 174, 2021. https://doi.org/10.1016/j.jnca.2020.102886.
10. S. Nakamoto, "Bitcoin: a peer-to-peer electronic cash system", (2008) Available at: https://bitcoin.org/bitcoin.pdf.
11. B. Bhushan, C. Sahoo, P. Sinha and A. Khamparia. "Unification of blockchain and Internet of Things (BIoT): requirements, working model, challenges and future directions", *Wireless Networks*, 2020. Doi: 10.1007/s11276-020-02445-6.
12. B. Bhushan, P. Sinha, K.M. Sagayam and J. Andrew. (2021). "Untangling blockchain technology: A survey on state of the art, security threats, privacy services, applications and future research directions", *Computers & Electrical Engineering*, 90, p. 106897. Doi: 10.1016/j.compeleceng.2020.106897.
13. S. Saxena, B. Bhushan and M.A. Ahad. "Blockchain based solutions to secure IoT: background, integration trends and a way forward", *Journal of Network and Computer Applications*, 2021, p. 103050. Doi: 10.1016/j.jnca.2021.10305.

14. A.K. Haque, B. Bhushan and G. Dhiman. "Conceptualizing smart city applications: Requirements, architecture, security issues, and emerging trends", *Expert Systems*, 2021. Doi: 10.1111/exsy.12753.

15. A. Kumar, K. Abhishek, B. Bhushan and C. Chakraborty. "Secure access control for manufacturing sector with application of ethereum blockchain", *Peer-to-Peer Networking and Applications*, 2021. Doi: 10.1007/s12083-021-01108-3.

16. D. Hong-Ning, Z. Zibin and Y. Zhang, "Blockchain for Internet of Things: a survey", *IEEE Internet of Things Journal*, Vol. 6, No. 5, Oct. 2019.

17. R. Ramaguru, M. Sindhu, and M. Sethumadhavan, "Blockchain for the Internet of Vehicles", In: Singh M., Gupta P., Tyagi V., Flusser J., Ören T., Kashyap R. (eds) *Advances in Computing and Data Sciences. ICACDS 2019. Communications in Computer and Information Science*, Vol 1045. Springer, Singapore.

18. H. Mhamdi, A. Zouinkhi and H. Sakli, "Multi-agents system of vehicle services based on blockchain", In: 20th International Conference on Sciences and Techniques of Automatic Control and Computer Engineering (STA), Monastir, Tunisia, 2020, pp. 291–296.

19. P. Tasca and C.J. Tessone, "A taxonomy of blockchain technologies: principles of identification and classification", *Ledger*, 4. Doi: 10.5195/ledger.2019.140.

20. D. Hong-Ning, Z. Zibin and Y. Zhang, "Blockchain for Internet of Things: a survey", *IEEE Internet of Things Journal*, Vol. 6, No. 5, Oct. 2019, pp. 8076-8094, Oct. 2019, doi: 10.1109/JIOT.2019.2920987.

21. N. Szabo, "Smart contracts: formalizing and securing relationships on public networks", *First Monday*, Vol. 2, No. 9-1, Sep. 1997, https://doi.org/10.5210/fm.v2i9.548

22. S. Wang, Y. Yuan, X. Wang, J. Li, R. Qin and F. -Y. Wang, "An Overview of Smart Contract: Architecture, Applications, and Future Trends," 2018 IEEE Intelligent Vehicles Symposium (IV), 2018, pp. 108-113, doi: 10.1109/IVS.2018.8500488.

23. I. Riabi, H. K. B. Ayed and L. A. Saidane, "A survey on blockchain based access control for Internet of Things", In: *15th International Wireless Communications & Mobile Computing Conference (IWCMC)*, Tangier, Morocco, 2019, pp. 502–507.

24. Othman, S.B., Bahattab, A.A., Trad, A. et al. Confidentiality and Integrity for Data Aggregation in WSN Using Homomorphic Encryption. *Wireless Pers Commun* 80, 867–889 (2015). https://doi.org/10.1007/s11277-014-2061-z

25. R. Jabbar, N. Fetais, M. Krichen and K. Barkaoui, "Blockchain technology for healthcare: enhancing shared electronic health record interoperability and integrity", In: *2020 IEEE* International Conference on Informatics, IoT, and Enabling Technologies (ICIoT), Doha, Qatar ,2020, pp. 310–317.

26. S. Bingqing, J. Guo, and Y. Yang. "MedChain: efficient healthcare data sharing via blockchain", *Applied Sciences*, Vol. 9, No. 6, p. 1207, 2019.

27. A. Azaria, A. Ekblaw, T. Vieira and A. Lippman, "MedRec: using blockchain for medical data access and permission management", In: 2016 2nd International Conference on Open and Big Data (OBD), Vienna, Austria, 2016, pp. 25–30.

28. Y. Yang et al., "Medshare: a novel hybrid cloud for medical resource sharing among autonomous healthcare providers", *IEEE Access*, Vol. 6, pp. 46949–46961, 2018.

29. K. Fan, et al. "Medblock: efficient and secure medical data sharing via blockchain", *Journal of Medical Systems,* Vol. 42, No. 8, p. 136, 2018.

30. K. Syeda, et al, "Trusted Remote Patient Monitoring using Blockchain-based Smart Contracts", Springer Nature Switzerland AG 2020 L. Barolli et al. (Eds.): BWCCA 2019, LNNS 97, pp. 765–776, 2020.

31. A. Ullah Khan, et al, "*Enhanced Decentralized Management of Patient-Driven Interoperability Based on Blockchain*", Springer Nature Switzerland AG 2020. L. Barolli et al. (Eds.): BWCCA 2019, LNNS 97, pp. 815–827, 2020.

32. A. Khatoon. "A blockchain-based smart contract system for healthcare management", *Electronics* Vol. 9, p. 94, 2020.
33. A.F. Hussein, N. ArunKumar, G. Ramirez-Gonzalez, E. Abdulhay, J.M.R.S. Tavares and V.H.C. de Albuquerque. "A medical records managing and securing blockchain based system supported by a genetic algorithm and discrete wavelet transform", *Cognitive Systems Research*, Vol. 52, pp. 1–11, 2018.
34. B. O. Soufiene, A. A. Bahattab, A. Trad, and H. Youssef. "Lightweight and confidential data aggregation in healthcare wireless sensor networks", *Trans. Emerging Tel. Tech.*, Vol. 27, pp. 576–588, 2016. doi: 10.1002/ett.2993.
35. H. Zhao, Y. Zhang, Y. Peng and R. Xu. "Lightweight backup and efficient recovery scheme for health blockchain keys", In: Proceedings of the 2017 IEEE 13th International Symposium on Autonomous Decentralized System (ISADS), Bangkok, Thailand, 22–24 March 2017, pp. 229–234.
36. X. Zhang and S. Poslad, "Blockchain Support for Flexible Queries with Granular Access Control to Electronic Medical Records (EMR)", 2018 IEEE International Conference on Communications (ICC), 2018, pp. 1–6, doi: 10.1109/ICC.2018.8422883.
37. R. Guo, H. Shi, Q. Zhao and D. Zheng, "Secure attribute-based signature scheme with multiple authorities for blockchain in electronic health records systems", *IEEE Access*, Vol. 6, pp. 11676–11686, 2018, Doi: 10.1109/ACCESS.2018.2801266.
38. A. Al Omar, M.S. Rahman, A. Basu and S. Kiyomoto. "MediBchain: a blockchain based privacy preserving platform for healthcare data", In: Wang G., Atiquzzaman M., Yan Z., Choo KK. (eds) *Security, Privacy, and Anonymity in Computation, Communication, and Storage. SpaCCS 2017. Lecture Notes in Computer Science*, Vol. 10658. Springer, Cham, 2017. Doi: 10.1007/978-3-319-72395-2_49.
39. X. Yue, et al. "Healthcare data gateways: found healthcare intelligence on blockchain with novel privacy risk control", *Journal of Medical Systems*, Vol. 40, p. 218, 2016. Doi: 10.1007/s10916-016-0574-6.
40. B.O Soufiene, A.A. Bahattab, A. Trad and H. Youssef. "RESDA: robust and efficient secure data aggregation scheme in healthcare using the IoT", In: *The International Conference on* Internet of Things, Embedded Systems and Communications (IINTEC 2019), HAMMAMET, Tunisia from 20–22 December 2019.
41. A. Clauson, A. Breeden, C. Davidson, K. Mackey, "Leveraging blockchain technology to enhance supply chain management in healthcare: an exploration of challenges and opportunities in the health supply chain", *Blockchain in Healthcare Today*™ ISSN 2573-8240 online Doi: 10.30953/bhty.v1.20.
42. S.B. Othman, A.A. Bahattab, A. Trad and H. Youssef, "PEERP: an priority-based energy-efficient routing protocol for reliable data transmission in Healthcare using the IoT", In: *The 15th International Conference on Future Networks and Communications (FNC)*, Leuven, Belgium, August 9–12, 2020.
43. R. Casado-Vara, A. González-Briones, J. Prieto, and J.M. Corchado. Smart Contract for Monitoring and Control of Logistics Activities: Pharmaceutical Utilities Case Study. In: Graña M. et al. (eds) International Joint Conference SOCO'18-CISIS'-18-ICEUTE'18. SOCO'18-CISIS'18-ICEUTE'18 2018. Advances in Intelligent Systems and Computing, vol 771. Springer, Cham. https://doi.org/10.1007/978-3-319-94120-2_49. 2019.
44. R. Raj, N. Rai and S. Agarwal, "Anticounterfeiting in Pharmaceutical Supply Chain by establishing Proof of Ownership," TENCON 2019 – 2019 IEEE Region 10 Conference (TENCON), 2019, pp. 1572–1577, doi: 10.1109/TENCON.2019.8929271.
45. F. Jamil, L. Hang, K. Kim and D. Kim, "A novel medical blockchain model for drug supply chain integrity management in a smart hospital", *Electronics* Vol. 8, No. 5, p. 505, 2019.

46. M. Benchoufi, R. Porcher, and P. Ravaud. Blockchain protocols in clinical trials: Transparency and traceability of consent. F1000Res. 2017 Jan 23; 6:66. doi: 10.12688/f1000research.10531.5. PMID: 29167732; PMCID: PMC5676196.
47. M. Benchoufi and P. Ravaud. "Blockchain technology for improving clinical research quality", *Trials* Vol. 18, p. 335, 2017.
48. I. Radanović and R. Likić. "Opportunities for use of blockchain technology in medicine", *Applied Health Economics and Health Policy*, Vol. 16, pp. 583–590, 2018. Doi: 10.1007/s40258-018-0412-8.
49. M.A. Engelhardt. "Hitching healthcare to the chain: an introduction to blockchain technology in the healthcare sector", *Technology Innovation Management Review*, Vol. 7, pp. 22–34, 2017.
50. J.M. Roman-Belmonte, H. De la Corte-Rodriguez, E.C.C. Rodriguez-Merchan, H. la Corte-Rodriguez and E. Carlos Rodriguez-Merchan. "How blockchain technology can change medicine", *Postgraduate Medical Journal*, Vol. 130, pp. 420–427, 2018.
51. S.B. Othman, A. Ali Bahattab, A. Trad and H. Youssef. "LSDA: lightweight secure data aggregation scheme in healthcare using IoT", In: *ACM -10th International Conference on Information Systems and Technologies*, Lecce, Italy. June 2020.
52. P. Mytis-Gkometh, P.S. Efraimidis, E. Kaldoudi and G. Drosatos. "Notarization of knowledge retrieval from biomedical repositories using blockchain technology", In: *IFMBE Proceedings*; Springer Nature: Basingstoke, UK, Vol. 66, 2017, pp. 69–73.
53. Y. Zhuang, L.R. Sheets, Z. Shae, Y.W. Chen, J.J.P. Tsai and C.R. Shyu. "Applying blockchain technology to enhance clinical trial recruitment", In: *AMIA Annual Symposium Proceedings AMIA Symposium*, 2019, pp. 1276–85.
54. Y. Zhuang, L. Sheets, X. Gao, Y. Shen, Z.Y. Shae, J.J.P. Tsai and C.R. Shyu. "Development of a blockchain framework for virtual clinical trials", In: *AMIA Annual Symposium Proceedings*, 2021 Jan 25, 2020, pp. 1412–1420, PMID: 33936517; PMCID: PMC8075489.

11 Blockchain for IoT-Based Healthcare
Overview of Security and Privacy Issues

Ben Othman Soufiene
Prince Laboratory Research

Faris. A. Almalki
Taif University

Hedi Sakli
University of Gabes
EITA Consulting

CONTENTS

11.1 INTRODUCTION

In recent years, the coming out of the Internet of Things (IoT) has taken a significant impact on science and technology [1]. The IoT is defined as a network of identifiable and unique elements that communicate without human interaction using IP connectivity [1]. These items can perceive, control, analyze, and make decisions independently, as well as in collaboration with other objects [2]. At the end of 2019, there were around 9.5 billion connected IoT devices, according to IoT Analytics estimates [3]. The concept of the IoT is evolving exponentially and covering more and more domains every day [4]. It will change the way we live and work by making different aspects of life smart. Through the development of new applications in fields such as smart homes, smart health, smart cities, industry 4.0, Wireless Sensor Networks (WSN), smart agriculture, and others, IoT has the potential to introduce and establish a smart world [5]. The interested reader is referred to [1–20] for a deeper understanding of the IoT.

Healthcare 4.0 is a combination between the IoT and modern Information and Communication Technologies [6]. The Smart health plays an important role in health applications by integrating sensors and actuators into patients' bodies for monitoring and follow-up. The global IoT medical device market is expected to grow at a compound annual growth rate of 4.5%, reaching $409.5 billion in 2025 [7]. The IoT is used in healthcare to monitor the physiological status of patients. On-board sensors can collect information directly from the patient's body and transmit it to the physician. These collected information can be stored, processed, and make it available to doctors to give a consultation at any time and from any devices that are connected to the Internet (e.g., Smartphone or Tablet) [8–15]. Further, the doctor is alerted in real time of any sudden change concerning the condition of his patient, as well as take actions like advising patients, and interrogate the sensors to have the current values. This technology can fully isolate the patient from the hospital's centralized system while yet allowing them to communicate with their physician. A remote medical surveillance system employing IoT is depicted in Figure 11.1.

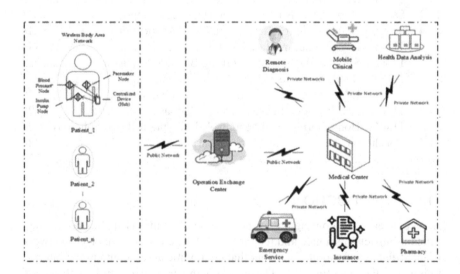

FIGURE 11.1   IoT-based healthcare monitoring architecture.

The IoT deploys a very large number of small intelligent devices to collect detailed information about the environment [10]. Despite miniaturization and reducing the manufacturing cost, these devices generally have limited resources in terms of power transmission, data processing, bandwidth, storage capacity, and energy. However, the transmission and reception operations consume a large part of the energy of the node devices [11]. Unsurprisingly, when it comes to evaluate the performance of a sensor network, service life is probably the most important metric, especially since the most low-power devices have a limited lifetime, besides continuous battery replacement of thousands of these devices deployed in areas with difficult access is often impractical and even impossible [12]. Therefore, energy consumption is a key challenge in sensors. To this end, several approaches have been proposed to conserve the energy resource at the sensory level and overcome the challenges inherent in its limitation [13].

Many other issues have been explored in relation to IoT, one of the most significant is the security issue [14]. The existence of a huge network with a big number of interconnected devices will almost certainly suggest a variety of attack and eavesdropping scenarios that could endanger those entities and their users [15]. The threat posed by these Internet-connected Things affects not only IoT systems, but the entire ecosystem, including websites, applications, social networks, and servers. In the healthcare application using IoT, we add more devices to our clothes and bodies, more personal information will be collected. As the number of IoT devices grows at an exponential rate, so do the technological and security challenges [16]. For example, an attack may rationally modify a drug dose that would kill or have catastrophic health consequences for a certain patient. Furthermore, the healthcare devices can be remotely exploited through the many communications medium (e.g., Wi-Fi, Zigbee, Bluetooth, 6LowPAN, and NFC). The attackers can easily eavesdrop on the communication channel in this instance and obtain the transmitted data [17]. It is critical to develop new security frameworks that prevent hostile or unauthorized objects from getting access to IoT systems, reading, or altering the data collected [18].

The purpose of this chapter is to review the current literature on the challenges and approaches to security and privacy in IoT-based healthcare applications. To demystify the roots of dangers in IoT, we introduce and categorize the IoT security threat categories as well as defense techniques in order to provide the reader with the security necessary background for a better understanding of this area. We present taxonomy of IoT attacks as well as an analysis of IoT security concerns at various tiers. We also give security requirements taxonomy depending on the goals of the assaults. Then, we present the solutions to increase IoT security. The remainder of this paper is organized as follows: We give a full taxonomy of current security and privacy attacks on healthcare systems in Section 11.2. The security needs a taxonomy of healthcare systems, which is provided in the next section. In Section 11.4, we look at some of the existing ways to secure healthcare systems that have been offered by researchers. Finally, we conclude the paper in Section 11.5.

11.2 THE SECURITY ATTACKS IN IOT-BASED HEALTHCARE APPLICATIONS

As mentioned previously, the present healthcare equipment and applications do not meet security and privacy standards. The attackers can use many components of healthcare systems to carry out unwanted operations [19]. To carefully incorporate security needs into IoT systems, it is first required to investigate IoT vulnerabilities and attacks. An attack is an attempt to break an encryption scheme, and a successful attack implies that the security of the data encrypted under this scheme has been compromised [20]. In this section, we discuss several types of attacks on different parts of healthcare systems (e.g., sensor, device, and network) and how attackers can undermine the security and privacy of targeted healthcare systems. A detailed summary is given in Table 11.1

11.3 SECURITY REQUIREMENTS IN IOT-BASED HEALTHCARE APPLICATIONS

We divide IoT security requirements into three categories based on the aims of IoT attacks shown in Section 11.2: data security, communication security, and device security. Table 11.2 summarizes the security requirements.

11.4 SECURITY SOLUTIONS IN IOT-BASED HEALTHCARE APPLICATIONS

One of the hottest study topics in healthcare system-based IoT is security, which has drawn many researchers from academia, business, and standardization bodies. There has been a slew of solutions aimed at addressing IoT security issues to date. To improve IoT security, several new technologies and methodologies were presented. In the following subsections, we discuss different existing security measures for healthcare systems by categorizing into six broad categories, including Fog Computing, Software-defined Networking, Blockchain, Lightweight Cryptography, Homomorphic and Searchable Encryption, and Machine Learning.

11.4.1 Fog Computing-Based Solutions

Fog computing has been introduced as a new paradigm for extending Cloud computing's processing resources. At the network's edge, it provides storage, processing, and networking/communication [20]. Fog computing is made up of fog nodes that are placed near IoT devices and connected to a cloud server. Because IoT devices have limited resources, fog nodes can help protect IoT settings by providing authentication, privacy preservation, and encryption. Several security schemes to protect healthcare system-based IoT using fog computing are available in the literature. A state-of-the-art review is outlined in this subsection. Hassen et al. [21] proposed a home hospitalization system by combining IoT applications like fog computing and cloud computing. The goal of the study was to propose a

TABLE 11.1
The Security Attacks for IoT-Based Healthcare

Attacks	Description	Security goals	Target Layers	PA	AA	IA	EA	HA	SA
Sybil attack [21]	Sybil attack is the generation of multiple fake identities by a malicious device.	Authentication Privacy	Multi-layer		✓		✓		
DoS attack [22]	DoS attacker can break down the network and block exchanging messages between devices.	Authentication Availability Confidentiality Integrity	Multi-layer		✓	✓			
DDos attack [20]	This attack oversends requests or messages to the target node with the intention to make this node busy and disable it.	Authentication Availability Confidentiality Integrity	Multi-layer		✓	✓			
MITM attack [21]	MITM attacker eavesdrops to the communication between legitimate devices. It behaves like one of them to reply to the other with false information.	Confidentiality Integrity Non-repudiation	Transport-Layer		✓	✓			
Black hole attack [23]	The Black Hole Attack is a kind of denial of service, in which the attacker drops all the data packets.	Authentication Availability Confidentiality Integrity	Network layer		✓	✓			
Wormhole attack [23]	In this attack, two or more malicious devices linked by a low-latency communication channel form a tunnel to transfer packets. Data gathered by attackers will be sent to the other end of the wormhole to influence devices existing close to these tunneled nodes.	Authentication Availability Confidentiality Integrity	Network layer	✓	✓				

(Continued)

TABLE 11.1 (Continued)
The Security Attacks for IoT-Based Healthcare

Attacks	Description	Security goals	Target Layers	PA	AA	IA	EA	HA	SA
				\multicolumn{6}{Attack Types}					
Gray hole attack [25]	The gray hole attack can be defined as a particular variation of the black hole attack with unpredictable behavior.	Authentication Availability Confidentiality Integrity	Network layer		✓		✓		
Spoofing attack [22]	An attacker uses spoofing to provide fake information about the location of nodes.	Authentication Privacy	Physical layer	✓					
Timing attack [21]	Through Timing attack, malicious node adds additional time to receive message to delay it. Therefore, messages will not be distributed at the normal time which makes them useless.	Integrity			✓				
Jamming attack [24]	Jamming attack is a type of DOS attack in which a malicious node generates a noise to interfere with the radio frequencies used by devices.	Availability	Physical layer		✓		✓		
Replay attack [21]	Replay attack, also known as playback attack, consists of replaying the transmission of old valid messages and injecting them into the network.	Authentication Integrity Non-repudiation	Multi-layer		✓				
Masquerading attack [23]	In this attack, a spiteful node is hidden using a spoofing identity and produces false messages in the network.	Authentication Non-repudiation	Multi-layer		✓				
Illusion attack [19]	The malicious node transmits false traffic warning messages to its neighbors. Normal devices will follow the fake traffic messages received which changes their behaviors and causes illusion in the network.	Authentication Integrity	Applications layer				✓		

(Continued)

TABLE 11.1 (*Continued*)
The Security Attacks for IoT-Based Healthcare

Attacks	Description	Security goals	Target Layers	Attack Types					
				PA	AA	IA	EA	HA	SA
Social attack [17]	The main idea of social attack is to alter the behavior of normal devices in the network using immoral messages.	Authentication Integrity	Network layer		✓	✓			
Spamming attack [21]	Consuming the network bandwidth and increasing the transmission latency in the network are the principal aims of the spamming attack.	Authentication Availability Confidentiality Integrity	Network layer			✓			
Malware attack [24]	The Malware attack is software produced to gain access or damage the network.	Availability Confidentiality	Network layer		✓	✓			✓
Eavesdrop attack [21]	Eavesdrop attack is an attack, which threatens confidentiality in IoT aimed to get unauthorized access to obtain confidential information which must be inaccessible to malicious nodes.	Confidentiality	Physical layer	✓					

AA, Active Attacks; EA, External Attackers; HA, Hardware Attacks; IA, Internal Attackers; PA, Passive Attacks; SA, Software Attacks.

TABLE 11.2

The Security Requirements for IoT-Based Healthcare

Features		Description
Data security	Confidentiality [3]	Only authorized persons or entities should have access to device information, system settings, and healthcare data. Before accessing any healthcare-related confidential information, these entities must be authorized. However, existing healthcare devices, such as an insulin pump communication route, can be eavesdropped on to obtain patient data and device-related information.
	Integrity [4]	Integrity is achieved when exchanged messages are protected against unauthorized modifications. It is a process of transmitting data from devices, applications, or infrastructure in a secure manner without the falsification of the original data.
	Privacy [6]	The concealing of personal information as well as the power to control what occurs with it are all examples of privacy. During data collection, transmission, and storage, data privacy must be considered. Many practical solutions to the problem of data privacy have been offered. Anonymization-based solutions, pseudo-random number generators, block ciphers, and stream ciphers are examples of these techniques.
Communication security	Authentication [8]	The authentication is the mechanism of verifying whether someone or something is who (or what) it is declared for allowing access to resources in an information system that prevents unauthorized access to a program, system, network, or device, only authenticated peers can participate in the process. There are two kinds of authentication mechanism which are Node authentication for whose has a right of accessing into network information and Message authentication to guarantee its integrity and privacy by authenticating it.
	Access control [12]	Access control is a security element that checks whether people and systems have permission to perform operations on other systems and resources. The access control algorithms are divided into five distinct types: role-based, organization-based, capability-based, attribute-based, and trust-based algorithms.
	Non-repudiation [4]	Different procedures are performed by a healthcare system, and this procedure is normally kept private in an access log. Any changes to this log should be traced and monitored, and only confirmed users should make them. To hide their tracks, the attackers may seek to remove these logs. Many resource-constrained medical equipment does not have a log in place, and attackers may try to gain access to the system without leaving any traces.
Device security	Trust [8]	The process of making decisions about communicating with unknown entities is known as trust management. In order to secure an IoT system, it is required to engage with trusted IoT devices to prevent rogue nodes from doing undesirable actions. There are two types of trust management techniques: deterministic trust and non-deterministic trust.
	Availability [16]	In normal and emergency scenarios, the healthcare system's service should always be available to authorized users for accessing device systems and patient data. In the availability network, the information shall be available 24 by 7 to the authentic users for preventing several attacks in the network.

smart-based model for usage in the healthcare system during a coronavirus pandemic. Pham et al. [23] conducted another study to build the "Cloudbased smart home environment (CoSHE)", which aided in the health assessment and monitoring of patients in order to provide them with healthcare at home. Tuli et al. [24] aimed to investigate the utility of fog computing systems for the development of a framework called Health fog for deep learning and real-time analysis of heart disorders. The study was effective in developing the Health Fog model's system architecture in conjunction with the IoT system. Table 11.3 summarizes these several works.

11.4.2 SOFTWARE DEFINED NETWORKING-BASED SOLUTIONS

Because of the programmability and intelligence, it has put into the network, Software Defined Networking (SDN) is a new paradigm that has transformed the world of networking. Correspondingly, in an SDN-based network, there exist a data plane, a control plane, and a monitoring plane [26]. Each of these functional planes has its unique challenge in reducing or protecting their corresponding resources. Software-defined networking enables healthcare organizations to take advantage of virtualization, resulting in increased network agility and lower total cost of ownership. As a result of its design, SDN provides security advantages [27]. Because the SDN controller can see all network data at the same time, it is easier to spot unexpected behavior in network traffic created by an intruder. Once a new danger has been identified, operators can instantly design new software to assess and address the vulnerability, rather than waiting for an operating system or application software update for manufacturer-proprietary devices. Several security schemes to protect healthcare system-based IoT using Software Defined Networking are available in the literature. In IoT applications, the SDN can be an excellent solution for key management [28], identity management, authentication, confidentiality, and intrusion detection. The authors demonstrated an OpenFlow SDN architecture for IoT devices in [29]. The suggested architecture incorporates IoT gateways that are managed to detect assaults and anomalies in order to figure out which devices are malfunctioning and which nodes in the network are affected. Aydeger et al. in [30] proposed an MTD (Moving Target Defense) mechanism based on SDN for defending against specific DDoS attacks known as Crossfire. Table 11.3 summarizes these several works.

11.4.3 BLOCKCHAIN-BASED SOLUTIONS

Many other issues have been explored in relation to IoT, one of the most significant is the security issue. The existence of a huge network with a big number of interconnected devices will almost certainly suggest a variety of attack and eavesdropping scenarios that could endanger those entities and their users. As previously stated, typical security measures cannot be directly applied to IoT devices due to their physical constraints in terms of processing and storage. Furthermore, mutual authentication and authorization between the device/user and the IoT

TABLE 11.3

Comparison of Some IoT Security Solutions

Solutions (References)	Challenges						
	Computation	Communication	Memory	Mobility	Heterogeneity	Scalability	QoS
Fog computing							
[20]	+	−	+	+	−	−	−
[21]	‡	+	+	−	+	−	+
[22]	‡	‡	‡	−	−	+	+
[23]	+	−	−	+	+	+	−
[24]	+	−	+	+	−	+	+
[25]	‡	+	‡	¦	+	−	+
SDN							
[26]	+	+	+	+	−	−	+
[27]	+	+	+	−	+	+	−
[28]	‡	−	−	+	−	−	+
[29]	‡	¦	−	−	+	+	−
[30]	+	‡	+	−	−	+	+
[31]	+	‡	+	+	−	+	+
[32]	‡	+	+	‡	−	−	‡
Blockchain							
[33]	+	‡	‡	−	−	¦	+
[34]	+	‡	+	−	+	−	−
[35]	‡	−	+	+	−	−	+
[36]	‡	¦	+	−	−	−	−
[37]	‡	‡	+	‡	¦	+	+

(Continued)

TABLE 11.3 (Continued)
Comparison of Some IoT Security Solutions

Solutions (References)		Computation	Communication	Memory	Mobility	Heterogeneity	Scalability	QoS
					Challenges			
Lightweight cryptography	[3]	+	++	-	+	-	-	+
	[4]	+	+	+	+	-	+	-
	[6]	+	++	-	+	+	-	+
	[8]	++	+	+	+	+	+	-
	[11]	++	+	+	+	+	-	+
	[12]	++	+	-	++	+	-	-
Machine learning	[38]	++	++	+	+	-	-	+
	[39]	++	-	-	+	-	+	-
	[40]	+	-	+	+	+	-	-
	[41]	++	++	-	+	-	+	+
	[42]	++	+	+	-	+	+	-
	[43]	++	+	+	++	+	-	-
HE and SE	[44]	+	+	+	-	+	+	+
	[45]	+	-	-	+	-	-	-
	[46]	+	-	+	+	++	+	-
	[47]	++	+	+	+	-	-	+
	[48]	+	-	-	-	+	+	-
	[49]	++	+	+	-	+	-	+

++Good; +Average; –Poor (limited) and ––Bad.

system must be performed in line with preset security regulations before a device or user can access IoT services. The proposed security measures, on the other hand, must consider the restricted resources of IoT devices. The major issues can be solved by blockchain technology [32]. Researchers are increasingly turning to blockchain-based security frameworks to protect healthcare data from unauthorized parties. To ensure the security of communication in IoT-based healthcare applications, the authors in [31] present an effective multilayer authentication protocol and a secure session key generation mechanism for wireless body area networks (WBANs). In [32], the authors have proposed a medical data storage scheme based on blockchain technology in order to ensure the secure storage and sharing of personal medical data. To enable safe communication in healthcare applications, Deebak et al. [33] proposed a Secure and Anonymous Biometric Based User Authentication Scheme (SAB-UAS) based on ECC and cryptographic hash function. Table 11.3 summarizes these several works.

11.4.4 LIGHTWEIGHT CRYPTOGRAPHY-BASED SOLUTIONS

Cryptographic solutions are all the security services that cryptography gave. Cryptography awards various security techniques and can provide confidentiality, authentication, and integrity and many other benefits in the healthcare application using IoT. To achieve these security services, cryptography uses different methods such as encryption/decryption method, Keys generation method, hash functions [3], and digital signature. The lightweight cryptographic techniques can be adopted to achieve key security requirements including confidentiality, integrity, and authentication [4]. Many approaches based on Cryptography were built to detect and block attacks in the healthcare application using IoT. In [6], the authors proposed a framework named MADAR against Dos attack. Madar can resist Dos attack that effects the communication using the combination of ID-based signature schemes and self-generated pseudonym. It can also detect Dos attack, which attacks the communication based on the use of the strength-alterable message-specific puzzle. Kiho et al. [8] introduced a key management protocol based on group signature to ensure authentication in protecting healthcare system-based IoT. Utilizing this concept, the devices having the same group of signatures can securely communicate. The authors in [10] used the hash function to build a HCPA-GKA scheme for healthcare system-based IoT. The group key management mechanism distribution for devices is done through the Chinese Remainder Theorem (CRT). IT can be updated when a device accedes and quits the group. Table 11.3 summarizes these several works.

11.4.5 ARTIFICIAL INTELLIGENCE-BASED SOLUTIONS

Machine learning (ML) is a data analytics technology that allows healthcare systems to learn from data and perform specific tasks like anomaly detection, behavior analysis, and more. There are two main kinds of ML: supervised and unsupervised learning. Supervised learning occurs when humans manually categorize training data as harmful or genuine, and then feed that data into an algorithm to develop a model with "classes" of data against which the traffic being analyzed is compared [38]. Unsupervised learning avoids the use of training data and manual labeling in favor of grouping comparable pieces of data into classes and then classifying them based on data coherence within each class and data modularity between classes [39]. ML is used to create complicated algorithms that defend networks and systems, including IoT devices. The research community has investigated ML techniques to detect assaults on healthcare systems [40]. A decision tree approach was utilized by Saeedi et al. to detect malicious assaults in healthcare devices in [41]. Vhaduri et al. used support vector machine (SVM) characteristics to detect the illegal access to a healthcare device and its acquired data using multiple physiological and behavioral indicators such as calorie burn, average step counts, and minute heart rate [42]. HealthGuard, an ML-based security framework presented by Newaz et al. to detect hostile behaviors in a connected healthcare system [43]. HealthGuard collects vital signs from various healthcare equipment and applies ML algorithms to connect changes in the patient's biological processes in order to discern between benign and malignant activity. Table 11.3 summarizes these several works.

11.4.6 Homomorphic and Searchable Encryption-Based Solutions

The advances in technology have now made it possible to monitor heart rate, body temperature, and sleep patterns; continuously track movement; record brain activity using IoT devices. Classical encryption techniques have been used very successfully to protect data in transit and in storage [44]. However, the process of encrypting data also renders it unusable in computation. Recently developed Fully Homomorphic Encryption (FHE) techniques improve on this substantially. Unlike classical methods, which require the data to be decrypted prior to computation, homomorphic methods allow data to be simultaneously stored or transferred securely and used in computation [45]. However, FHE imposes serious constraints on computation, both arithmetic (e.g., no divisions can be performed) and computational (e.g., multiplications become much slower), rendering traditional statistical algorithms inadequate. Secure search over encrypted data stored on a cloud server is possible using searchable encryption (SE). Asymmetric SE, symmetric SE, and attribute-based SE are examples of SE techniques [46]. Several security schemes to protect healthcare system-based IoT using homomorphic encryption and SE are available in the literature. Almalki et al. [8] propose EPPDA: An Efficient and Privacy-Preserving Data Aggregation Scheme with authentication for IoT-based healthcare applications. EPPDA verifies data integrity during data aggregation and forwarding processes so that false data can be detected as early as possible at the verification and authorization phase. In another work, Helen et al. [46] highlight Enhanced MAC-based secure delay-aware Healthcare Monitoring System (E-MHMS) for WBAN systems. The proposed solution ensures secure and efficient data aggregation, where data are classed into three types: critical data, nearly critical, and normal data. First, Base Station (BS) sends keys to all authorized nodes. Mahender et al. [48] shade the light on a new contribution called "Escrow-Free Identity-based Aggregate Sign-encryption scheme to secure data transmission (EF-IDASC)" to assure the privacy-preserving access control on the Internet-of-Medical-Things (IoMT). Table 11.3 summarizes these several works.

11.5 CONCLUSION

The IoT-based healthcare offers continuous health monitoring, especially elderly people and patients who are suffering from chronic diseases, which leads medical teams and/or health services to faster and more accurate responses to patients. Indeed, due to multiple design faults and a lack of effective security measures in healthcare equipment and applications, the healthcare industry based on IoT is increasingly confronting security challenges and threats. The consequences of inadequate security in the healthcare system can be, for example, some health records may contain information about the address, name, and family details that can be used to infer or reveal the patients' identities to unauthorized users causing privacy compromise. This overview is meant to act as a knowledge base that will provide unique insight to assist users and administrators in placing themselves and their organizations in ways that are consistent with their overall objectives, mission, and vision for exceptional results.

REFERENCES

1. Goyal S., Sharma N., Bhushan B., Shankar A., Sagayam M. (2021) IoT enabled technology in secured healthcare: applications, challenges and future directions. In: Hassanien A. E., Khamparia A., Gupta D., Shankar K., Slowik A. (eds) *Cognitive Internet of Medical Things for Smart Healthcare. Studies in Systems, Decision and Control*, vol 311. Springer, Cham. Doi: 10.1007/978-3-030-55833-8_2.
2. Bhushan, B., & Sahoo, G. (2020). Requirements, protocols, and security challenges in wireless sensor networks: an industrial perspective. *Handbook of Computer Networks and Cyber Security*, 683–713. https://doi.org/978-3-030-22277-2_27.
3. Othman, S. B., Bahattab, A. A., Trad, A., & Youssef, H. (2019). LSDA: lightweight secure data aggregation scheme in healthcare using IoT. *10th International Conference on Information Systems and Technologies*, Lecce, Italy, Dec 28, 2019– Dec 30, 2019, Tunisia. https://doi.org/10.1145/3447568.3448530.
4. Othman, S. B., Bahattab, A. A., Trad, A. et al. (2015). Confidentiality and integrity for data aggregation in WSN using homomorphic encryption. *Wireless Pers. Commun.* 80, 867–889. Doi: 10.1007/s11277-014-2061-z.
5. Soufiene, B. O., Bahattab, A. A., Trad, A., & Youssef, H. (2019). RESDA: robust and efficient secure data aggregation scheme in healthcare using the IoT. *2019 International Conference on Internet of Things, Embedded Systems and Communications (IINTEC)*,Tunis, Tunisia, pp. 209–213, Doi: 10.1109/IINTEC48298.2019.9112125.
6. Onesimu, J. A., Karthikeyan, J. & Sei, Y. (2021). An efficient clustering-based anonymization scheme for privacy-preserving data collection in IoT based healthcare services. *Peer-to-Peer Net. Appl.* 14, 1629–1649. Doi: 10.1007/s12083-021-01077-7.
7. Almalki, F. A., & Soufiene, B. O. (2021). EPPDA: an efficient and privacy-preserving data aggregation scheme with authentication and authorization for IoT-based healthcare applications. *Wireless Commun. Mobile Comput.* 2021, Article ID 5594159, 18 pages. Doi: 10.1155/2021/5594159.

8. Arul, R., Al-Otaibi, Y. D., Alnumay, W. S. et al. (2021). Multi-modal secure healthcare data dissemination framework using blockchain in IoMT. *Pers Ubiquit Comput.* Doi: 10.1007/s00779-021-01527-2.

9. Kumar, M., & Chand, S. (2020, Oct.). A secure and efficient cloud-centric internet-of-medical-things-enabled smart healthcare system with public verifiability. *IEEE Int. Things J.* 7(10), 10650–10659. Doi: 10.1109/JIOT.2020.3006523.

10. Almalki, F. A., Othman, S. B., Almalki, F. A., & Sakli, H. (2021). EERP-DPM: energy efficient routing protocol using dual prediction model for healthcare using IoT. *J. Healthcare Eng.* 2021, Article ID 9988038, 15 pages. Doi: 10.1155/2021/9988038.

11. soufiene, B. o., Bahattab, A. A., Trad, A., & Youssef, H. (2020). PEERP: an priority-based energy-efficient routing protocol for reliable data transmission in healthcare using the IoT, *Procedia Comput. Sci.* 175, 373–378. Doi: 10.1016/j.procs.2020.07.053.

12. Goyal, S., Sharma, N., Kaushik, I., & Bhushan, B. (2021). Blockchain as a solution for security attacks in named data networking of things. In *Security and Privacy Issues in IoT Devices and Sensor Networks*, 211–243. Doi: 10.1016/B978-0-12-821255-4.00010-9.

13. Saxena, S., Bhushan, B., & Ahad, M. A. (2021). Blockchain based solutions to secure IoT: background, integration trends and a way forward, *J. Net. Comput. Appl.* 181, 103050, Doi: 10.1016/j.jnca.2021.103050.

14. Haque, A. K., Bhushan, B., & Dhiman, G. (2021). Conceptualizing smart city applications: requirements, architecture, security issues, and emerging trends. *Expert Syst.* Doi: 10.1111/exsy.12753.

15. Kumar, A., Abhishek, K., Bhushan, B., & Chakraborty, C. (2021). Secure access control for manufacturing sector with application of ethereum blockchain. *Peer-to-Peer Net. Appl.* Doi: 10.1007/s12083-021-01108-3.

16. Saxena, S., Bhushan, B., & Ahad, M. A. (2021). Blockchain based solutions to secure IoT: background, integration trends and a way forward. *J. Net. Comput. Appl.* 103050. Doi: 10.1016/j.jnca.2021.10305.

17. Bhushan, B., Sahoo, C., Sinha, P., & Khamparia, A. (2020). Unification of blockchain and Internet of Things (BIoT): requirements, working model, challenges and future directions. *Wireless Net.* Doi: 10.1007/s11276-020-02445-6.

18. Bhushan, B., Sinha, P., Sagayam, K. M., & Andrew, J. (2021). Untangling blockchain technology: a survey on state of the art, security threats, privacy services, applications and future research directions. *Comput. Elect. Eng.* 90, 106897. Doi: 10.1016/j.compeleceng.2020.106897.

19. Paul, A., Pinjari, H., Hong, W.-H., Seo, H. C., & Rho, S. (2018). Fog computing-based IoT for health monitoring system. *J. Sens.* 2018, Article ID 1386470, 7 p. Doi: 10.1155/2018/1386470.

20. Kraemer, F. A., Braten, A. E., Tamkittikhun, N., & Palma, D. (2017). Fog computing in healthcare–a review and discussion. *IEEE Access*, 5, 9206–9222. Doi: 10.1109/ACCESS.2017.2704100.

21. Awaisi, K. S., Hussain, S., Ahmed, M., Khan, A. A., & Ahmed, G. (2020, Jun.). Leveraging IoT and fog computing in healthcare systems. *IEEE Int. Things Magaz.* 3(2), 52–56. Doi: 10.1109/IOTM.0001.1900096.

22. Ijaz, M., Li, G., Lin, L., Cheikhrouhou, O., Hamam, H., & Noor, A. (2021). Integration and applications of fog computing and cloud computing based on the Internet of Things for provision of healthcare services at home. *Electronics*, 10, 1077. Doi: 10.3390/electronics10091077.

23. Qi, Q., & Tao, F. (2019). A smart manufacturing service system based on edge computing, fog computing, and cloud computing. *IEEE Access*, 7, 86769–86777. Doi: 10.1109/ACCESS.2019.2923610.

24. Fu, J., Liu, Y., Chao, H., Bhargava, B. K., & Zhang, Z. (2018, Oct.). Secure data storage and searching for industrial IoT by integrating fog computing and cloud computing. *IEEE Trans. Indus. Inform.* 14(10), 4519–4528. Doi: 10.1109/TII.2018.2793350.
25. Wang, T., & Chen, H. (2017). SGuard: a lightweight SDN safe-guard architecture for DoS attacks. *China Commun.* 14(6), 113–125, Doi: 10.1109/CC.2017.7961368.
26. Wang, T., Chen, H., Cheng, G., & Lu, Y. (2018). SDNManager: a safeguard architecture for SDN DoS attacks based on bandwidth prediction. *Secur. Commun. Net.* 2018, Article ID 7545079, 16 p. Doi: 10.1155/2018/7545079.
27. Wang, T., & Chen, H. (2021). A lightweight SDN fingerprint attack defense mechanism based on probabilistic scrambling and controller dynamic scheduling strategies. *Secur. Commun. Net.* 2021, Article ID 6688489, 23 p. Doi: 10.1155/2021/6688489.
28. Shu, Z., Wan, J., Li, D. et al. (2016). Security in software-defined networking: threats and countermeasures. *Mobile Net. Appl.* 21, 764–776. Doi: 10.1007/s11036-016-0676-x.
29. Ahvar, E., Ahvar, S., Raza, S. M., Manuel Sanchez Vilchez, J., & Lee, G. M. (2021). Next generation of SDN in cloud-fog for 5G and beyond-enabled applications: opportunities and challenges. *Network*, 1, 28–49. Doi: 10.3390/network1010004.
30. Li, Y., Su, X., Ding, A. Y., Lindgren, A., Liu, X., Prehofer, C., Riekki, J., Rahmani, R., Tarkoma, S., & Hui, P. (2020). Enhancing the Internet of Things with knowledge-driven software-defined networking technology: future perspectives. *Sensors*, 20, 3459. Doi: 10.3390/s20123459.
31. Kamboj, P., Khare, S. & Pal, S. (2021). User authentication using blockchain based smart contract in role-based access control. *Peer-to-Peer Net. Appl.* Doi: 10.1007/s12083-021-01150-1.
32. Patil, P., Sangeetha, M. & Bhaskar, V. (2021). Blockchain for IoT access control, security and privacy: a review. *Wireless Pers. Commun.* 117, 1815–1834. Doi: 10.1007/s11277-020-07947-2.
33. Mubarakali, A. (2021). An efficient authentication scheme using blockchain technology for wireless sensor networks. *Wireless Pers. Commun.* Doi: 10.1007/s11277-021-08212-w.
34. Ren, Y., Zhao, Q., Guan, H. et al. (2020). A novel authentication scheme based on edge computing for blockchain-based distributed energy trading system. *J. Wireless Com. Net.* 2020, 152. Doi: 10.1186/s13638-020-01762-w.
35. Andola, N., Raghav, Yadav, V. K. et al. (2021). SpyChain: a lightweight blockchain for authentication and anonymous authorization in IoD. *Wireless Pers. Commun.* 119, 343–362. Doi: 10.1007/s11277-021-08214-8.
36. Kuzlu, M., Fair, C. & Guler, O. (2021). Role of Artificial Intelligence in the Internet of Things (IoT) cybersecurity. *Discov. Int. Things* 1, 7. Doi: 10.1007/s43926-020-00001-4.
37. Meneghello, F., Calore, M., Zucchetto, D., Polese, M., & Zanella, A. (2019, Oct.). IoT: Internet of Threats? a survey of practical security vulnerabilities in real IoT devices. *IEEE Int. Things J.* 6(5), 8182–8201. Doi: 10.1109/JIOT.2019.2935189.
38. Farivar, F., Haghighi, M. S., Jolfaei, A., & Alazab, M. (2020, Apr.). Artificial Intelligence for detection, estimation, and compensation of malicious attacks in nonlinear cyber-physical systems and industrial IoT *IEEE Trans. Indus. Inform.* 16(4), 2716–2725. Doi: 10.1109/TII.2019.2956474.
39. Wang, S., & Qiao, Z. (2019). Robust pervasive detection for adversarial samples of Artificial Intelligence in IoT environments. *IEEE Access*, 7, 88693–88704. Doi: 10.1109/ACCESS.2019.2919695.
40. Liang, F., Hatcher, W. G. Liao, W., Gao, W., & Yu, W. (2019). Machine learning for security and the Internet of Things: the good, the bad, and the ugly. *IEEE Access*, 7, 158126–158147. Doi: 10.1109/ACCESS.2019.2948912.

41. Kumar, M., & Chand, S. (2021). MedHypChain: a patient-centered interoperability hyperledger-based medical healthcare system: Regulation in COVID-19 pandemic. *J. Net. Comput. Appl.*, 179, 102975. Doi: 10.1016/j.jnca.2021.102975.

42. Li, J., Jin, J., Lyu, L., Yuan, D., Yang, Y., Gao, L., & Shen, C. (2021). A fast and scalable authentication scheme in IOT for smart living, *Fut. Gener. Comput. Syst.* 117, 125–137. Doi: 10.1016/j.future.2020.11.006.

43. Sharmila, A. H., & Jaisankar, N. (2020). E-MHMS: enhanced MAC-based secure delay-aware healthcare monitoring system in WBAN. *Cluster Comput.* 23, 1725–1740. Doi: 10.1007/s10586-020-03121-2.

44. Sangeetha Priya, N., Sasikala, R., Alavandar, S. et al. (2018). Security aware trusted cluster based routing protocol for wireless body sensor networks. *Wireless Pers. Commun.* 102, 3393–3411. Doi: 10.1007/s11277-018-5374-5.

45. Haseeb, K., Islam, N., Saba, T., Rehman, A., & Mehmood, Z. (2020). LSDAR: a light-weight structure based data aggregation routing protocol with secure internet of things integrated next-generation sensor networks. *Sustain. Cities Soc.* 54, 101995. Doi: 10.1016/j.scs.2019.101995.

46. Sachin, D., Chinmay, C., Jaroslav, F., Rashmi, G., Arun, K. R., & Subhendu, K. P. (2021). SSII: secured and high-quality steganography using intelligent hybrid optimization algorithms for IoT. *IEEE Access*, 9, 1-16. Doi: 10.1109/ACCESS.2021.3089357.

47. Chinmay, C., & Arij, N. A. (2021). Intelligent Internet of Things and advanced machine learning techniques for COVID-19. *EAI Endorsed Trans. Pervasive Health Technol.* 1–14. Doi: 10.4108/eai.28-1-2021.168505.

48. Chinmay, C., & Rodrigues, J. J. (2020). A comprehensive review on device-to-device communication paradigm: trends, challenges and applications, *Springer: Int. J. Wireless Personal Commun.* 114, 185–207. Doi: 10.1007/s11277-020-07358-3.

49. Chinmay, C. (2019, Apr.). Performance analysis of compression techniques for chronic wound image transmission under smartphone-enabled tele-wound network. *Int. J. E-Health Med. Commun. (IJEHMC)*, IGI Global, 10(2), 1–20.

12 Effective Management of Personal Health Records using Blockchain Technology

Jacek Klich
Cracow University of Economics

CONTENTS

12.1 INTRODUCTION

As is presented in this book, blockchain technology (BT) is widely used in the healthcare sector. It is perceived as an appropriate response to structural changes in healthcare systems fuelled – among others – by the rapid development of tele-health, telemedicine, and mobile health (mHealth). BT allows the delivery of healthcare services in a secure, reliable, trustful, traceable, tamper-proof, transparent, and decentralized manner (Ahmad et al. 2021). Radanović and Likić (2018) identify six applications of BT in healthcare: quality control, drug supply chain management, public health, health insurance and procurement policies, medical education, biomedical research, and electronic health records (EHRs) which are the topic of this chapter.

DOI: 10.1201/9781003224075-12

Blockchain also impacts considerably the healthcare industry and healthcare systems, which are documented in the most recent systematic literature review (Hussien et al. 2021). This impact can be analysed from the Fourth Industrial Revolution perspective because BT is an important part of it (Kimani et al. 2020). In other words, it is worth looking at the relationship between BT and health as a whole.

12.1.1 MOTIVATION

This relationship is complex and multidimensional and can be observed in numerous fields and at different levels. The complexity of this relationship is very vividly shown on interactive maps (called Transformation Maps) created by the World Economic Forum (WEF) and its Strategic Intelligence. They identify fields and areas of BT impact on healthcare systems and show their interconnectedness on three maps. The first such map where blockchain is the central component (a point of departure) identifies eight areas/factors impacted directly by BT, such as *Blockchain and Leveraging Data, Blockchain and Cryptocurrency Climate Impact, Smart Contracts and Automation, Blockchain and Digital Identity, Decentralized Governance and New Models, Tokenization and Digital Assets, Blockchain, Security and Interoperability,* and *Blockchain Policy, Regulation and Law.*

Category: *Blockchain and Leveraging Data* is then linked to ten areas/phenomena out of which two, i.e., *Precision Medicine* and *Future of Health and Healthcare* represent components of the healthcare system.

As shown on the second map, the *Future of Health and Healthcare* is directly connected to five areas/factors: *Sustainability of Healthcare Systems, Healthcare Technology, Preparing for and Responding to Epidemics, Enabling Access to Health,* and *Preserving Health.*

The third interactive map focuses on *Precision Medicine.* Here, *Precision Medicine* is linked directly to nine areas/factors: *Avoiding Disparities, Ethics and Legality, Multi-omics Science, A Precise Approach to Prevention, Data into Action, A New Way to Probe DNA, The Cost of Precision Medicine, Redefining Health and Disease,* and *Preparing for Precision.*

12.1.2 MAJOR CONTRIBUTION

This exhausting presentation of the impact of BT on healthcare showed on transformation maps of WEF has a dual purpose. Firstly, it illustrates the complexity of the issue as well as the multidimensional and multilateral relations between blockchain and health and healthcare systems, and secondly to indicate the added value of this chapter. In terms of the latter, one may observe that *Blockchain, Security, and Operability* is linked neither to *Precision Medicine* nor to *Future of Health and Healthcare,* which are the crucial elements of the healthcare system. This missing link is elaborated in this chapter since security and interoperability are the most important issues as far as PHRs are concerned. Consequently, one may conclude that the chapter contributes to the WEF model sketched above.

12.1.3   CHAPTER ORGANIZATION

The goal of this chapter is to identify the key challenges for the implementation of BT to PHRs as identified in more recent publications. The main findings are presented in three areas: technical developments, legal challenges, and social challenges. The findings build a platform for reflection on the future of BT in PHRs. The results create a foundation for anticipating future directions of blockchain developments in the context of PHR. This is accompanied by the identification of key success factors for the effective implementation of BT in PHR. Conclusions end the chapter.

12.2   REVIEW OF THE LITERATURE

PHRs can be perceived as constitutive elements of healthcare systems. Although an effective flow of information is essential in every sector of the economy, it has double importance in healthcare which is virtually based on the exchange of information between health professionals and patients and where quick access to reliable information in many cases means life. Because the medical information gets in volume and comes from diversified sources, this leads to the development of digitized platforms. Researching on them, Flaumenhaft and Ben-Assuli (2018) distinguish between the PHR and the electronic medical/health record (EMR/EHR).

The EHR is usually defined as a repository of patient data kept in a digital form by different healthcare providers. An EHR consists of a retrospective, current, and also prospective information regarding the patient's medical condition. The information usually includes demographic characteristics, documentation of encounters with healthcare providers (i.e., primary physician, community clinic, and hospital), or a patient's health history, including immunization plans, diagnosis, laboratory reports, etc. The European Commission to foster the cross-border exchange of medical information defined EHR as consisting of at least five components: Patient Summary, ePrescription/eDispensation, Laboratory results, Medical imaging and reports, and Hospital discharge reports (Commission Recommendation on a European Electronic Health Record exchange format).

The notion of PHR is older than EHR because personal health information in paper-based records has been kept for decades (if not centuries). Over the last few decades, PHR has undergone a radical change because of the fast development of digitalization and health information technology. There is no clear consensus regarding the exact definition of PHR so one can find various definitions in the literature (Flaumenhaft and Ben-Assuli 2018).

In this chapter, PHR is understood as a private application where data comes from multiply sources (including EHR from various healthcare providers) accessed through the Internet and entered by the patient and is freely and easily accessible by patients 24/7. PHR's goal is to offer individual patients free and full access to their personal health information and to allow them to exercise control over this information. This means that PHR is driven by the patient who may access, provide, manage, and share his/her personal health information. One may maintain that PHR is a patient-centred tool leveraging patients' engagement and involvement. It also allows the self-management of ongoing healthcare. PHR – like EHR – may include medical history and related information but also information generated and collected by patients themselves such as weight, health, and lifestyle habits such as diet, exercise, activity logs, and stress levels. PHR may contain alerts and reminders for assisting in disease management and monitoring, especially for chronic diseases like diabetes (where glucose levels monitoring and data storage are essential) (Chen et al. 2021; Sheela and Priya 2022). The latter functions are gaining in importance leveraged by better access to broadband Internet, implementation of 3G, 4G, and 5G systems, a growing number of biomedical sensors, various mobile devices (especially smartphones and related applications), and development of mHealth (Wang et al. 2020a). Taking into account the current stage of development of digitalization as well as in communication technologies, one may consider PHR as an electronic PHR (ePHR) and, therefore, use these two terms interchangeably.

The administration and disposal of health records depend largely on the chosen architecture of the place health records are stored. Following Alsahafi and Gay (2018) typology, the architecture of ePHR can be grouped into three models: (1) standalone or web-based ePHR, (2) tethered ePHR, and (3) integrated/unified ePHR. In the first model, patients are responsible for creating and maintaining their health information; thus, all administrative decisions are in their hands. In the second model, the executive power of patients/consumers is smaller because they are only granted access to the information stored by a healthcare provider. The third model responds to the growing number of medical data because it enables the gathering and viewing of health information from multiple sources. As such, it could be used regionally as well as at the national level (Alsahafi and Gay 2018).

Comparing EHR to PHR one may indicate that EHR is structured, keyed, kept, and managed by healthcare providers. It may only contain information from a single healthcare provider. Opposite to EHR, PHR is kept and managed by the patient and might encompass health information from different sources, mainly healthcare providers, but also – in the growing scale – monitoring devices (mHealth) and the Internet at large.

12.2.1 Method

To review, assess, and synthesize publications proposing to utilize the blockchain to PHRs, a structured literature search on the topic was used. Databases such as ScienceDirect, EBSCOhost (including Health Source – Consumer Edition and MEDLINE), OECD iLibrary, Open Knowledge Repository, Scopus, and Web of Science were searched and a combination of the following terms: PHRs, benefits, healthcare, challenges, security, and trust was used. Although the time frame used in the search was 2019–2021, a few earlier publications were also analysed. The study selection process was performed in two steps. In the first step, after the elimination of duplications (the results of a search came from six databases indicated above), the titles were checked against the goal of the chapter. Then, in the second step, abstracts of all publications chosen in the first step were studied and compared with the chapter's goal. Finally, 86 publications were selected for analysis. As occurred later, not all of them matched with the topic and goals of the chapter.

12.2.2 RESULTS

The results will not be presented in a formal academic manner as in the case of a classic systematic review on BT in healthcare (Agbo et al. 2019), i.e., without tables and graphs. Also, the structure will not mirror the standard style. Consequently, the findings are presented on two levels: general and specific.

12.2.2.1 General Observations

General observations can be presented in just three points:

- Widespread EHR adoption originates, among others, from substantial investment and increased financial incentives to implement EHRs even in mid-income countries.
- Gaining in importance are also PHRs. Their rising value is leveraged by fast mobile health (mHealth) development and the growing number of various sensory devices.
- Blockchain implementation to EHR and PHR gets positive assessments in the vast majority of publications. Among the benefits from block-chain are: access control (Hasselgrena et al. 2020; McGhin et al. 2019; Tandona et al. 2020; Dagher et al. 2018; Nguyen et al. 2021; Singh et al. 2021; Ogundoyin and Kamil 2021; Wang et al. 2021), interoperability (Gordon and Catalini 2018; Sreenivasan and Chacko 2020; Margheri et al. 2020), security (Tariq et al. 2020; Shi et al. 2020; Tseng et al. 2021; Gimenez-Aguilar et al. 2021; Shamshad et al. 2020), and privacy protection (Hussien et al. 2021; Agbo et al. 2019; Tandona et al. 2020; Sookhak et al. 2021; Saxena and Verma 2020; Antwi et al. 2021; Mohanta et al. 2019; Soni and Singh 2021; Axon et al. 2018; Feng et al. 2019; Badr et al. 2018; Al Omar et al. 2019; Ul Hassan et al. 2020; Attarian and Hashemi 2021; Hathaliya and Tanwar 2020; Bhavin et al. 2021; Jeet and Kang 2020).

Other classifications of benefits originating from BT are presented by Abu-elezz et al. (2020) who distinguish between patient-related and organizational-related benefits. Personalized healthcare, security and authorization, patients' health data tracking, and patient's health status monitoring belong to the first category, while health information exchange, pharmaceutical supply chain, clinical trials, and medical insurance management belong to the second category (Abu-elezz et al. 2020).

It is worth stressing that there is a limited number of publications exploring the limitations of blockchain in general (Jeet and Kang 2020; Abu-elezz et al. 2020; Negro-Calduch et al. 2021) and concerning PHR in particular. This issue will be further developed in subsection three below.

12.2.2.2 Specific Observations

Departing from (and further elaborating on) the typology of strategic risks of blockchain adoption proposed by Malhotra et al. (2021), one may identify three fields where the more detailed findings from our review can be placed. There are technical, legal, and social issues. Below *legal* and *social* ones are titled "challenges" since reporting on the appropriate findings nearly automatically lead us to future and necessary actions needed to address the identified problems.

12.2.2.2.1 Technical Developments

BT is continuously developing, thus several publications are presenting new improvements and ideas in this respect. These new propositions have different names. In the articles cited below, one can find "a new model", "a new system", "a new architecture", "a new framework", "a new concept", "a new mechanism", "a new scheme", "a new structure", or "a new platform".

Starting from "new models", we may refer to Chen et al. (2021) who present as they call it "a complete medical information system model" and a data collection system based on the Internet of Things (IoT). This system has an anonymous medical data sharing scheme based on cloud servers and a proxy re-encryption algorithm. This helps to improve the security of private medical data sharing.

Unlike the previous one, the second model developed by Roehrs et al. (2019) integrates distributed health records using BT and openEHR interoperability standard following the OmniPHR architecture model. The model was tested using a dataset of more than forty thousand adult patients from two hospital databases. As reported by the authors, the blockchain used in the prototype achieved 98% availability (Roehrs et al. 2019).

Kanwa et al. (2020) have acknowledged that there is always a trade-off between privacy and utility in data publishing, proposing an extended privacy model called "1: M MSA-(p, l)-diversity". Experimental results show that the model is efficient.

The last model reviewed, presented by Mohsin et al. (2019), is a hybrid biometric pattern model combining radio frequency identification and finger vein (FV) biometric features to increase security. The results from the evaluation showed that a high-resistance verification framework is protected against spoofing and brute-force attacks. The model had an advantage over the benchmark.

Moving to new systems one may start from a system proposed by Chelladura et al. (2021). It is a patient-centric system aimed at mastering integrity management. The system launches smart contracts in respect to registration, health record creation, and storage, to secure storage, update permission, access at emergencies, data sharing permission, and viewership permission contracts. The article shows how BT can be further developed.

Another system to implement EHRs using BT to make EHRs more secure and private is presented by Sharma and Balamurugan (2020). It is using cryptographic techniques and decentralization (classic BT traits) and maintains a balance between data privacy and data accessibility.

The next system developed by Kumar and Chand (2021) is called by the authors "a state-of-the-art privacy preserving medical data sharing system based on Hyperledger Fabric". Its name is MedHypChain. The authors maintain that MedHypChain achieves confidentiality, anonymity, traceability, and unforgeability. The MedHypChain – which is a response to SARS-CoV-2 pandemic – allows the patient to manage health-related information in the blockchain and the performance of MedHypChain in latency time, execution time, and throughput achieved positive results. As marketized in the article, a comparison of MedHypChain with related blockchain-based healthcare systems revealed that MedHypChain needs minimum computation and communication costs and achieves all security features, such as authenticity, scalability, and access control.

Equally competitive (at least in the eyes of the authors) seems to be a permissioned blockchain-based healthcare data sharing system based on Istanbul Byzantine Fault Tolerant (IBFT) consensus algorithm and Interplanetary File System (IPFS) developed by Shuaib et al. (2022). The performance of the system evaluated and compared based on transaction latency, throughput, and failure rate showed that it performs better than other systems. The results also showed that the decentralized file system provides better security than existing traditional centralized database systems.

The next new system developed by Hussein et al. (2018) was designed primarily to protect patient's privacy and security. The system is supported by a Discrete Wavelet Transform and a Genetic Algorithm technique. It allows requesting data only when the users' cryptographic keys and identities are confirmed. The authors maintain that the system is robust, efficient, immune, and scalable.

A similar goal was set by Wang et al. (2020b) for their GuardHealth system, described by the authors as an "efficient, secure and decentralized Blockchain system for data privacy preserving and sharing". GuardHealth offers confidentiality, authentication, data preserving, and data sharing when handling sensitive information. We also learn from the article that experiment results show that the system is applicable for the smart healthcare system.

The last of the reviewed systems is developed by Huang et al. (2021). It is a blockchain-based eHealth system called BCES. It allows auditing the manipulation of EHRs, which is a very sensitive issue. In BCES, each legitimate query manipulation of data consumers and legitimate outsourcing manipulation are written into the blockchain as a transaction for permanent storage. This, in turn, ensures traceability. The attribute-based proxy re-encryption is used in this system, which allows discovering any behaviour that threatens the integrity of EHRs by the auditor.

There were two proposals where the term "architecture" was used. The first one by Amour et al. (2021) making the inventory of available applications presents the architecture of "uTakeCare", an open-source application designed to keep people at risk (especially elderly people and people suffering from co-morbidities) safe from the SARS-CoV-2 pandemic. The article develops also on the ethical and legal issues of this application, which is rather unusual for technically focused publications.

The second one, written by Bebortta and Senapati (2021), deals with a secure architecture for the acquisition and distribution of healthcare information, especially through sensory devices. The authors argue that the architecture adds more ubiquity, reliability, and traceability to the healthcare sector.

Next on the list of identified sources is an article by Miyachi and Mackey (2021) on a modular hybrid privacy-preserving framework. The authors illustrate (using three different models) how blockchain can enhance healthcare information management by enabling sharing, sovereignty, and enhanced trust.

Hardin and Kotz (2021) present their *Amanuensis*, which is a concept for a secure, integrated healthcare data system that leverages blockchain and Trusted Execution Environment (TEE) technologies to achieve information provenance for mobile health (mHealth) data. In *Amanuensis*, participating organizations form a consortium to share responsibility for verifying data integrity and enforcing access policies for data stored in private data silos. The consortium is an interesting concept that will certainly be further developed in the future.

The next in line is *Medi-Block*, a blockchain-based and distributed authentication mechanism process and network architecture developed by Singh et al. (2021). It is advertised as a tamperproof and anonymous identity management model for medical record sharing for hospitals and patients. It utilizes the concept of bilinear mapping for the authentication phase and eliminates third-party trust issues. It is based on a two-way authentication between the hospital and the patients. The authors present how a blockchain platform based on BAN logic can enable medical data sharing while also meeting security requirements during the authentication phase.

Benil and Jasper (2020) propose a new scheme called *the Elliptical Curve Certificateless Aggregate Cryptography Signature* scheme (EC-ACS) for the public verification and auditing in the Medical Cloud Server (MCS). It is aimed at securing EHR using authorized BT. They use Elliptic Curve Cryptography (ECC) to encrypt medical data and the Certificateless Aggregate Signature scheme (CAS) to generate the digital signature for sharing and storing data in cloud storage. All these are designed to promote security and trust among the users.

A novel data transmission structure named *HBRSS* for high-security data transmission and data processing in insecure cloud environments and channels developed by Xie et al. (2021) crowns the presentation of identified publications on new technical solutions concerning blockchain, EHR, and PHR. *HBRSS* offers an improved partial homomorphic encryption algorithm improving privacy. The experimental results indicate larger key-space and lower power consumption compared with some encryption algorithms.

Efforts to prevent transmission of the SARS-CoV-2 virus led Bandara et al. (2021) to develop *Connect*, a blockchain empowered digital contact tracing platform that can leverage information on positive cases and notify people in their immediate proximity, which would thereby reduce the rate at which the infection could spread.

Finishing the presentation of the most recent technical developments in respect of BT, it must be acknowledged that the results presented above do not meet the condition of completeness. Also, their assessment can be questioned as done by an outsider, i.e., not by an IT expert who explains – partly – why extracts from abstracts are often cited above.

Nevertheless, the content presented above can be treated as sufficiently illustrative to show the most recent achievements in improving the BT usage in EHR and PHR. The vast majority of them are aimed at increasing security, trust, and privacy protection. This means that even existing BT can guarantee all the above, there is always room for improvement.

12.2.2.2.2 Legal Challenges

Contrary to the rich literature on new technical developments in BT, the literature on the legal and social determinants of the use of BT in the healthcare sector is relatively modest. There are a limited number of publications related to legal regulations in the context of BT usage in EHR and PHR.

Among the publications identified in this search, items are dealing with classic issues like legal provisions and data protection as well as with newly emerging ones like ownership rights to PHR.

General Data Protection Regulation (GDPR) which is a basic in countries of the European Union was intensively discussed in the literature. In Article 4(5) GDPR one may find the definition of pseudonymization. The question was whether the GDPR expands the scope of personal data through the term "pseudonymization". Mourby et al. (2018) argue that "pseudonymization" will not expand the category of personal data. They insist that the meaning of pseudonymization is not intended to determine whether data are personal data. They also argue that all data falling within the definition in Article 4(5) GDPR are personal data. This, in turn, leads to the question about the protection of this personal data.

Among the constantly discussed topics is effective data protection. The issue is complicated mainly because it is regulated on various levels (regional and international) and regulations to guide the safety and privacy of sensitive health records differ substantially between regions and states. Examples of these regulations are the Health Insurance Probability and Accountability Act (HIPPA) and the GDPR mentioned above. These two were analysed by Shuaib et al. (2021a) within the context of blockchain-based EHR system compliance with HIPPA and GDPR. As expected, the authors concluded that there are many gaps and inconsistencies.

The results of a systematic literature search by Pool et al. (2020) revealed that the failures and successes in data protection and their impacts depend upon contextual and causal mechanisms. Among contextual factors, one may find systems, users, tasks, services, and geographic elements while among casual mechanisms unauthorized access, device theft, loss, and sharing, lack of cyber-hygiene, and data protection concerns for failures, trust-building activity, secure and law compliant platforms, and perceived data protection. Their conclusion is predicted and rather trivial: they argue that for effective mHealth interventions data breaches must be mitigated and remediated.

Nalin et al. (2019) notice that nowadays more and more health data must be exchanged between European Union member states. It is difficult partly because each member state has a different national regulatory framework as well as a different national healthcare structure. The authors address this challenge via the epSOS ("Smart Open Services for European Patients") project. They present the landscape of the evolving eHealth infrastructure for cross-border health data exchange in Europe and illustrate challenges, open issues, and limitations through a specific case study describing how Italy is approaching its adoption and accommodates the identified barriers. One may learn that the secure and reliable flow of medical information among the EU member states remains a considerable challenge.

BT introduces a very interesting thread to the discussion of property rights of medical information contributing to the debate in the literature, especially concerning the ownership of PHRs. This is especially interesting and important in the USA where ownership and ownership rights possess the highest social, political, and legal value in the entire world. Under the law, patients have legal privacy, security, and accuracy rights related to their health information. As Schneider and Scheibling (2019) indicate, once this information is documented (in either written or electronic form) and the healthcare provider owns the media in which the information is stored, it gains the property right of possession of data. Now, when a blockchain-based platform helps patients resume ownership of their data and they can manage its use, the issue of the ownership right to PHR causes controversy. This is partly because – as Schneider and Scheibling (2019) calculate – PHRs generate some economic value. The approximation of added value within the context of ownership, markets, privacy, quality, and innovation in respect to PHRs done by the authors revealed that each PHR owner can generate some value. In other words, where PHR transactions take place, the owners, the life sciences companies, and local economies can generate total economic value at $2,107 per capita ($620, $343, and $1,144, respectively). Even such rough estimations put a new light on the problem of PHR ownership rights.

The latter takes on additional value if it is remembered that patients, as primary owners of the medical data, do not receive any benefits from their property unlike secondary data owners (such as Facebook and Twitter which are getting financial benefits either by reselling these data to third entities or by generating statistical analysis). This inequality inspired Bataineh et al. (2020) to develop a two-sided market-based platform for monetizing patients' data and to get financial benefits from their ownership. The authors formally prove that their concept is a realistic solution and can be implemented.

The above-mentioned publications and the issues they address can be placed within a broader framework proposed by Malgieria and Custers (2018) who noticed that the data-driven economy is based upon the commodification of digital identities. They share Schneider's and Scheibling's opinion that the personal data of individuals represents a monetary value but individuals do not seem to be fully aware of the monetary value in their data and tend to underestimate their economic power. The authors search on how EU legislation is addressing the emerging issue of propertization and monetization of personal data. They propose models allowing for quantification of the value of personal data. They show that the monetary value of personal data can be quantified, and consequently, the value of the property rights can be estimated. The most intriguing from their research is the conclusion that their models are incompatible with EU data protection law. This, in turn, raises the question about possible modifications of the EU legislation.

This pessimistic assessment coincides with the negative assessment of the legal regulations regarding the use of blockchain in the supply chain presented by Nir Kshetri (2021). He describes regulations affecting the use and attractiveness of BT in supply chains and shows how poor law enforcement and lawlessness in some countries can make the implementation process of blockchain projects difficult. The latter means that the growing PHR resources represent an increasing market value (in monetary term), so a clear definition of property rights of personal medical records and owner's rights (*ius utendi, fruendi at abutendi*) will have to be precisely defined and then efficiently executed.

12.2.2.2.3 Social Challenges

As described in the Introduction, BT affects societies (and – *ipso facto* – each of us) in many ways. Interestingly enough, publications aimed at researching the impact of BT are outperformed by those focused on technical aspects of BT.

Among the publications dealing with social aspects of BT, two groups deserve special attention. One is formed by healthcare professionals, mainly physicians (and their attitude toward digitalization and EHRs), and the second are patients.

The first group is portrayed in the book written by Eric Topol (2012), a medical doctor, and published in 2012. What struck in Topol's book (keeping in mind that it was written by a practicing medical doctor) is his critical assessment of the US healthcare system's readiness to implement EHRs. As we can learn "Of more than 3,000 American hospitals surveyed in 2009, only 1.5 per cent had fully electronic health records and health information technology (HIT) systems, and these were largely confined to large teaching hospitals in big cities" (Topol 2012, 143). Taking into account that the US healthcare system is highly fragmented "The average person in the United States age sixty-five or older receives care from seven physicians spread through four organizations each year" (Topol 2012, 144) to integrate IT systems is a considerable challenge. In addition to this, "…hundreds of companies, hospitals, and physician practices have developed proprietary, unconnected software for EHRs. Taken together, we get fragmentation to an exponential level" (Topol 2012, 144). The development of EHRs could help, but Eric Topol opts for the electronic PHR. The rapid development of the IoT and Big Data support such a choice. Topol feels somewhat uncomfortable with the growing digitalization of healthcare systems and with EHR because individual physician–patient relations are suffering. The physician pays more attention to typing (preparing a medical record) than to the patient. In the end, both physicians and patients feel uncomfortable (Topol 2012, 150). One may question the above opinions indicating that it took place nearly a decade ago and both the IT infrastructure in hospitals and physicians' attitude could change substantially. Unfortunately, there is no evidence for this. Quite to the contrary, the physicians (as well as hospitals and other healthcare providers) are rather reluctant to share medical information with patients and are even more reluctant to make any changes in the medical records. This is supported by Chen et al. (2019) findings. The authors showed that most data in EHR remain unchanged once they are placed in the system. To what extend this reluctance applies to the usage of BT remains unknown.

When compared to physicians and EHRs, patients are only slightly more active with managing their PHRs. As indicated earlier, patients are partly aware of the value of their PHRs and the opportunities they have as the owners of medical records. Heister and Yuthas (2020) follow this direction envisioning potential impacts that may result from self-sovereign ownership of medical data. Self-sovereign ownership is an interesting concept assuming the patient's full autonomy and the possession of information and data enabling him/her to make rational decisions. The term "self-sovereign" appears also in the next article under review, where Shuaib et al. (2021b) develop on secure and reliable identity. They develop a concept of self-sovereign identity, which can be used to provide user control and secure identity. Although technical, this proposal indicates a growing role by the PHR owners and underlines the role of an individual.

While the above-mentioned publication possesses a rather theoretical value, the work of Esmaeilzadeh (2021) has an empirical focus. The author conducted an online survey on the use of various personal health devices to improve health status and/or achieve health goals. As expected, the results showed that IT identity is a complicated and multidimensional construct. The identity verification process leads toward fostering IT identity and encouraging individuals to engage in beneficial kind of behaviours. This research contributes to a better understanding of outcomes of mobile health, which is still not well researched yet.

Another empirical research on a patient's preferences was done by Avram et al. (2018) who assessed 590 cardiology patients' preferences regarding the use of personal information in the context of sharing this information with the national health databases. The results showed that the majority of responders (80.3%) would grant researchers access to health administrative databases for screening and follow-up. This generally positive result notwithstanding, one may indicate a potential bias because cardiological diseases have (comparatively speaking) more neutral character than, for example, venereal, psychiatrical, or chronic diseases. It would be also interesting to check how the responders perceive the value of this personal information.

This paragraph indicates that PHR as a social phenomenon is only partially researched and there are dozens of questions remaining unanswered.

12.3 ANTICIPATED TRENDS IN THE FUTURE OF BLOCKCHAIN TECHNOLOGY IN PHRS

Combined results from this concise review of the most current publications on BT can be generalized and extrapolated as future trends. The anticipated trends can be synthesized as follows:

- There is enough ground to maintain that BT will be further expanding in the healthcare sector. Even the above concise review of the literature on the technical developments in respect to BT implementation to PHR shows how fast is the speed of BT expansion just in one field, i.e., PHR. One may extend this to EHR and to medical information in general to see further opportunities for BT in the healthcare sector.
- This expansion will be propelled by the expansion of eHealth and mHealth accompanied and leveraged by the fast development of bio-medical sensors, the IoT, and electronic devices. Also, the development of personalized medicine will support BT (Abul-Husn and Kenny 2019). The current SARS-CoV-2 pandemic shows that eHealth can substantially help with fighting against COVID-19. One may also expect that in the post-COVID-19 era, e-consultations, e-subscriptions, and other eHealth applications will be getting in scope and importance. Even more perspective is the rapid development of various biomedical sensors used – among others – in monitoring, for example, cardiological and diabetes patients. Parallel to this is fast-growing number of various IoT applications. One should notice that unlike in the past when PHRs were tightly connected to health problems of a given person, nowadays PHR can also be applied to healthy individuals using spa and fitness facilities, active in sports, i.e., jogging, walking, swimming, hiking, and biking. The plethora of electronic devices and Wi-Fi technologies allow to record and store individual information which must be properly protected.
- The sources/databases of health data will be more dispersed and differentiated. As indicated above, personalized information will be leveraged by the development of IoT leading to a growing number of sources of information. These sources will be highly heterogeneous and spread in the net.
- Interoperability will be gaining in importance. Due to the above-mentioned heterogeneity of sources and information stored, interoperability will become a strategic factor. Here both cutting edge hardware and proper software will be the key success factors.
- The health information deposited in and obtained from various sources/databases other than administered by healthcare providers (i.e., EHRs) will have a growing share in PHRs. This goes in line with and results from the comments presented in item 2 above. Again one may stress here that the development of IoT will lead to the growing amount of personal data concerning people with good health status.

- Although security and privacy issues are successfully addressed by BT, there will still be needed for further improvement in this respect. Although BT allows for secure transfer and storage of individual medical records, it does not guarantee full protection. This, in turn, means that security and privacy issues always will be top priorities forcing continuous mastering of BT and other technologies aimed at security and privacy protection.
- Patients will be more aware of the market value of medical information they possess and manage. This, in turn, may lead toward the creation of platforms where information from PHR could be traded. It is not the question "if" but "when". Even if the supply of PHR information is moderate (assuming that individuals are rather reluctant to sell the data), the demand side of the market will make such an option feasible. Parallel to this could be unofficial, not registered and – most probably – illegal trade.

12.4   KEY SUCCESS FACTORS FOR EFFECTIVE IMPLEMENTATION OF BT IN PHR

As rightly concluded by Radanović and Likić "…the academic literature is still considerably deficient regarding potential blockchain uses in healthcare systems" (Radanović and Likić 2018, 589). This is partly because BT remains *in statu nascendi* and is rapidly developing. Consequently, the first is to know well this phenomenon, which means constant monitoring BT development. The second is to study the process of BT implementation into healthcare, in general, and PHRs, in particular. As concluded by Balasubramanian et al. "…to date, no comprehensive, evidence-based effort has been made to understand the readiness of this sector (i.e. healthcare, JK) for blockchain adoption" (Balasubramanian et al. 2021, 1). Such an assessment is shared by Kouhizadeh et al. (2021) who investigated blockchain adoption barriers.

The common denominator for the activities indicated above is **knowledge**, so it is sufficient, more practical knowledge about both cut edge technical achievements and about effective implementation practices, which can be named the first key success factor in introducing BT to the healthcare sector.

The second key success factor can be named **a clear, comprehensive legal regime** on national and international (vide the European Union) levels. As it is documented in the chapter, a barrier to BT implementation is a lack of clarity on blockchain regulations and laws (Balasubramanian et al. 2021).

The third key success factor is **adequate resources** (human and capital) since BT requires considerable investments

Last but not least is the **political and social acceptance and support** for the implementation of BT in the healthcare sector.

12.5   CONCLUSIONS

This chapter has shown that BT is unavoidable in healthcare, in general, and in EHRs and PHRs, in particular. The chapter contributes to filling the gap in the interactive WEF maps, where Blockchain, Security, and Operability are not linked to the Future of Health and Healthcare. This missing link is elaborated here since security and interoperability are the most important issues of PHR. The chapter shows that BT allows for the solving of security and privacy problems of PHR. One must stress, however, that there is still room for improvement since a vast majority of publications cited above deal with further improvements of security and privacy in the forms of new models, systems, architectures, frameworks, concepts, mechanisms, schemes, structures, and platforms. Security and privacy are gaining in importance due to the growing share of mHealth and eHealth in healthcare systems. As the SARS-CoV-2 pandemic shows, eHealth possesses great potential and can substitute (with certain limitations) healthcare services provided traditionally, i.e., face-to-face interactions between physicians and patients. The latter refers first of all to primary care, but also some specialist care services can be offered online. Due to its nature, BT receives the greatest attention from IT specialists and technicians. Due to BT nature, this is natural but one may notice that the legal and social dimensions of blockchain should also be researched. This refers first of all to the execution of property rights to PHRs and confidential medical and medical-related individual/patient data.

REFERENCES

Abu-elezz, I., Hassan, A., Nazeemudeen, A., Househ, M., and Abd-alrazaq, A. 2020. The benefits and threats of blockchain technology in healthcare: a scoping review. *International Journal of Medical Informatics* 142: 104246. Doi: 10.1016/j.ijmedinf.2020.104246.

Abul-Husn, N.S., and Kenny, E.E. 2019. Personalized medicine and the power of electronic health records. *Cell* 177(1): 58–69. Doi: 10.1016/j.cell.2019.02.039.

Agbo, C.C., Mahmoud, Q.H., and Eklund, J.M. 2019. Blockchain technology in healthcare: a systematic review. *Healthcare* 7(2). Doi: 10.3390/healthcare7020056.

Ahmad, R.W., Salah, K., Jayaraman, R., Yaqoob, I., Ellahham, S., and Omar, M. 2021. The role of blockchain technology in telehealth and telemedicine. *International Journal of Medical Informatics* 148: 104399. Doi: 10.1016/j.ijmedinf.2021.104399.

Al Omar, A., Bhuiyan, Z. A., Basu, A., Kiyomoto, S., and Rahman, M.S. 2019. Privacy-friendly platform for healthcare data in cloud based on blockchain environment. *Future Generation Computer Systems* 95: 511–521. Doi: 10.1016/j.future.2018.12.044.

Alsahafi, A.Y., and Gay, B.V. 2018. An overview of electronic personal health records. *Health Policy and Technology* 7(4): 427–432. Doi: 10.1016/j.hlpt.2018.10.004.

Amour, L., Quiniou, M., Tucci-Piergiovanni, S., Bourak, H., and Souihi, S. 2021. uTakeCare: unlock full decentralization of personal data for a respectful decontainment in the context of COVID-19: toward a digitally empowered anonymous citizenship. In *Data Science for COVID-19. Volume One: Computational Perspectives*, eds U. Kose, D. Gupta, V.H.C. de Albuquerque, and A. Khanna, 231–253. San Diego, CA: Academic Press.

Antwi, M., Adnane, A., Ahmad, F., Hussain, R., ur Rehman, M.H., and Kerrache, C.A. 2021. The case of hyperledger fabric as a blockchain solution for healthcare applications. *Blockchain: Research and Applications* 2(1):100012. Doi: 10.1016/j.bcra.2021.100012.

Attarian, R., and Hashemi, S. 2021. An anonymity communication protocol for security and privacy of clients in IoT-based mobile health transactions. *Computer Networks* 190: 107976. Doi: 10.1016/j.comnet.2021.107976.

Avram, R., Marquis-Gravel, G., Simard, F. et al. 2018. Understanding the patient perspective on research access to national health records databases for conduct of randomized registry trials. *International Journal of Cardiology* 262: 110–116. Doi:10.1016/j.ijcard.2017.12.074.

Axon, L., Goldsmith, M., and Creese, S. 2018. Privacy requirements in cybersecurity applications of blockchain. *Advances in Computers* 111: 229–278. Doi: 10.1016/bs.adcom.2018.03.004.

Badr, S., Gomaa, I., and Abd-Elrahman, E. 2018. Multi-tier blockchain framework for IoT-EHRs systems. *Procedia Computer Science* 141: 159–166. Doi: 10.1016/j.procs.2018.10.162.

Balasubramanian, S., Shukla, V., Sethi, J.S., Islam, N., and Saloum, R. 2021. A readiness assessment framework for Blockchain adoption: a healthcare case study. *Technological Forecasting and Social Change* 165: 120536. Doi: 10.1016/j.techfore.2020.120536.

Bandara, E., Liang, X., Foytik, P. et al. 2021. A blockchain empowered and privacy preserving digital contact tracing platform. *Information Processing & Management* 58(4): 102572. Doi: 10.1016/j.ipm.2021.102572.

Bataineh, A.S., Mizouni, R., Bentahar, J., and El Barachi, M. 2020. Toward monetizing personal data: a two-sided market analysis. *Future Generation Computer Systems* 111:435–459. Doi: 10.1016/j.future.2019.11.009.

Bebortta, S., and Senapati, D. 2021. A secure blockchain-based solution for harnessing the future of smart healthcare. In *IoT-Based Data Analytics for the Healthcare Industry Techniques and Applications Intelligent Data-Centric Systems*, eds S. K. Singh, R. S. Singh, A.K. Pandey, S.S. Udmale, and A. Chaudhary, 167–191. San Diego, CA: Academic Press.

Benil, T., and Jasper, J. 2020. Cloud based security on outsourcing using blockchain in E-health systems. *Computer Networks* 178: 107344. Doi: 10.1016/j.comnet.2020.107344.

Bhavin, M., Tanwar, S., Sharma, N., Tyagi, S., and Kumar, N. 2021. Blockchain and quantum blind signature-based hybrid scheme for healthcare 5.0 applications. *Journal of Information Security and Applications* 56: 102673. Doi: 10.1016/j.jisa.2020.102673.

Chelladura, U., Pandian, S., and Ramasamy, K. 2021. A blockchain based patient centric EHR storage and integrity management for e-health systems. *Health Policy and Technology.* Journal Pre-proof. Doi: 10.1016/j.hlpt.2021.100513.

Chen, L., Lee, W-K., Chang, C-C., Choo, K-K.R., and Zhang, N. 2019. Blockchain based searchable encryption for electronic health record sharing. *Future Generation Computer Systems* 95: 420–429. Doi: 10.1016/j.future.2019.01.018.

Chen, M., Malook, T., Rehman, A.U. et al. 2021. Blockchain-enabled healthcare system for detection of diabetes. *Journal of Information Security and Applications* 58: 102771. Doi: 10.1016/j.jisa.2021.102771.

Chen, Z., Xu, W., Wang, B., and Yu, H. 2021. A blockchain-based preserving and sharing system for medical data privacy. *Future Generation Computer Systems* 124:338–350. Doi: 10.1016/j.future.2021.05.023.

Commission Recommendation on a European Electronic Health Record exchange format (C(2019)800) of 6 February 2019. https://digital-strategy.ec.europa.eu/en/library/recommendation-european-electronic-health-record-exchange-format (accessed June 18, 2021).

Dagher, G.G., Mohler, J., Milojkovic, M., and Marella, P.B. 2018. Ancile: privacy-preserving framework for access control and interoperability of electronic health records using blockchain technology. *Sustainable Cities and Society* 39: 283–297. Doi: 10.1016/j.scs.2018.02.014.

Esmaeilzadeh, P. 2021. How does IT identity affect individuals' use behaviors associated with personal health devices (PHDs)? An empirical study. *Information & Management* 58(1): 103313. Doi: 10.1016/j.im.2020.103313.

Feng, Q., He, D., Zeadally, S., Khan, M.K., and Kumar, N. 2019. A survey on privacy protection in blockchain system. *Journal of Network and Computer Applications* 126: 45–58. Doi: 10.1016/j.jnca.2018.10.020.

Flaumenhaft, Y., and Ben-Assuli, O. 2018. Personal health records, global policy and regulation review. *Health Policy* 122: 815–826. Doi: 10.1016/j.healthpol.2018.05.002.

Gimenez-Aguilar, M., de Fuentes, J.M., Gonzalez-Manzano, L., and Arroyo, D. 2021. Achieving cybersecurity in blockchain-based systems: a survey. *Future Generation Computer Systems* 124: 91–118. Doi: 10.1016/j.future.2021.05.007.

Gordon, W.J., and Catalini, C. 2018. Blockchain technology for healthcare: facilitating the transition to patient-driven interoperability. *Computational and Structural Biotechnology Journal* 16: 224–230. Doi: 10.1016/j.csbj.2018.06.003.

Hardin, T., and Kotz, D. 2021. Amanuensis: information provenance for health-data systems. *Information Processing & Management* 58(2): 102460. Doi: 10.1016/j.ipm.2020.102460.

Hasselgrena, A., Kralevska, K., Gligoroski, D., Pedersen, S.A., and Faxvaag, A. 2020. Blockchain in healthcare and health sciences -a scoping Review. *International Journal of Medical Informatics* 134: 104040. Doi: 10.1016/j.ijmedinf.2019.104040.

Hathaliya, J.J., and Tanwar, S. 2020. An exhaustive survey on security and privacy issues in Healthcare 4.0. *Computer Communications* 153: 311–335 Doi: 10.1016/j.comcom.2020.02.018.

Heister, S., and Yuthas, K. 2020. The blockchain and how it can influence conceptions of the self. *Technology in Society* 60: 101218. Doi: 10.1016/j.techsoc.2019.101218.

Huang, H., Sun, X., Xiao, F., Zhu, P., and Wang, W. 2021. Blockchain-based eHealth system for auditable EHRs manipulation in cloud environments. *Journal of Parallel and Distributed Computing* 148: 46–57. Doi: 10.1016/j.jpdc.2020.10.002.

Hussein, A.F., Kumar, N.A., Ramirez-Gonzalez, G., Abdulhay, E., Tavares, J.M.R.S., and de Albuquerque, V.H. 2018. A medical records managing and securing blockchain based system supported by a Genetic Algorithm and Discrete Wavelet Transform. *Cognitive Systems Research* 52: 1–11. Doi: 10.1016/j.cogsys.2018.05.004.

Hussien, H.M., Yasin, S.M, Udzir, N.I., Ninggal, M.I.H., and Salman, S. 2021. Blockchain technology in the healthcare industry: trends and opportunities. *Journal of Industrial Information Integration* 22: 100217. Doi: 10.1016/j.jii.2021.100217.

Jeet, R., and Kang, S.S. (2020). Investigating the progress of human e-healthcare systems with understanding the necessity of using emerging blockchain technology. *Materials Today: Proceedings*, In Press. Available online 19 November 2020. Doi: 10.1016/j.matpr.2020.10.083.

Kanwa, T., Anjuma, A., Malik, S.U.R., et al. 2020. A robust privacy preserving approach for electronic health records using multiple dataset with multiple sensitive attributes. *Computers & Security* 105: 102224. Doi: 10.1016/j.cose.2021.102224.

Kimani, D., Adams, K., Attah-Boakye, R., Ullah, S., Frecknall-Hughes, J., and Kim. J. 2020. Blockchain, business and the fourth industrial revolution: whence, whither, wherefore and how? *Technological Forecasting and Social Change* 161: 120254. Doi: 10.1016/j.techfore.2020.120254.

Kouhizadeh, M., Saberi, S., and Sarkis, J. 2021. Blockchain technology and the sustainable supply chain: theoretically exploring adoption barriers. *International Journal of Production Economics*, 231: 107831. Doi: 10.1016/j.ijpe.2020.107831.

Kshetri, N. 2021. Policy, legal, and ethical implications. In *Blockchain and Supply Chain Management*, ed. N. Kshetri, 193–220. Amsterdam: Elsevier.

Kumar, M., and Chand, S. 2021. MedHypChain: a patient-centered interoperability hyperledger-based medical healthcare system: regulation in COVID-19 pandemic. *Journal of Network and Computer Applications* 179: 102975. Doi: 10.1016/j.jnca.2021.102975.

Malgieria, G., and Custers, B. 2018. Pricing privacy – the right to know the value of your personal data. *Computer Law & Security Review* 34(2):289–303. Doi: 10.1016/j.clsr.2017.08.006.

Malhotra, A., O'Neill, H., and Stowell, P. 2021.Thinking strategically about blockchain adoption risks and risk mitigation. *Business Horizons*. Journal Pre-proof. Doi: 10.1016/j.bushor.2021.02.033.

Margheri, A., Masi, M., Miladi, A., Sassone, V., and Rosenzweig, J. 2020. Decentralised provenance for healthcare data. *International Journal of Medical Informatics* 141: 104197. Doi: 10.1016/j.ijmedinf.2020.104197.

McGhin, T., Choo, K-K. R., Liu, C.Z., and He, D. 2019. Blockchain in healthcare applications: research challenges and opportunities. *Journal of Network and Computer Applications* 135: 62–75. Doi: 10.1016/j.jnca.2019.02.027.

Miyachi, K., and Mackey, T.K. 2021. hOCBS: a privacy-preserving blockchain framework for healthcare data leveraging an on-chain and off-chain system design. *Information Processing & Management* 58(3): 102535. Doi: 10.1016/j.ipm.2021.102535.

Mohanta, B.K., Jena, D., Panda, S.S., and Sobhanayak, S. 2019. Blockchain technology: a survey on applications and security privacy challenges. *Internet of Things* 8: 100107. Doi: 10.1016/j.iot.2019.100107.

Mohsin, A.H., Zaidan, A.A., Zaidan, B.B. et al. 2019. Based blockchain-PSO-AES techniques in finger vein biometrics: a novel verification secure framework for patient authentication. *Computer Standards & Interfaces* 66: 103343. Doi: 10.1016/j.csi.2019.04.002.

Mourby, M., Mackey, F., Elliot, M. et al. 2018. Are 'pseudonymised' data always personal data? Implications of the GDPR for administrative data research in the UK. *Computer Law & Security Review* 34: 222–233. Doi: 10.1016/j.clsr.2018.01.002.

Nalin, M., Baroni, I., Faiella, G. et al. 2019. The European cross-border health data exchange roadmap: case study in the Italian setting. *Journal of Biomedical Informatics* 94: 103183. Doi: 10.1016/j.jbi.2019.103183.

Negro-Calduch, E., Azzopardi-Muscat, N., Krishnamurthy, R.S., and Novillo-Ortiz, D. 2021. Technological progress in electronic health record system optimization: systematic review of systematic literature reviews. *International Journal of Medical Informatics* 152: 104507. Doi: 10.1016/j.ijmedinf.2021.104507.

Nguyen, G.N., Le Viet, N.H., Elhoseny, M., Shankar, K., Gupta, B.B., and Abd El-Latif, A.A. 2021. Secure blockchain enabled Cyber–physical systems in healthcare using deep belief network with ResNet model. *Journal of Parallel and Distributed Computing* 153:150–160. Doi: 10.1016/j.jpdc.2021.03.011.

Ogundoyin, S.O., and Kamil, I.A. 2021. PAASH: a privacy-preserving authentication and fine-grained access control of outsourced data for secure smart health in smart cities. *Journal of Parallel and Distributed Computing* 155:101–119. Doi: 10.1016/j.jpdc.2021.05.001.

Pool, J., Akhlaghpour, S., and Fatehib, F. (2020). Towards a contextual theory of Mobile Health Data Protection (MHDP): a realist perspective. *International Journal of Medical Informatics* 141: 104229. Doi: 10.1016/j.ijmedinf.2020.104229.

Radanović, I., and Likić, R. 2018. Opportunities for use of blockchain technology in medicine. *Applied Health Economics and Health Policy* 16:583–590. Doi: 10.1007/s40258-018-0412-8.

Roehrs, A., da Costa, C.A., da Rosa Righi, R. et al. 2019. Analyzing the performance of a blockchain-based personal health record implementation. *Journal of Biomedical Informatics* 92: 103140. Doi: 10.1016/j.jbi.2019.103140.

Saxena, D., and Verma, J. K. 2020. Blockchain for public health: technology, applications, and a case study. In *Computational Intelligence and Its Applications in Healthcare*, eds J.K. Verma, S. Paul, and P. Johri, 53–61. San Diego, CA: Academic Press.

Schneider, J., and Scheibling, C. 2019. Estimating the market value of personal health records: the case of individual data ownership. *Value in Health* 22(3): S788. Doi: 10.1016/j.jval.2019.09.2061.

Shamshad, S., Mahmood, K., Kumari, S., and Chen, C-M. 2020. A secure blockchain-based e-health records storage and sharing scheme. *Journal of Information Security and Applications* 55: 102590. Doi: 10.1016/j.jisa.2020.102590.

Sharma, Y., and Balamurugan, B. 2020. Preserving the privacy of electronic health records using blockchain. *Procedia Computer Science* 173: 171–180 Doi: 10.1016/j.procs.2020.06.021.

Sheela, K., and Priya, C. 2022. Blockchain-based security & privacy for biomedical and healthcare information exchange systems. *Materials Today: Proceedings*. In Press. Available online 8 May 2021. Doi: 10.1016/j.matpr.2021.04.105.

Shi, S., Hea, D., Li, L., Kumar, N., Khane, M.K., and Choof, K-K.R. 2020. Applications of blockchain in ensuring the security and privacy of electronic health record systems: a survey. *Computers & Security* 97: 101966. Doi: 10.1016/j.cose.2020.101966.

Shuaib, K., Abdella, J., Sallabi, F., and Serhani, M.A. 2022. Secure decentralized electronic health records sharing system based on blockchains. *Journal of King Saud University - Computer and Information Sciences*. In Press. Available online 14 May 2021. Doi: 10.1016/j.jksuci.2021.05.002.

Shuaib, M., Alam, S., Alam, M.S., and Nasir, M.S. 2021a. Compliance with HIPAA and GDPR in blockchain-based electronic health record. *Materials Today: Proceedings*. In Press. Available online 24 March 2021. Doi: 10.1016/j.matpr.2021.03.059.

Shuaib, M., Alam, S., Alam, M.S., and Nasir, M.S. 2021b. Self-sovereign identity for healthcare using blockchain. *Materials Today: Proceedings*, In Press, Available online 27 March 2021. Doi: 10.1016/j.matpr.2021.03.083.

Singh, C., Chauhan, D., Deshmukh, S.A., Vishnu, S.S., and Walia, R. 2021. Medi-block record: secure data sharing using blockchain technology. *Informatics in Medicine Unlocked* 4: 100624. Doi: 10.1016/j.imu.2021.100624.

Soni, M., and Singh, D.K. 2021. Blockchain-based security & privacy for biomedical and healthcare information exchange systems. *Materials Today: Proceedings*. In Press. Available online 26 February 2021. Doi: 10.1016/j.matpr.2021.02.094.

Sookhak, M., Jabbarpour, M.R., Safa, N.S., and Yu, F.R. 2021. Blockchain and smart contract for access control in healthcare: a survey, issues and challenges, and open issues. *Journal of Network and Computer Applications* 178: 102950. Doi: 10.1016/j.jnca.2020.102950.

Sreenivasan, M., and Chacko, A. M. 2020. Interoperability issues in EHR systems: research directions. In *Data Analytics in Biomedical Engineering and Healthcare*, eds K. C. Lee, P. Samui, S. Sekhar Roy, and V. Kumar, 13–28, San Diego, CA: Academic Press.

Tandona, A., Dhir, A., Islam, A.K.M.N., and Mäntymäki, M. 2020. Blockchain in healthcare: a systematic literature review, synthesizing framework and future research agenda. *Computers in Industry* 122: 103290. Doi: 10.1016/j.compind.2020.103290.

Tariq, N., Qamar, A., Asim, M., and Khan, F.A. 2020. Blockchain and smart health-care security: a survey. *Procedia Computer Science* 175: 615–620. Doi: 10.1016/j.procs.2020.07.089.

Topol, E. 2012. *The Creative Destruction of Medicine. How the Digital Revolution Will Create Better Health Care.* New York: Basic Books.

Tseng, F-M., Palma Gil, E.I.N., and Lu, L.Y.Y. 2021. Developmental trajectories of block-chain research and its major subfields. *Technology in Society* 66: 101606. Doi: 10.1016/j.techsoc.2021.101606.

Ul Hassan, M., Rehmani, M.H., and Chen, J. 2020. Differential privacy in blockchain technology: a futuristic approach. *Journal of Parallel and Distributed Computing* 145: 50–74. Doi: 10.1016/j.jpdc.2020.06.003.

Wang, J., Han, K., Alexandridis, A. et al. 2020a. A blockchain-based eHealthcare system interoperating with WBANs. *Future Generation Computer Systems* 110: 675–685. Doi: 10.1016/j.future.2019.09.049.

Wang, W., Huang, H., Xue, L., Li, Q., Malekian, R., and Zhang, Y. 2021. Blockchain-assisted handover authentication for intelligent telehealth in multi-server edge com-puting environment. *Journal of Systems Architecture* 115: 102024. Doi: 10.1016/j.sysarc.2021.102024.

Wang, Z., Luo, N., and Zhou, P. 2020b. GuardHealth: blockchain empowered secure data management and graph convolutional network enabled anomaly detection in smart healthcare. *Journal of Parallel and Distributed Computing* 142: 1–12 Doi: 10.1016/j.jpdc.2020.03.004.

Xie, H., Zhang, Z., Zhang, Q., Wei, S., and Hu, C. 2021. HBRSS: providing high-secure data communication and manipulation in insecure cloud environments. *Computer Communications* 174: 1–12. Doi: 10.1016/j.comcom.2021.03.018.

13 Interoperability, Anonymity and Privacy Issues in Blockchain for Healthcare Systems

Avinash Kumar, Abhishek Bhardwaj, and Trisha Bhowmik
Sharda University

Ahmed J. Obaid
Kufa University

Muzafer Saracevic
University of Novi Pazar

Tanmayee Prakash Tilekar
ISAC India

CONTENTS

DOI: 10.1201/9781003224075-13

13.1 INTRODUCTION

Healthcare records are becoming larger and more complex with the advent of big data, but they are not yet optimized. It is common to find duplicate records that use the same identifiers and names. These records are stored on diverse networks and directories of medical architecture [1]. As medical data are highly sensitive, data security becomes more vital to prevent security breaches and unlawful activities. In case unauthorized users gain access to patient's information, the information can be sold to adversary or leaked from the hospital. The patient's individual information could be exposed in the public domain [2,3]. In order to successfully manage healthcare, it is essential to protect patient's data. Distributed networks, which contain tamper prone more personal and sensitive data, can be protected using blockchain technology. The only way to update or add transactions to a blockchain is through a hash value; this also ensures that standing transactions cannot be altered [4].

The pharmaceutical industry has now become a vital asset of any nation as it ensures the proper availability of medicines and other essential elements for hospitals. The pharmaceutical industries are now evolving as a combination of traditional and modern industrial concepts [5,6]. These industries have very complex working environments. It is very important to optimize, control, and monitor pharmaceutical industries for secure and sustainable work. Blockchain is a very secure technology that can work for supply chain (SC) as well as data integrity management. The use of blockchain in the case of pharmaceutical industries will bring various solutions that could achieve the integrity and security of the industry [7,8]. Blockchain has a very specified data structure. Also, it can be efficiently used for tracing and monitoring. The use of blockchain would help to make the pharmaceutical industries more reliable by ensuring data integrity while in transit and in storage. This paper tries its best to cover the vital aspects of blockchain that would enhance the pharmaceutical industry.

In summary, the major contributions of this paper are as follows:

- This work presents the evolution of the healthcare and pharmaceutical industries.
- This work presents the blockchain contribution for tackling the healthcare ecosystem and its relevancy related to traceability and monitoring.
- This work scrutinizes various critical challenges in the healthcare and pharmaceutical industries and their solutions using blockchain.

- This work presents various approaches that blockchain can handle in pharmaceutical-based SC industries.
- This work presents state-of-art solution using blockchain for data sharing and interoperability in the healthcare and pharmaceutical industries.

The remainder of the paper is organized as follows: Section 13.2 represents the evolution of healthcare. Section 13.3 describes the role of blockchain. Section 13.4 presents critical challenges faced by the healthcare and pharmaceutical industries and their solution using blockchain. Section 13.5 presents implementing blockchain in the healthcare and pharmaceutical industries. Finally, healthcare SC has been covered in Section 13.5, followed by the conclusion and future research directions in Section 13.6.

13.2   HEALTHCARE AND ITS EVOLUTION

The quality of life is improving because of the escalating development of the healthcare sector, and therefore, it has significant social importance. The healthcare area resolves the real health issues and, in turn, helps to improve the quality of life [9]. The healthcare system has been progressed in a very significant manner by using the computer to perform tasks, such as sharing consistent information, association in clinical training and diagnosis, a computerized healthcare record system, and analysis in Big Data [10–12].

The healthcare system has developed and helped make the pharmaceutical industry more competitive, overcoming numerous challenges [13]. For the better management of healthcare records, users (e.g., physicians, social workers, and nurses) can provide higher quality care to their patients. Through computers, various methods can be used to help organize and manage the information necessary for patient care [11,13,14].

The previously stored data in the computer can give important medical information about the status of the patients. These data can be organized and used to investigate epidemics as well as medical facilities of different areas. The researchers of different fields use these data to understand spectacles and overcome specific challenges [11]. Since the information refers to the personal information of patients, this must be handled with confidentiality. Patients' personal information leaking to the public may have a negative impact on healthcare institutions' reputations [11]. In order to avoid unethical or embarrassing situations, patients' clinical information must be protected and prevented from being disclosed.

Blockchain technology has motivated various researchers and professionals to find solutions for creating a safer, more reliable healthcare system [12,15,16]. In addition to the immutability, transparency, and reliability of blockchains, other factors can mitigate privacy and integrity issues related to patient data in healthcare [15,17]. Healthcare systems based on blockchains still face difficulties that need to be overcome [18]. It is hard to trace the interrelation behind the information accessibility since the core features of the network are unspecified [19]. Controlling and managing drugs distribution is one of the many ways the blockchain can be applied, and this can be achieved by implementing blockchain through all the phases of the SC [20–22]. In addition to combating drug counterfeiting, blockchain can be helpful in preventing pharmaceutical product diversion and theft [21]. A notable fact is that according to Dash et al. [23], the International Business Machine Corporation (IBMC)-based study shows that about 16% of healthcare administrators are planning to implement blockchain as a solution in their work environment. Moreover, above 56% of healthcare executives are planning to implement blockchain on a priority basis. In a word, blockchain can function in various healthcare field situations and has been spired [24]. It is necessary to analyse its subsequent strengths, weaknesses, opportunities, and threats. Specifically, this technology has uncovered many key points that can bring privacy and security in future technologies [25]. Babenko et al. [25] briefly discussed these systems' benefits and limitations by providing a brief, methodical evaluation of the field, the implemented search constraints surveyed by a brief discussion, and some interrelated work to the topic. The Internet of Things (IoT) technology with blockchain is also used very effectively in the area of healthcare. Cai et al. [26] discussed the Decentralised Applications (DApps) with numerous distribution scenarios in specific cryptocurrencies and inspected some essential features of blockchain. It provides an in-depth analysis of current blockchain works related to healthcare. In contrast, this study provides a comprehensive overview of implementation of blockchain in a wide variety of places and describes its possibilities.

13.3 ROLE OF BLOCKCHAIN TECHNOLOGY

An advanced technology named blockchain was initiated around the year 2008 cryptocurrencies [27,28]. Recently, blockchain performs some precise tasks in healthcare, government, finance, transport, and other areas. Users' assets can be recorded more efficiently and securely using this new technology [18]. Rouhani et al. [29] surveyed that it can also be understood as a Peer-to-Peer (P2P) network based on the idea of the distributed ledger and can be conceived of as a decentralized technology. The blockchain data structure can link blocks in chronological order by linking each block with a cryptographic hash pointer to the origin block. As a result, the Merkle tree (MT) groups' transactions within blocks are distributed among nodes [30].

The cryptocurrencies like bitcoin, litecoin, and Ethereum are made accessible to the general public [28]. These ideas have led to the development of other types of cryptocurrency and blockchain-based technologies. Hoy et al. [31] classified the advanced blockchain technology as blockchain 1.0, 2.0, and 3.0. The first part of the blockchain is characterized by the arrival of cryptocurrencies like bitcoin with Berentsen [28] and their launch simultaneously with the emergence of simple asset transfer systems. As Blockchain 2.0 emerges, innovative agreements are visible [32], and new ways of using it are discovered, such as loans, real estate funds, and other investments. The evolutionary stage of blockchain is blockchain 3.0, which applies to finance and other segments of society such as science, pharmaceutical, and the arts. Decentralization, immutability, distributed ledger, transparency, privacy, and intelligent contacts are the features of Blockchain [33,34].

The arrival of cryptocurrencies like bitcoin and Ethereum has increased interest in blockchain and intelligent ledger research. Blockchain technology accumulates and shares data distributed in a reliable and absolute manner that does not require intermediaries for data sharing. It does not require transactional confirmation to be centralized [35,36]. In blockchains, transparency makes it simpler to access ledger-based transactions across networks; the network can connect to different computing power from multiple nodes, so its calculation speed is breakneck [37]. Various techniques and facilities are included in the blockchain. These are described in brief.

- **Hash Cryptography**: Blockchains add transactions using SHA256 hashes. The National Security Agency (NSA) created this one, and it has 64 characters codes as well as one-way cryptography, deterministic functions, enhanced computation, and the avalanche effect to endure collisions. Hash algorithms also need to be deterministic.
- **Distributed P2P Network**: Distribute and update data across many users. Transactions are transmitted over the network.
- **Consensus Protocol**: Blockchain networks have an individual consensus protocol, which determines which users are permitted to make transactions.
- **Immutable Ledger**: A blockchain network records all transactions, and the shared ledger cannot be accessed or modified by third parties.
- **Mining**: The rewards are determined by hash values derived from nonce values, and in order to achieve and obtain them, miners must have high computational power.

A blockchain network can be duplicated to another different location so that healthcare data can be shared with scholars, partner facilities, or other concerned organizations, such as insurance providers. Blockchain is a network of tethered computers that share data and ensure its accuracy, reliability, and consistency. So, a blockchain can be populated at one location and distributed at another or additional locations on the same network. In addition, these new locations transmit the data across the entire network, eventually allowing location access to the latest data, which is distributed to everyone across the entire network.

13.3.1 Types of Blockchain Network

There are several distinct blockchain groups, each with its characteristic, which reflects the network behaviour. In terms of the features of blockchain, Gautam et al. [38] described the classification of blockchain. The types of blockchain are enumerated below.

- **Public Blockchain**: Transparency of transactions is maintained across all nodes. Any node in the network can validate a blockchain transaction by using consensus mechanisms. Network administrators do not need to grant permission to this node. Nodes within a network of this type can communicate and work together at an unprecedented level. Cryptocurrencies such as Bitcoin and Ethereum are examples of such networks [34].

- **Permissioned Blockchain**: Nodes in this network are allowed to join the structure only with prior authorization by an organization, which also controls their transactions [34]. Since the authentication process is required to access content on this network, it provides a higher degree of confidentiality. The Multichain Platform (MP) is an example of this type of platform [39].

- **Consortium Blockchain**: Permissioned blockchain shares some of their features since a group manages them and joining this network requires authentication. It is characterized by a minimal number of validating nodes that can validate a transaction through predefined features. In such networks, validating transactions requires mutual consent among the chosen nodes, creating a novel block and finishing the procedure [40].

13.3.2 VALIDITY PROCESS IN BLOCKCHAIN

The blockchain is used in many algorithmic implementations, where algorithms, like proof-of-work (PoW), define the blockchain validation process as mining [28]. A consensus algorithm determines the rules that the nodes must follow in order to validate the blocks. It follows the order in which the transactions should be carried out to ensure the validation nodes receive satisfactory responses from all of them. The blocks can be inserted into the chain based on these decisions [40,41]. Blockchain has become more dependable networks to consensus protocols designed to validate blocks. The analysis of healthcare blockchain requires the following vital protocols that are mentioned below.

- **PoW**: In this authentication process, several nodes solve a cryptographic puzzle (i.e., the miners). The nodes can create a valid block for creating a transaction and validating it by finding a solution. It is also important to note that certain PoW implementations, such as Bitcoin, provide a reward to the prize winner [28]. In case of healthcare, it could be used to check the valid transactions.

- **Proof of Stake**: Participation in the network is considered when choosing the validations. This node will determine block authenticity by validating more blocks that has more coins [42,43]. This can identify if the node involved is a valid user or an intruder in the healthcare system.

- **Practical Byzantine Fault Tolerance (PBFT)**: Nodes in this system are divided into two types, clients and servers. The PBFT takes various processes to validate a transaction such as the customer node requests a transaction from the provider node. The service provider node broadcasts the deal to whether or not it should be accepted. The node broadcasts a readiness message after having acceptance of transaction from the server node. In this case, as long as many nodes approve the transaction, it goes into the "confirmation alert", after the nodes confirm the transaction, they transmit a message to the other nodes to verify their actions and at the end the sender receives a response, whether the transaction is valid or not [43,44].

13.3.3 BLOCKCHAIN FOR HEALTHCARE ECOSYSTEM

In the healthcare industry, blockchain adoption has been divided into various phases. In the initial phase, blockchain is accessible directly to healthcare providers; existing healthcare Information Technology (IT) systems track and store all clinical data. The Application Program Interface (API) for the blockchain network transmits a variety of patient data using patient's IDs. Smart contracts allow inward transfers to be executed in the blockchain system. A patient public ID, which is not personal information, is used in every transaction on the blockchain network. An immutable ledger links the blocks together. Then, a unique identifier is assigned to each transaction. So, the health provider initiates the mining process or query processing via the APIs. Among the information available in the database of blocks are only non-identifiable characteristics of patients, including gender, age, and illnesses. New insights are uncovered by analyzing clinical data. Finally, a patient may also choose to share a private key with their healthcare provider if he/she wishes to disclose their identity. So, the data of patients can be accessed by the provider, who can then provide care or solutions for the symptoms that have been identified. Anyone without the patient's private key cannot access the data, so it remains confidential.

13.3.4 BLOCKCHAIN IN PHARMACEUTICALS: CHALLENGES AND OPPORTUNITIES

Blockchain is a multidisciplinary notion that makes it more proficient for applying in several areas, even though blockchain poses multiple limitations and challenges [18]. There are several kinds of research going on to diminish or overcome the effect of these factors. In the healthcare sector, blockchain technology faces many challenges, and some are mentioned below.

13.3.4.1 Throughput

In healthcare systems, there is always a high probability of throughput as there will always be an increased quantity of data dealings and nodes that increase checks in the network pipeline and ultimately cause network bottleneck. Throughput is a common problem in blockchain embedded healthcare systems because the network needs fast access if not provided; this might poorly affect an analysis that could save human life [31].

13.3.4.2 Latency

Latency in the system can be proven detrimental for it as validating a block might take 10 minutes and that can be an ideal time frame for a successful attack on the system [45]. The delays in any medical examination can drastically affect its results that compel healthcare systems' assessment in regular intervals.

13.3.4.3 Security

Security can be conceded if any object or entity can take hold of 51% of the network's computational ability [45]. Security is an essential aspect for the healthcare systems of which they must always take care because losing security will become a reason for losing credibility.

13.3.4.4 Resource Consumption

Requirement of the immense amount of energy for embedding blockchain in the system impairs investors' severe loss of resources. The energy usage by this technology is mainly due to the mining process. The real threat to the investor for the blockchain is that several devices need monitoring and a regular supply of power. However, this technology might also produce a heavy load on the existing systems and can avail a real threat to the already used resources. Managing the cost of embedding is one of the biggest problems for organizations [46].

13.3.4.5 Centralization

The architecture of blockchain is not centralized, but some methods try to centralize miners, which condenses the reliability of the network. Centralization makes the network vulnerable as the central node can be attacked, and all its information can be retrieved by cyber-attacks.

13.4 CRITICAL CHALLENGES AND BLOCKCHAIN-BASED SOLUTIONS

The United States of America (USA) has the most prominent healthcare industry globally and gets a business of about $1.7 trillion each year and in current times, the annual expenditure of an average Americans on healthcare is nearly $10,739, which is the highest compared to the rest of the countries [47]. The healthcare sector takes about 18% of the Growth Domestic Product (GDP) of America [47]. According to the projections based on the current scenario, the healthcare sector will take up to 20% of America's GDP in 2027 [48]. Many new approaches are in development and are being implemented in healthcare systems to improve the quality of life and enhance the growth of medical infrastructure.

The healthcare sector is altering various modifications due to several challenges and problems with the rapidly advancing technology. Earlier, this sector was usually an alliance of big pharma organizations and well-trained medical professionals. However, now this sector is taken over by tech giants that intend to implement technology with the existing system. These tech giants may use various tactics and methods to optimize the profit using technology and minimize the value of invested resources. The goals for these newly formed alliances have shifted, and now they are focusing more on consumer's health. One of the factors that fail the existing healthcare system is that the system focuses more on symptoms and tries to treat after a person gets sick but not prevent the root cause.

The other tactic of tech giants is introducing wearables that monitor a person's health regularly on many parameters like body temperature, heart rate, walking steps, and much more by using many sensors. The data collected by all these sensors is then evaluated and can be used to predict person's sleeping habits, food habits, and a set of behaviours. Many software are developed and used by these companies to fulfill the aim of improving patients' life. This software monitors our daily activities and suggests precautionary guidance published by digital health researchers [48].

In the current scenario of the pandemic, the companies like Apple and Google are trying to launch an all-inclusive Bluetooth-based opt-in interaction tracing technology [49]. This Bluetooth protocol aims to implement whole contact tracing by sharing consumer data, tracking distinct movements, and tracking specific interactions between trailed users and their health data [49].

Technological advancements to improve healthcare must reflect real needs from the various viewpoints of consumers, patients, and be reactive to inimitable challenges that the healthcare sector faces compared to other sectors. Investors actively search for optimization of business using blockchain. These explorations' solutions result in lowering initial costs, improving patient results, and allowing better usage of data related to healthcare [50]. Blockchain is actively embedded in healthcare systems these days in a survey conducted by IBM on over 200 life sciences executives in 18 nations [50].

It was observed that in every ten respondents, more than seven think that blockchain is going to help them overcome unproductive bureaucratic methods and inheritance systems that work as a barrier in their way of becoming innovative and adaptive [51]. One of the most significant health insurance companies, Anthem, announced in 2019 that it is going to use blockchain for storing the healthcare data of over 40 million patients [52].

13.4.1 DATA COLLECTION AND STORAGE

Technologies developed for monitoring healthcare that includes wearables such as digital wrist bands produce enormous data related to an individual's health. All the essential and critical data-driven decisions need to be made using data that has been adequately managed and safely retrieved from the sources. The current healthcare structure also produces data by standard day-to-day actions of conducting business and providing facilities.

Usually, a person visits various healthcare providers in a lifespan and hence, the healthcare data of that person remains dispersed in many providers systems. In a large number of cases, the data is retained by providers in their means, and they often fragment data trail that eventually decays the ease in the process of access for patients. Big data obtained from the healthcare sector is generally categorized in three ways: large volume, diversity, and speed. The three basic categories are non-uniform, have numerous variables, and require a real-time data analysis. The data obtained is generally inaccessible, unregulated, or scattered across systems and difficult to comprehend, use, and share [53].

The histories of patients are still stored on paper and in scattered locations that eventually make the healthcare sector very incompetent in a rapidly developing world. These paper records are not appropriate for synchronized care and for reducing common medical mistakes [47]. Nowadays, the collection of healthcare data is done by digital means at various points. It becomes necessary to retrieve the collected data to get the best out of it without confounding the procedure. The healthcare sector is encountering a critical challenge of having an inability to store and share big data efficiently and with reasonable resource expenditure [54]. Achieving data portability and distributed data compatibility is essential while operating across various systems [55].

The data that requires authentication and consent about data coherence, blockchain technology is a perfect fit. Blockchain can have a better use to secure big data that has multiple access points, and several parties can access it. The critical and necessary data becomes unbreachable using blockchain [56]. The problems faced by the healthcare industry are record-keeping and collecting continuous stable growth of business dealings, and for these blockchain is a sturdy solution.

Open consumer transactions can find blockchain more of their use, where the importance of older data is minimalistic, and data grows steadily and continuously [57]. The data records contain genetic information and personal healthcare history is considered for applying blockchain to provide high standard security. The healthcare organizations can implement blockchain to store specific information about patient's history and help doctors access these data through the network provided to them [58].

13.4.2 DATA SHARING AND INTEROPERABILITY

The non-efficient exchangeability gives rise to two types of problems. The first common problem is recognizing patients when healthcare organizations do not allow the exchange of information with another network. Secondly, information blocking occurs because patients have to go through many tests and check-ups repetitively [59]. The efficient healthcare system can only be in everyday practice when collectively recognized identifiers for patients and laws against information blocking will be introduced at a basic level. Furthermore, exchangeability matters, especially in an epidemic like the coronavirus. The sudden outbreak of the pandemic revealed the current position of the healthcare system, and it disclosed the critical need for full-bodied data-sharing infrastructure.

A robust infrastructure can help in streamlining the communication between patients and organizations, easing the flow of data that is manageable and avoids public health threats. A person visiting a doctor who might not be his primary care physician must have easy access to his history of medical records. Additionally, refining the healthcare data flow would allow doctors to accomplish remote monitoring and telemedicine consulting that permits patients to keep their primary care physicians conversant of their healthcare history [60]. In present times, the mounting number of coronavirus infectants, valuable and transparent data, including data on patients' signs and symptoms that have risk becomes most important.

The lack of exchangeability in the present healthcare system got more highlighted in this pandemic [60]. A centralized IT system preserves healthcare histories digitally and makes sharing problematic. It is exhausting, laborious, and costly to appeal, send, obtain, and accumulate a patient's medical information. The healthcare data administration industry has been slower to develop solution because of regulatory constraints fragmented patient's records and discordant backends. Data transmission, recovery, and investigation are problematic because of the absence of an alliance between medical data storage systems. Thus, patients are limited in their ability to interact with their medical records because most data are housed in silo databases [54].

Introducing blockchain technology to healthcare could help share medical information significantly more efficiently and end the lack of exchangeability issue in the industry. The hash identification (ID) can be an exclusive identifier for patients employing the authorized medical blockchain. The hash of an ID makes it unique and ensures the user's authenticity. The patients would choose their healthcare providers to whom they would disclose their respective decryption keys. The health ecosystem could become more secure, private, and interoperable and put patients at its centre [61]. The healthcare records that are precise, current, and inclusive will significantly benefit patients and providers.

13.4.3 Securing Data and Managing

The security breaches of patient health records have alarming concerns about patient data and privacy. The company named Beazley reported an increase of 45% cyber-attack using ransomware over healthcare and pharmaceutical industries [62]. The healthcare records are increasingly being hacked, and medical data is breached. The report found that in 2017, more than 350 data breaches had been reported in the medical sector, up from below 20 in 2009 [63]. The Department of Health and Human Services (DHHS) data shows that thirteen million total medical records were uncovered in 2018 due to data breaches in the healthcare industries [64]. In 2016, there were more than 27 million records of patients affected by health data breaches, averaging one per day [65]. The Unity Point Health hospital network was hacked in 2018, revealing the sensitive medical information of 1.4 million patients and hackers stole lab test results, treatments, and social security numbers from patient records with their insurance information [66].

The IT infrastructure of most healthcare organizations is ageing, often vulnerable to ransomware and other cyber-attacks. Various healthcare and pharmaceutical companies save their vital health-related data as well as information in their centralized location [54]. A medical organization's massive amount of data often makes them the prime target of sophisticated cyber-attacks. If a provider loses access to a patient's medical records and other essential data, it can cause the organization to lose millions of dollars. The healthcare sector invests in advanced security technologies such as encrypting data and leveraging artificial intelligence to prevent breaches before they become serious. The data security and patient privacy concerns have increased and the number of cyber-attacks has risen, IT security has become a vital issue to be tackled.

A blockchain-based system can provide several benefits for the security and management of medical data [66]. It protects private data from being misused and can curb threats. In addition to making data immutable, blockchain encrypts and make it impossible to decrypt. Each transaction is initiated by a unique private identification key. The transactions are authorized by a private identification key known exclusively to the user. As a result, unlike today's data access technologies, healthcare providers would only be permitted access to patient's medical information with direct access to the blockchain record [55]. The healthcare facilities can provide cost-effective care by improving data collaboration between providers.

The accurate diagnosis results in the successful treatment of the disease. It is possible for patients to keep their information safe and secure while still sharing it with the service providers of their choice using blockchain. The credentials prove who owns a medical record. They act as the security check against counterfeiting [67]. The Business Intelligence and Strategy Research (BIS) conducted a recent study that noted that by 2025, the healthcare industry can save as much as $100 billion annually by implementing blockchain [68]. In addition to saving money on breaches, operations, IT, misappropriation fraud, and insurance cover fraud, the savings will improve the overall quality of life. The reports suggest that approximately six billion dollars could be generated by 2025 [68].

13.5   HEALTHCARE SUPPLY CHAIN

SC logistics in healthcare consists of several procedures, different teams involved, and the movement of medicines, surgical kits, and other different products that healthcare providers use on a daily basis. On exploring SC vulnerabilities in the healthcare sector, the healthcare managers can propose measures to reduce those vulnerabilities. The global health investments can increase by identifying weak areas and focusing resources on targeted health outcomes. The SC in healthcare have numerous benefits such as improving processes, utilizing resources efficiently, serving employees, and effectively treating patients. In order to meet objectives, hospitals should use integrated SC that ensures operation and department of hospitals are adequately linked in the SC. An example of a SC is a back-end computer program that helps to integrate all different steps in the manufacturing process. SC implementation ensures that medicine and products are available at the right time, inventory is minimized, patients are given maximum care, all departments are coordinated to minimize human error and minimize medication errors.

13.5.1   BLOCKCHAIN FOR SUPPLY CHAIN

Blockchain technology allows pharmaceutical companies to track raw components, materials, or compounds from a source to a patient at every point of transition

[69]. The medical and health-related SC can also be protected using blockchain for pharmaceutical research data and information. SC security is improved by blockchain, as it improves the capability to identify medical products' origins and authenticity [70–72]. Moreover, blockchain allows us to track and detect the full scope of difficulties associated with pharmaceutical treatments, which has become more prevalent over the past several decades. Pharmaceutical industry data is shared using blockchain-based technology in a more trusted manner. In addition, Modum.io, a Swiss firm with sensors and technology of blockchain, improves SC productivity [73]. MODSense system can guarantee an accurate reading of the recorded temperatures and ensure stakeholders to get information about the actual handling of a specific product during transit [73]. In addition to medical supplies, vaccines transportation, trials of clinical, samples of medications, and perishable foods, the blockchain solution can benefit a wide range of other products.

The pharmaceutical SC claims, the solution enabled a higher level of efficiency and security by identifying product locations faster than usual [74]. As a certification agent for shared data and information, blockchain has the potential to convince SC managers to adopt this technology for use in SC management. The research on blockchain related to SC management is still in its infancy, so investigating possible applications for this technology is worth investigating. The companies must demonstrate quantitatively what advantages can be gained before a blockchain-enabled SC can be implemented in industries. In this respect, the trust in blockchain still relies on the trust of partner companies. The data that companies send to the blockchain can still be counterfeited or incorrected in advance. In order for blockchain to deliver high performance, accurate or counterfeit data about demand and inventory have to be shared between actors in the SC.

13.5.2 Pharmaceutical Traceability using Blockchain

In order to reduce data breaches related to cost, procedure, and IT, the reducing fake numbers of traditional solutions to trace medications within the SC is typically centralized and costly. The central authority is able to modify data without informing other shareholders because there is little transparency across the participants of the SC. The blockchain-based solution, on the other hand, offers data security, transparency, immutableness, provenance, and authentication of transaction records.

Blockchain technology facilitates the transaction of information across a decentralized, immutable ledger used to record many kinds of business transactions. Although transparent and traceable terms are used interchangeably, they serve various different purposes. SC transparency refers to the openness of top-level information. A detailed SC map would include the apparatuses of the product, the facility locations, and the suppliers' names. Traceability, on the other hand, involves selecting specific components to trace, defining common ideals to communicate with associates, identifying proper procedures for producing and gathering accurate information, selecting a platform to accumulate data, and making the necessary decisions regarding data sharing mechanism. Despite the differences between transparency and traceability, these concepts are linked together because accessing detailed information requires a comprehensive study of the SC. In this regard, several existing pharmaceutical drug tracking and tracing solutions make use of the cryptographic properties of the blockchain.

Ingraham et al. [75] gave an overview of healthcare issues, blockchain-based approaches were described, although there were no details or examples. Nageswar et al. [76] discussed how blockchain technology could be used in pharmaceutical SC. Dindarian et al. [77] projected a traceability system by utilizing Ethereum as an anti-counterfeiting tool. Smart contracts are used in the proposed solution, yet implementation or evaluation is lacking, leaving the contribution unclear. Stevens et al. [78] developed an integrated, secure drug traceability system, Drug Ledger (DL), which imitates the practical transactions governing the SC while maintaining the identity and confidentiality of stakeholder traceability information while not compromising the security of the system.

Data structures using Unspent Transaction Outputs (UTXOs), including that of the package, repackage, and unpack, a DL, complete its workflow. Studies have shown concerns with respect to the UTXO data structure, which is prone to bugs, comes with high storage charge, and uses little state space [79]. Jamil et al. [80] proposed a solution for tracking drugs in the medical SC, utilizing hyperledger technology and it is a more efficient system with minor latency increases throughput and fewer funds. However, their solution was not systematically tested and applied in a small-scale environment.

The hyper ledger technology failed to provide an appropriate solution for scalability [81]. McKee et al. [82] had similar concerns for his method of analysis as well. Concurrent with the development of Bitcoin, a private blockchain was developed to hash specific data for the purpose of securing transactions. It is impossible to manipulate the private keys associated with each product because each blockchain maintains its own permanent record. This system was created to prevent any errors in the product transfer process and ensure complete transparency throughout the SC.

The pharmaceutical SC has also been the subject of a number of ongoing projects exploring the use of distributed ledgers in order to achieve traceability. Arsene et al. [83] involved a global collaboration among companies such as IBM, Cisco, Intel, Bloomberg, and Blockstream. Each drug is assigned a timeframe, allowing it to be traced back to its origin and manufacturer. Le et al. [84] conducted an examination of using blockchain to offer a solution compliant with the DSSA regulatory framework to enhance interoperability around the globe.

13.5.3 Pharma Supply Chain Tracker using Blockchain

It is found that the stakeholder can use a front-end layer of software that is called a DApp that is connected through an API like Infura, Web3, and JSON RPC to the blockchain and storage system. Stakeholders can call pre-authorized functions through smart contracts and access data files through decentralized storage systems. As a final step, they will interact with the on-chain capitals to obtain relevant data, such as logs, Inter-Planetary File System (IPFS) hashes, and transactions. The following points provide more information on each system component.

- Pharmacies, manufacturers, distributors, and regulatory agencies such as the Food and Drug Administration (FDA) are stakeholders. In smart contracts, the participants are each assigned a particular function based on their roles in the SC. On-chain resources (OR) such as log information and history are readily accessible to ensure that SC transactions can be tracked. Furthermore, they have access to IPFS information, including images of drug lots and information leaflets.
- A decentralized storage system allows SC transaction data to be publicly accessible, reliable, and secure using low-cost off-chain storage [85]. Each uploaded file is generated with a unique hash value stored on the company's server. Those hashes are then deposited on the blockchain and retrieved via the smart contract when any changes occur to those uploaded files using hashing technology.
- A blockchain SC is deployed by using Ethereum Smart Contracts (ESC) and using smart contract, and the participants can access SC information and track the antiquity of transactions. The intelligent contract regulates the hashes on the decentralized storage server and thus keeps track of the history of transactions. Furthermore, the smart contract defines the functions of each stakeholder and grants admittance to these functions to authorized parties through the use of modifiers. Modifiers add additional features or restrictions to functions in order to enhance or decorate them.
- SC deployment is handled through ESC. It allows participants to retrieve information about the SC because the smart contract enables them to access the history of transactions and manages the hashes. In addition, the smart contract defines the responsibilities of various stakeholders. The participants with authorizations have access to these functions via modifiers. Modifiers are used to enhance a component by adding more features or by imposing restrictions. A smart contract can also handle transactions like trade drug lots or boxes.
- Logs and events are stored in OR by smart contracts so they can be tracked. The enrolment and documentation system serves as an OR to link participants' Ethereum addresses to a decentralized way for storing human-readable text.

Integrating the system components can allow the user to verify the drug's history in real time, eliminating real-time tracking requirements. The user will only need to check the drug's authenticity and confirm the drug is released from a reputable manufacturer with the proposed solution. It is possible to implement several technologies to track the location of a drug lot in real time. The smart containers enabled with IoT are equipped with sensors for continuous monitoring and tracking of the containers from their initial point to their destination. Global

Positioning System (GPS) receivers seek to determine its location, a temperature sensor to monitor its temperature, and a pressure sensor, sensitive to any openings or closings of its container [86].

13.6 CONCLUSION AND FUTURE RESEARCH DIRECTIONS

Blockchain is one of the most revolutionary underlying technologies in the field of healthcare today. Data collection and verification are automatized and provide error-free, immutable, and tamper-resistant data, assuring that cybercrime attempts are reduced. Data can also be aggregated from a variety of sources and can be viewed in a secure manner. In addition, blockchain is fault-tolerant and supports distributed data. Healthcare is one of the most significant applications of blockchain technology, which is a relatively new field. Several applications of this technology have been developed in healthcare, including sharing medical information, managing drug SC, and monitoring patients. Using blockchain technology, we can decentralize operations and manage security efficiently and with fidelity. In this paper, an in-depth analysis is conducted to suggest blockchain technology as one of the concrete solutions for securing and tracing data in healthcare and pharmaceutical industries. The paper begins with current advancements in the field of blockchain-embedded healthcare systems. The paper also presents various cyber-attacks that are prevailing in healthcare and pharmaceutical industries.

Finally, numerous future guidelines in the context of blockchain in the medical industry are outlined. This work is predicted to assist as a knowledge base and orderly standard for future research in integrating blockchain, IoT devices, and connected technology to healthcare systems. The healthcare and pharmaceutical industries are now rapidly adopting modern technologies, and hence it requires more security and traceability. This paper provides various parameters that could be used to carry future research work.

REFERENCES

1. Peng, S. (2021). Convergence of blockchain and big data. *Blockchain for Big Data*, 79–108. Doi: 10.1201/9781003201670-4.
2. Olnes, S., & Jansen, A. (2021). Blockchain technology as information infrastructure in the publicsector. *Public Administration and Information Technology*, 19–46. Doi: 10.1007/978-3-030-55746-1_2.
3. Huck, S., & Weizsacker, G. (2015). Markets for leaked information. *SSRN Electronic Journal*. Doi: 10.2139/ssrn.2684769.
4. Morabito, V. (2017). Blockchain value system. *Business Innovation Through Blockchain*, 21–39. Doi: 10.1007/978-3-319-48478-5_2.
5. Ramasamy, L. K., & Kadry, S. (2021). Combination of blockchain and IIOT. *Blockchain in the Industrial Internet of Things*. Doi: 10.1088/978-0-7503-3663-5ch7.
6. Haque, A. K., Bhushan, B., & Dhiman, G. (2021). Conceptualizing smart city applications: requirements, architecture, security issues, and emerging trends. *Expert Systems*. Doi: 10.1111/exsy.12753.

7. Bhushan, B., Khamparia, A., Sagayam, K. M., Sharma, S. K., Ahad, M. A., & Debnath, N. C. (2020). Blockchain for smart cities: a review of architectures, integration trends and future research directions. *Sustainable Cities and Society*, 61, 102360. Doi: 10.1016/j.scs.2020.102360.

8. Goyal, S., Sharma, N., Bhushan, B., Shankar, A., & Sagayam, M. (2020). IoT enabled technology in secured healthcare: applications, challenges and future directions. *Cognitive Internet of Medical Things for Smart Healthcare*, 25–48. Doi:10.1 007/978-3-030-55833-8_2.

9. Roman-Belmonte, J. M., De la Corte-Rodriguez, H., & Rodriguez-Merchan, E. C. (2018). How blockchain technology can change medicine. *Postgraduate Medicine*, 130(4), 420–427. Doi: 10.1080/00325481.2018.1472996.

10. Khan, I. R., & Baig, M. A. (2021). Managing medical supply chain using blockchain technology. *Blockchain for Healthcare Systems*, 149–158. Doi: 10.1201/9781003141471-10.

11. Sosa García, J. O. (2020). Atención de pacientes Con covid-19 en el consultorio médico. *Revista Conamed*, 25(S1), 4–14. Doi: 10.35366/97343.

12. Xia, Q., Sifah, E. B., Asamoah, K. O., Gao, J., Du, X., & Guizani, M. (2017). MeDShare: trust-less medical data sharing among cloud service providers via blockchain. *IEEE Access*, 5, 14757–14767. Doi: 10.1109/access.2017.2730843.

13. Maji, U., Mandal, R., Bhattacharya, S., & Priya, S. (2021). An IoT-based remote health monitoring system for smart healthcare. *Research Anthology on Telemedicine Efficacy, Adoption, and Impact on Healthcare Delivery*, 455–473. Doi: 10.4018/ 978-1-7998-8052-3.ch024.

14. Bell, L., Buchanan, W. J., Cameron, J., & Lo, O. (2018). Applications of blockchain within healthcare. *Blockchain in Healthcare Today*, 1. Doi: 10.30953/bhty.v1.8.

15. Al Omar, A., Rahman, M. S., Basu, A., & Kiyomoto, S. (2017). MediBchain: a blockchain based privacy preserving platform for healthcare data. *Security, Privacy, and Anonymity in Computation, Communication, and Storage*, 534–543. Doi: 10.1007/978-3-319-72395-2_49.

16. Dubovitskaya, A., Xu, Z., Ryu, S., Schumacher, M., & Wang, F. (2017). How blockchain could empower ehealth: an application for radiation oncology. *Data Management and Analytics for Medicine and Healthcare*, 3–6. Doi: 10.1007/978-3-319-67186-4_1.

17. Mackey, T., Bekki, H., Matsuzaki, T., & Mizushima, H. (2019). Examining the potential of blockchain technology to meet the needs of 21st-century Japanese health care: viewpoint on use cases and policy (Preprint). Doi: 10.2196/preprints.13649.

18. Swan, M. (2018). Blockchain economic networks: economic network theory— systemic risk and blockchain technology. *Business Transformation through Blockchain*, 3–45. Doi: 10.1007/978-3-319-98911-2_1.

19. Feng, Q., He, D., Zeadally, S., Khan, M. K., & Kumar, N. (2019). A survey on privacy protection in blockchain system. *Journal of Network and Computer Applications*, 126, 45–58. Doi: 10.1016/j.jnca.2018.10.020.

20. Kshetri, N. (2018). 1 Blockchain's roles in meeting key supply chain management objectives. *International Journal of Information Management*, 39, 80–89. Doi: 10.1016/j.ijinfomgt.2017.12.005.

21. Mackey, T. K., & Nayyar, G. (2017). A review of existing and emerging digital technologies to combat the global trade in fake medicines. *Expert Opinion on Drug Safety*, 16(5), 587–602. Doi: 10.1080/14740338.2017.1313227.

22. Cundell, D. R. (2017). Culturing the empathic health professional: challenges and opportunities. *Healthcare Transformation*, 2(2), 71–83. Doi: 10.1089/ heat.2017.29043.drc.

23. Dash, S., Gantayat, P. K., & Das, R. K. (2021). Blockchain technology in Healthcare: opportunities and challenges. *Intelligent Systems Reference Library*, 97–111. Doi: 10.1007/978-3-030-69395-4_6

24. Dujak, D., & Sajter, D. (2018). Blockchain applications in supply chain. *Smart Supply Network*, 21–46. Doi: 10.1007/978-3-319-91668-2_2.

25. Babenko, K. (2020). SWOT-analysis of the territory as a prerequisite for the a strategic vision formation of its economic development. *Ekonomika Ta Derzhava*, 6, 126. Doi: 10.32702/2306-6806.2020.6.126.

26. Cai, W., Wang, Z., Ernst, J. B., Hong, Z., Feng, C., & Leung, V. C. (2018). Decentralized applications: the blockchain-empowered software system. *IEEE Access*, 6, 53019–53033. Doi: 10.1109/access.2018.2870644.

27. Buckley, J. J. (2018). Theory of the fuzzy controller: a brief survey. *Cybernetics and Applied Systems*, 293–307. Doi: 10.1201/9781482277180-15.

28. Biswal, A., & Bhushan, B. (2019). Blockchain for Internet of Things: architecture, consensus advancements, challenges and application areas. *2019 5th International Conference on Computing, Communication, Control and Automation (ICCUBEA)*. Doi: 10.1109/iccubea47591.2019.9129181.

29. Rouhani, S., & Deters, R. (2021). Data trust framework using blockchain technology and adaptive transaction validation. *IEEE Access*, 9, 90379–90391. Doi: 10.1109/access.2021.3091327.

30. Kumar, A., Abhishek, K., Bhushan, B., & Chakraborty, C. (2021). Secure access control for manufacturing sector with application of ethereum blockchain. *Peer-to-Peer Networking and Applications*. Doi: 10.1007/s12083-021-01108-3.

31. Hoy, M. B. (2017). An introduction to the blockchain and its implications for libraries and medicine. *Medical Reference Services Quarterly*, 36(3), 273–279. Doi: 10.1080/02763869.2017.1332261.

32. Su, H., Guo, B., Lu, J., & Suo, X. (2021). Fully decentralized application model by peer-to-peer smart contract of blockchain. Doi: 10.36227/techrxiv.14074469.v1.

33. Preethi, D., Khare, N., & Tripathy, B. K. (2020). Security and privacy issues in blockchain technology. *Blockchain Technology and the Internet of Things*, 245–263. Doi: 10.1201/9781003022688-11.

34. Wang, H., Zheng, Z., Xie, S., Dai, H. N., & Chen, X. (2018). Blockchain challenges and opportunities: a survey. *International Journal of Web and Grid Services*, 14(4), 352. Doi: 10.1504/ijwgs.2018.10016848.

35. Bhushan, B., Sahoo, C., Sinha, P., & Khamparia, A. (2020). Unification of blockchain and Internet of Things (BIoT): requirements, working model, challenges and future directions. *Wireless Networks*. Doi: 10.1007/s11276-020-02445-6.

36. Kabra, N., Bhattacharya, P., Tanwar, S., & Tyagi, S. (2020). MudraChain: blockchain-based framework for automated cheque clearance in financial institutions. *Future Generation Computer Systems*, 102, 574–587. Doi: 10.1016/j.future.2019.08.035.

37. Rajnish, D. R. (2019). Securing healthcare records using blockchain technology. *SSRN Electronic Journal*. Doi: 10.2139/ssrn.3349590.

38. Gautam, S., Singal, P., & Sharma, G. (2020). Transforming healthcare with blockchain. *International Journal of Blockchains and Cryptocurrencies*, 1(1), 1. Doi: 10.1504/ijbc.2020.10032023

39. Barbieri, S. F., & Fortes Villas Boas, P. J. (2021). Blockchain in health technology assessment: a low cost solution in developing and transition countries using multichain. *Anais Online Do "Health Technology Research in Brazil: Challenges for the New Decade"*. Doi: 10.17648/htbr-2021-125080.

40. Saxena, S., Bhushan, B., & Ahad, M. A. (2021). Blockchain based solutions to secure IoT: background, integration trends and a way forward. *Journal of Network and Computer Applications*, 103050. Doi: 10.1016/j.jnca.2021.103050.

41. Bhushan, B., Sinha, P., Sagayam, K. M., & Andrew, J. (2021). Untangling blockchain technology: a survey on state of the art, security threats, privacy services, applications and future research directions. *Computers & Electrical Engineering*, 90, 106897. Doi: 10.1016/j.compeleceng.2020.106897.

42. Catalini, C., Jagadeesan, R., & Kominers, S. D. (2020). Markets for crypto tokens, and security under proof of stake. *SSRN Electronic Journal*. Doi: 10.2139/ssrn.3740654.

43. Li, K., Li, H., Wang, H., An, H., Lu, P., Yi, P., & Zhu, F. (2020). PoV: an efficient voting-based consensus algorithm for consortium blockchains. *Frontiers in Blockchain*, 3. Doi: 10.3389/fbloc.2020.00011.

44. Alfandi, O., Otoum, S., & Jararweh, Y. (2020). Blockchain solution for IoT-based critical infrastructures: byzantine fault tolerance. *NOMS 2020-2020 IEEE/IFIP Network Operations and Management Symposium*. Doi: 10.1109/noms47738.2020.9110312.

45. McGhin, T., Choo, K.-K. R., Liu, C. Z., & He, D. (2019). Blockchain in healthcare applications: research challenges and opportunities. *Journal of Network and Computer Applications*, 135, 62–75. Doi: 10.1016/j.jnca.2019.02.027.

46. Yli-Huumo, J., Ko, D., Choi, S., Park, S., & Smolander, K. (2016). Where is current research on blockchain technology? A systematic review. *PLOS One*, 11(10). Doi: 10.1371/journal.pone.0163477.

47. Hossian, M. (2021). Electronic medical record and electronic health record have potential to improve quality of care. *Academia Letters*. Doi: 10.20935/al1565.

48. Liu, T., & Mulherin, J. H. (2018). How has takeover competition changed over time? *Journal of Corporate Finance*, 49, 104–119. Doi: 10.1016/j.jcorpfin.2018.01.005.

49. Sharon, T. (2020). Blind-sided by privacy? Digital contact tracing, the Apple/Google API and Big Tech's newfound role as global health policy makers. *Ethics and Information Technology*. Doi: 10.1007/s10676-020-09547-x.

50. Clauson, K. A., Breeden, E. A., Davidson, C., & Mackey, T. K. (2018). Leveraging blockchain technology to enhance supply chain management in healthcare. *Blockchain in Healthcare Today*. Doi: 10.30953/bhty.v1.20.

51. Dhoolia, P., Chugh, P., Costa, P., Gantayat, N., Gupta, M., Kambhatla, N., Kumar, R., Mani, S., Mitra, P., Rogerson, C., & Saxena, M. (2017). A cognitive system for business and technical support: a case study. *IBM Journal of Research and Development*, 61(1). Doi: 10.1147/jrd.2016.2631398.

52. Shen, M., Zhu, L., & Xu, K. (2020). Secure homogeneous data sharing using blockchain. *Blockchain: Empowering Secure Data Sharing*, 39–59. Doi: 10.1007/978-981-15-5939-6_4.

53. Kamble, S. S., Gunasekaran, A., Goswami, M., & Manda, J. (2018). A systematic perspective on the applications of big data analytics in healthcare management. *International Journal of Healthcare Management*, 12(3), 226–240. Doi: 10.1080/20479700.2018.1531606.

54. Sharma, Y., Balamurugan, B., & Khan, F. (2020). Blockchain and big data in the healthcare sector. *Blockchain, Big Data and Machine Learning*, 207–231. Doi: 10.1201/9780429352546-9.

55. Yaeger, K., Martini, M., Rasouli, J., & Costa, A. (2019). Emerging blockchain technology solutions for modern healthcare infrastructure. *Journal of Scientific Innovation in Medicine*, 2(1). Doi: 10.29024/jsim.7.

56. Agbo, C., Mahmoud, Q., & Eklund, J. (2019). Blockchain technology in healthcare: a systematic review. *Healthcare*, 7(2), 56. Doi: 10.3390/healthcare7020056.

57. Cheng, E. C., Le, Y., Zhou, J., & Lu, Y. (2017). Healthcare services across China–on implementing an extensible universally unique patient identifier system. *International Journal of Healthcare Management*, 11(3), 210–216. Doi: 10.1080/20479700.2017.1398388.

58. Sahani, A., Priyadarshini, S. B. P., & Chinara, S. (2021). The role of blockchain technology and its usage in various sectors in the modern age. *Advances in Data Mining and Database Management*, 221–245. Doi: 10.4018/978-1-7998-6694-7.ch014.

59. Gordon, W. J., & Catalini, C. (2018). Blockchain technology for healthcare: facilitating the transition to patient-driven interoperability. *Computational and Structural Biotechnology Journal*, 16, 224–230. Doi: 10.1016/j.csbj.2018.06.003.

60. Oyeniran, O. I., & Chia, T. (2020). Novel coronavirus disease 2019 (COVID-19) outbreak in Nigeria: how effective are government interventions? *Ethics, Medicine and Public Health*, 14, 100515. Doi: 10.1016/j.jemep.2020.100515.

61. Paranjape, K., Parker, M., Houlding, D., & Car, J. (2019). Implementation considerations for blockchain in healthcare institutions. *Blockchain in Healthcare Today*, 2. Doi: 10.30953/bhty.v2.114.

62. Rangel, A. (2019). Why enterprises need to adopt 'need-to-know' security. *Computer Fraud & Security*, 2019(12), 9–12. Doi: 10.1016/s1361-3723(19)30127-7.

63. Lynch, J. (2017). Access to health records by the patient. *Health Records in Court*, 125–134. Doi: 10.1201/9781315382982-13.

64. Thompson, E. C. (2020). Hipaa security rule and cybersecurity operations. *Designing a HIPAA-Compliant Security Operations Center*, 23–36. Doi: 10.1007/978-1-4842-5608-4_2.

65. Chauhan, A. (2017). Youth barometer report -2017. *SSRN Electronic Journal*. Doi: 10.2139/ssrn.3333308.

66. Bouras, M. A., Lu, Q., Zhang, F., Wan, Y., Zhang, T., & Ning, H. (2020). Distributed ledger technology for ehealth identity privacy: state of the art and future perspective. *Sensors*, 20(2), 483. Doi: 10.3390/s20020483.

67. Oliver, S. (2000). Revolutionizing how we generate new knowledge: a challenge for librarians, health professionals, service users and researchers. *Health Libraries Review*, 17(1), 22–25. Doi: 10.1046/j.1365-2532.2000.00256.x.

68. Shukla, R., Thok, K., Alam, I., & Singh, R. (2020). Nanophytomedicine market: global opportunity analysis and industry forecast. *Nanophytomedicine*, 19–31. Doi: 10.1007/978-981-15-4909-0_2.

69. Motsi-Omoijiade, I., & Kharlamov, A. (2021). Blockchain for healthcare applications and use cases. *Blockchain and Public Law*, 157–190. Doi: 10.4337/9781839100796.00015.

70. Bocek, T., Rodrigues, B. B., Strasser, T., & Stiller, B. (2017). Blockchains everywhere - a use-case of blockchains in the pharma supply-chain. *2017 IFIP/IEEE Symposium on Integrated Network and Service Management (IM)*. Doi: 10.23919/inm.2017.7987376.

71. Kshetri, N. (2021). Healthcare and pharmaceutical industry supply chains. *Blockchain and Supply Chain Management*, 115–137. Doi: 10.1016/b978-0-323-89934-5.00008-8.

72. Abelseth, B. (2018). Blockchain tracking and Cannabis regulation: developing a permissioned blockchain network to track Canada's Cannabis supply chain. *Dalhousie Journal of Interdisciplinary Management*, 14. Doi: 10.5931/djim.v14i0.7869.

73. Muniandi, G. (2021). Blockchain-enabled balise data security for train control system. *IET Blockchain*. Doi: 10.1049/blc2.12003.

74. Hofmann, E., Strewe, U. M., & Bosia, N. (2017). Introduction—why to pay attention on blockchain-driven supply chain finance? *Supply Chain Finance and Blockchain Technology*, 1–6. Doi: 10.1007/978-3-319-62371-9_1.

75. Ingraham, A., & St. Clair, J. (2020). The fourth industrial revolution of health-care information technology: key business components to unlock the value of a blockchain-enabled solution. *Blockchain in Healthcare Today*. Doi: 10.30953/bhty. v3.139.

76. Nageswar, A. K., & Yellampalli, S. (2019). Distributed trust using blockchain for efficient pharmaceutical supply chain. *Global Supply Chains in the Pharmaceutical Industry*, 248–268. Doi: 10.4018/978-1-5225-5921-4.ch011.

77. Dindarian, A., & Chakravarthy, S. (2019). Chapter 7. Traceability of electronic waste using blockchain technology. *Issues in Environmental Science and Technology*, 188–212. Doi: 10.1039/9781788018784-00188.

78. Stevens, S. K. (2019). Tracing the food safety laws and regulations governing trace-ability: a Brief history of food safety and traceability regulation. *Food Traceability*, 13–26. Doi: 10.1007/978-3-030-10902-8_2.

79. Pérez-Solà, C., Delgado-Segura, S., Navarro-Arribas, G., & Herrera-Joancomartí, J. (2019). Another coin bites the dust: an analysis of dust in Utxo-based cryptocurren-cies. *Royal Society Open Science*, 6(1), 180817. Doi: 10.1098/rsos.180817.

80. Jamil, F., Hang, L., Kim, K. H., & Kim, D. H. (2019). A novel medical blockchain model for drug supply chain integrity management in a smart hospital. *Electronics*, 8(5), 505. Doi: 10.3390/electronics8050505.

81. Bougdira, A., Ahaitouf, A., & Akharraz, I. (2019). Conceptual framework for general traceability solution: description and bases. *Journal of Modelling in Management*, 15(2), 509–530. Doi: 10.1108/jm2-12-2018-0207.

82. McKee, E. D., Makela, E. F., & Scassa, E. T. (2018). Law and the "sharing econ-omy": regulating online market platforms. http://www.jstor.org/stable/10.2307/j. ctv5vdczv?refreqid=search-gateway.

83. Uddin, M. (2021). Blockchain medledger: hyperledger fabric enabled drug trace-ability system for counterfeit drugs in pharmaceutical industry. *International Journal of Pharmaceutics*, 597, 120235. Doi: 10.1016/j.ijpharm.2021.120235.

84. Le Gear, A. (2020). A blockchain supported solution for compliant digital security offerings. *Progress in IS*, 113–131. Doi: 10.1007/978-3-030-44337-5_6.

85. Dias, D., & Benet, J. (2016). Distributed web applications with IPFS, Tutorial. *Lecture Notes in Computer Science*, 616–619. Doi: 10.1007/978-3-319-38791-8_60.

86. Satpathy, A. (2020). Evolution of cloud-fog-IoT interconnection networks. *Cloud Network Management*, 3–14. Doi: 10.1201/9780429288630-1.

14 Blockchain in the Pharmaceutical Industry for Better Tracking of Drugs with Architectures and Open Challenges

Ayasha Malik
Noida Institute of Engineering Technology (NIET)

Neha Yadav
Babasaheb Bhimrao Ambedkar University

Jaya Srivastava
Noida Institute of Engineering Technology (NIET)

Ahmed J. Obaid
Kufa University

Muzafer Saracevic
University of Novi Pazar

CONTENTS

DOI: 10.1201/9781003224075-14

14.1   INTRODUCTION

Medication tampering has become a prime concern today, and it becomes vicious for public health that has an adverse effect on human health and medical treatment results. According to the World Health Organization (WHO) [1], tampered medication is an outcome of counterfeiting with the source and identity of the product. As per the WHO data, 15% of the medicines in developing nations and 1.5%–2.5% of medicines in developed nations are tampered with [2]. The tampered medicines have an adverse impact on all pharmaceutical stakeholders including hospitals, pharmacies, wholesale distributors, global health programs, and regulatory authorities all over the world. These medicines are fatal to humans. A big illegal drug market is functional behind the foresighted Pharmaceutical Supply Chain (PSC), these markets produce false and contaminated medicines by changing their ingredients, adding expired stock along with the fresh stock. This process is feasible only because of the lack of technology to track and verify the authenticity of the drug at every step in the supply chain. The delivery of fake Remdesivir injection during the covid-19 pandemics is a recent example of a counterfeit medication that took a toll on human lives [3].

The regions that are more susceptible to inauthentic drugs are Asia Pacific, Egypt, and Latin America. 40% of drugs manufactured and used as the reason for 1.7 million deaths every year [4]. In the region of Europe, the total number of cases that are based on counterfeit drugs became twice as compared to the last year [5]. A just now report prepared by a brilliant researcher of Europe emphasizes that the fake drug industry is now considered a more fruitful and profitable business because selling legal drugs is more difficult and its evaluated revenue fall equals about 8% in industry medicine sales to counting €16 billion each year [6]. The growth in purchasing and accessing drugs via online pharmacies and through illegal distribution channels makes it very challenging to make the safety of the product in the system of supply chain network. Likewise, clarity of limited data for stockpiles toward the supply chain network gives more opportunities for inauthentic actions to intrude the market [7]. Detection of drugs is an ability to distinguish the ingenuity and legitimacy of drugs that ensure all stakeholders detect and trace each transaction at every stage of the supply chain system. Regulations like the United States Drug Supply Chain Security Act (DSCSA) [8] demand for all drug supply chain stakeholders to apply reliable measures for better product tracking; the factual implementation of DSCSA will be in an incremental phased manner by the year 2025. The ever-growing demand for accessing the PSC through online access covers more ways to the agents for counterfeiting drugs, distribution of drugs by unauthorized dealers is also an add-on to drug counterfeit [9]. Lack of transparency and traceability also provides opportunities to drug counterfeiters.

Blockchain technology is a chain of blocks arranged in a distributed manner to assure the security, authenticity, transparency, and traceability of data it holds. The data stored on a blockchain is immutable [10]; it covers almost all spheres of life with its applications like banking, education, logistics, traffic management, identity management, electronic health record management, energy, trading, and many more [11]. Blockchain holds a promising future to track the PSC in order to get rid of tampered drugs. Blockchain technology is able to create a platform for allocated shared data for storage and share the transaction data between distinct supply chain systems of stakeholders that make sure the information will remain available to authorized groups, unchangeable, transparent, and kept secure with different cryptographic techniques [12,13]. So, providing a forward approach to trace, find, and manage authenticity in system supply chains of pharmaceuticals is very important. The major contributions of our research work are as follows:

- The paper deliberates the causes of how the industries of pharmaceutical take welfare from blockchain-based supply chain drug tracking systems.
- The paper uncovers all the important assistance that comes by using a blockchain-based solution for drug delivery as related to surviving solutions.
- The paper highlights three blockchain-based architectures named Hyperledger fabric, Hyperledger besu, and Ethereum for proper tracking of drug supply or uses in the pharmaceutical industry.
- The paper detects, estimates, and reversed some challenging problems that may hamper the effective organization of blockchain-based solutions to proper use and delivery of drugs.

The rest part of the paper is described as follows: Section 14.2 highlights the overview of blockchain technology including its feature and nature, and the comparison of blockchain categories is also deliberated. Furthermore, Section

14.3 highlights the overview of drug tracking in the pharmaceutical industry. Additionally, Section 14.4 enlightens the three blockchain-based drug tracking systems with their drug tracking flow. Moreover, three discussed blockchain-based architectures for drug tracking are compared on the basis of some parameters. Section 14.5 enlightens some challenges or limitations related to the blockchain adoption technologies that need to be described in order to facilitate drug tracking. Finally, Section 14.6 concludes with a conclusion and is followed by a future research direction.

14.2 OVERVIEW OF BLOCKCHAIN

Blockchain is the chain of blocks, each block containing information about transactions. The copy of the blockchain is shared with every computer/node in the network, which ensures the transparency of stored data. A blockchain network is formed by a set of these computers that are operating over a single protocol to adding newer blocks to the existing chain [14,15]. Thus, the network of the blocks of the blockchain is a distributed system that stored information of all past performed transactions and selects a protocol for working that validates the transactions, and arbitrates the transaction course, and determines all work of the network with its all participants. Thus, this network is known as a distributed, in such network, the data of every transaction is stored on each particular block working in it [16].

Mainly, there are three kinds of blockchain networks: public blockchain, private blockchain, and consortium blockchain. A public blockchain is open for everyone to join either as a user, minor, developer, or community member. It targets the general public as end-users, it is non-restricted and permissionless, and anyone having internet access can join the public blockchain network and become its node. Public blockchain examples are Bitcoin (BTC) and Ethereum (ETH) [17]. Private blockchains work in a restricted environment under the control of a single entity. Nodes having permission to join the network can only join the network of private blockchain; therefore, it is also called permission blockchain. Hyperledger and Ripple (XRP) are widely known examples of private blockchain. The consortium blockchain has the features of both public blockchain and private blockchain. Members from multiple organizations collaborate on a consortium blockchain network [18]. The present node controls the consensus mechanism in consortium blockchain. Differences between the three kinds of blockchain are shown in Table 14.1.

The selection of blockchain technology depends on the type of work at hand. For instance, accounting in small businesses is managed by other institutions, the other option for this scenario is to create a private blockchain network, in such network, distributed set of blocks named distributed ledger is only the source for true information. Although, in a scenario, within the supply chain system, the customer desire to go through everything for the product, the approach of consortium network will apply. Thus, the participants were able to read product data, but

TABLE 14.1

Difference between Blockchain's Categories

Property	Public [17]	Private [18]	Consortium [18]
Type of governance	Public	Single owner	Set of owners
Example	Ripple, Bitcoin, Ethereum	Hyperledger, Quorum	Multi-chain
Consensus algorithm	PoW, PoS, etc.	PoA, PBFT, etc.	Tendermint, etc.
Infrastructure	Highly decentralized	Distributed	Decentralized
Transaction reading	Any node	Any node/list of predefined node	Any node/list of predefined node
Immutability of data	Yes	Yes	Yes
Network scalability	High	Low to medium	Low to medium
Throughput of transaction	Low	High	High

make sure that only authentic participants, such as the vendor, the manufacturing, and the vendor for raw materials [19].

14.3 OVERVIEW OF DRUG TRACKING IN THE HEALTHCARE DOMAIN

The focus of this section is on issues related to drug traceability in the PSC. A PSC follows an end-to-end supply from collecting the raw material to supplying the final product to the end-user (patients). The main objective of the supply chain is to deliver correct and good quality drugs at the right time as the lives of people are at a safe stage. Many loopholes exist in the current PSC and also it lacks traceability and transparency. There is no clear ownership due to non-uniformity in stakeholders and also it makes verification of transactions more difficult. There is no single view of the whole system, which leads to the involvement of central authority to manage the whole system [20].

The PSC consists of a number of processes from storing, packing, unpacking, repacking, and several stakeholders from vendors, manufacturers, dealers, salespersons, drug stores, and patients, which makes drug traceability difficult. There are many factors that contribute to tampered drugs in the system of the supply chain; there are some examples of buying substandard drugs from other countries without taking the permission of administrative authority, bad manufacturing and storage custom, stealing, and leakage of inadequate drugs [21]. A huge number of remedies have been applied for improving the traceability and transparency of the supply chain like serialization, bar codes, Radio Frequency Identification (RFID), etc., but they all have some limitations when it comes to privacy, security, and transparency.

Wide use of blockchain is found in the supply chain, transport, logistics, and traffic control systems as it delivers an unchangeable, secure, verifiable, and

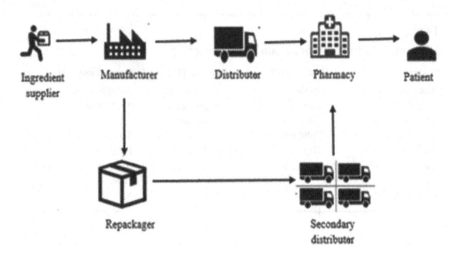

FIGURE 14.1   Relationship between stakeholders of the drug supply chain.

transparent environment to store transaction data among mistrusting stakehold-ers [22]. The main feature of blockchain is the connectivity of blocks containing transaction data with the previous block using a hash function. This ensures the immutability of the data and facilitates traceability. Blockchain technology pro-vides a structured and economical solution that can find many different types of drug tracking functions and approach to make sure of proper finding, tracking, and training. The benefit of blockchain technologies can be merged with already existing anti-fake solutions with RFID, Near Field Communication (NFC), Quality Risk and Compliance (QRC), and e-pedigree to deliver interoperable and improved integrated solutions [23]. Figure 14.1 shows the relationship between all the intermediate stakeholders in the supply chain system of the drug.

Blockchain technology permits an authorized private network to trail and track the events within the PSC and deliver the time-sealed history of every transaction. Samples of events consist of execution, owner, time, location of the transaction, and concerned stakeholders [24]. This maintains the reliability, integrity, validity, transparency, and security of drugs. This method depreciates the impediments in the drug system of the supply chain, enables collaboration among reciprocally mistrusted stakeholders, and creates a secure and tamper-proof distributed drug tracking system [25]. These edges provide standardization and directive oversight over numerous countries and drug restrictive authorities by shared knowledge exchange, to attain practical solutions supported by many regulators like Food and Drug Administration (FDA) and the European Medication Agency (EMA). In the next part, there is a comparison and explanation of three architectures of blockchain for product tracking within the PSC. The extended acceptance of blockchain technology-based explanation in the industry of pharmacy is distinctly based on some current projects that involved primary stakeholders as shown in Table 14.2.

TABLE 14.2

Traceability of Drugs Products Including Initials Participants Based on Blockchain

Products and Initials Participants [26]	Solutions Types Based on Blockchain [26]	Platform [26]
SAP multi-chain Merck, Ameri-source, Bergen, GSK, Amgen, Boehringer Ingellheim, McKesson, Novo Nordisk	Authentication of copies along with tracing of profitable revenues	Multi-chain
IBM, KPMG, Merck, Walmart ID Logiq	Proper tracking and authentication of intelligent medication management on a regular basis	Hyperledger private platform
Indiana university health, Wakemed health, and hospitals	Tracking of special medicine inside as well as outside of providers or networks	Private platform
Ledger Domain, University of California Los Angeles health	Provide detection and solution for extra or fake copies	Hyperledger
Medi Ledger-AmerisourceBergen, McKesson, drug manufacturer Genentech, Pizer, Gilead	Authentication and validation system for profitable revenues	Permission enterprise Ethereum
Trace Link above 25 participants (producer, suppliers, etc.)	A solution including digital recollections and interoperable	Hyperledger

14.4 ARCHITECTURES FOR DRUG TRACKING BASED ON BLOCKCHAIN

This section introduces and deliberates the construction of three blockchain architectures to meet the key requirements of drug tracking. These structures or architecture are based on three distinct platforms of blockchain: Hyperledger fabric, Hyperledger besu, and Ethereum. As it offers a high level of reliability, power allocation, clearness, confidentiality, safety, data reliability, arrangement, and failure as equated to other blockchain platforms. These are the major blockchain architecture that is used for generating an approved private/public blockchain in which producers, contributors, and end-users are recorded. The three structures and flow of transmission are defined in the succeeding subsections [27].

14.4.1 HYPERLEDGER FABRIC BLOCKCHAIN-BASED ARCHITECTURE

Hyperledger fabric blockchain-based architecture is a Distributed Ledger Technology (DLT) with a linked structural design that provides the max point of secrecy, robustness, and elasticity. It's a blockchain-based business DLT that employs smart agreements to impose confidence among numerous contributors. It does away with the idea of mining while retaining the benefits of a traditional cryptocurrency based on blockchain technology, like unassailability of the block, event's order, and protection of double-spending. Hyperledger fabric has been proven to provide higher transaction throughput, with thousands of transactions per second [28]. Hyperledger fabric is an excellent customer for complicated supply chain networks with numerous procedures and contributors because of these properties, as well as others that will be discussed further down. The adoption criterion for smart contracts is lower than for other technologies that use specific programming languages like Java, Go, and NodeJS [29]. The Hyperledger fabric blockchain-based drug tracking architecture is the first draught of a business-level supply chain system based on blockchain, in which dissimilar shareholders inside PSC remain recognized and associations among them are implemented by various stations to ensure an extreme level of secrecy, authority along with full protection of data. Hyperledger fabric is the first to introduce the concept of channels. Channels allow unlike shareholders in identical networks to separate their business logic and data privacy standards. It also delivers a protected and clear smash fault lenient deal gathering, confirming unavoidable event records, protected transmission, and dependable medical conversation among a group of distrustful shareholders. This contributes to the development of a standardized track attribution mechanism in PSC [30]. The suggested blockchain design employs a unique modular method to allow maximum points of tractability, adaptability, and anonymity. The architecture creates a restricted blockchain system in which the Health Authority (HA) uses the Membership Service Provider (MSP), a factor of the architecture to identify and register all participating organizations and their end-users. The MSP factor of Hyperledger fabric could provide the Certificate Authority (CA), or the provided CA can be an external such as the certificates of OpenSSL, in co-operation with active directory. The architecture requires the use of an MSP to produce a confidential atmosphere among distrustful parties [31].

Finally, the Ordering Service (OS) and peer nodes are at the heart of the Hyperledger fabric design. Hyperledger fabric peers maintain replicas of the ledger, run smart agreements (also known as chain code), endorse, and commit transactions. The operating system takes authorized transactions from client apps and organizes them as blocks with the endorsing parties' encrypted digital signs of the approving nobles, as well as lastly forwards these blocks to promising nobles into the system for the authentications in contrast to the authorization strategies [32]. Figure 14.2 shows the architecture of Hyperledger fabric blockchain-based architecture.

14.4.1.1 Drug Tracking Flow with Hyperledger Fabric Blockchain Architecture

A business deal proposal is given by the manufacturers, this proposal is shared with all the peers of the networks as per the endorsement policy of the blockchain. Endorsement policies are a pre-specified set of policies that specify the extent to which peers can sign/check every transaction. These transaction proposals are executed via a total number of nodules as specified in the endorsement policy. The outcomes of the transaction proposal, also known as endorsements, are shared with the endorsement peers' digital signature, Read/Write (RW) sets,

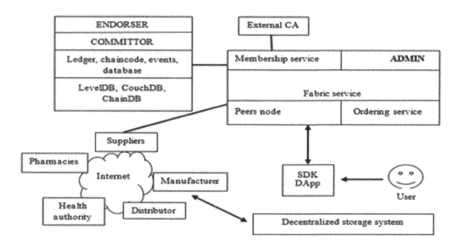

FIGURE 14.2 Hyperledger fabric blockchain-based architecture.

and then sent back to the user/client app as an acknowledgment of submission of the proposal. When enough responses reach the user app, it checks them to find whether RW sets are the same or not, to make sure that the blockchain is not up to date with the proposal and certification stages. After this, the user app will broadcast the proposals and their reactions inside a business note to the OS. For the proper estimation and maintaining of the implementation sequence of the business transaction that is forwarded by each channel, a consensus algorithm is used by the dispersed OS. The sorting facility sorts numerous transmissions of the drug in a block in chronological order and links the block hash to the previous block. Then, the operating system forwards all the freshly block to the foremost nodule on architecture. The task of the leader node is to use the conversation procedure to spread the block to further participating nodes in the organization. Top nodes are selected by the association then also received to the subscription facility. The endorsement is legal and agreeing by chaincode's certification strategy" is done by peers, also verifies that the RW set has not remained despoiled meanwhile the last verification. If some endorsements are unacceptable or do not match by RW set, then the operation is mentioned as illegal. Or, the record is efficient, in addition, all peers add transactions to the channel ledger in a predefined order to ensure accuracy. A valid transaction will update the state of the world. Invalid ones will remain in the ledger, but the world status will not be updated. Finally, the customer application that sends the deal offer will be informed through every peer on the system that the occurred business deal was successful [33–35].

14.4.2 HYPERLEDGER BESU BLOCKCHAIN-BASED ARCHITECTURE

To generate a licensed blockchain with private access for PSC, Hyperledger besu blockchain-based architecture permits the use of linked network accounts to create specific organizations and their users. Hyperledger besu uses an inherent

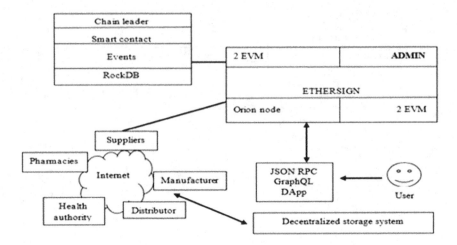

FIGURE 14.3 Hyperledger besu blockchain-based architecture.

infrastructure-based public key to digitally sign along with authentication of businesses deals/transactions, address of each nodule is used for the distinctive recognition of intermediate nodule. For distinction of stowage procedure, administration procedure, and logic of business, it is suggested to use EthSigner conjunction with Hyperledger besu blockchain-based architecture as a third-party supplier of wallet facility. After acceptance of the deal, EthSigner platform will use the stored private key to generate a signature and broadcast the business deal through a completely legal sign to the customer of Ethereum for the purpose of adding in the blockchain [36–38].

In order to preserve the dealings among the shareholders, a Private Transaction Manager (PTM) like Orion is used by the architecture. PTM, which complies with the Enterprise Ethereum Alliance (EEA) 42 customer specifications, allows the common logic of corporate in smart agreements to the remote and restricted count of contributors so that each business dealing and state related to these smart contracts is also private. Orion, the native besu of Hyperledger is a PTM [39]. Finally, in order to grant admittance to dissimilar consumers along with the access of their personal accounts in the system, it provides on-chain as well as off-chain permissions. Authorize the system to enable nodules and ledger permissions for access, and restrict network access to only specific nodes and accounts. In addition, the permission function of Hyperledger besu allows real-time suspension of accounts, denial of access to damaged smart contracts, and restriction of operations on the basis of required details of the group [40] (Figure 14.3 shows the Hyperledger besu blockchain-based architecture).

14.4.2.1 Drug Tracking Flow with Hyperledger Besu Blockchain-Based Architecture

This section describes exactly how to execute and communicate drug-related traceability transactions among dissimilar shareholders in the Hyperledger besu blockchain-based system. When organizational users want to perform transactions, they will initially send signed private transaction requests to Hyperledger besu Electronic Voting Machine (EVM) nodes through a Distributed Application (DApp). The signed transaction includes the recipient's address list or secrecy of the unique ID of the group, the source's address, transaction type, transaction medium, etc. To explain the confidentiality of the group, all intermediate nodes are recognized by Orion by a matchless confidential ID of the group. Orion uses a privacy group ID to store each private transaction. Nodes of Hyperledger besu blockchain-based architecture maintain the public world state of the blockchain and the private state of each privacy group. The private state contains data that is not shared in the globally replicated world state. The privacy group only allows one set of accounts/nodes to access certain data. The app operator interface performs transaction sending task by JSONRPC to Orion via Parathyroid Hormone (PTH). Orion allocates the transaction to further Orion nodules identified through the private group ID or the receiver's address. Once the Orion node receives the transaction, it stores it in the record of state also returns the hash function of the transaction to PTH. In addition to private transactions, PTM also created a privacy token for transmission of PMT that is excavated in the blocks of ledger and transmitted. The main-net transmission workstation on each node of a system will process the PMT and pass the transaction to the contract for execution on the node containing the consistent private pre-assembled smart agreements. The contract uses the transaction hash value to query Orion for private transactions and hand over the business deal to the reserved or private business deal workstation, it implements the deal and sends the RW processes to the reserved stage for updation of remaining contributing nodules. Nodules lacking pre-compiled contracts will disregard flagged transactions [41–43].

14.4.3 ETHEREUM-BASED ARCHITECTURE

Ethereum is unauthorized public blockchain technology, and it can be able to be edited by any person [44]. The smart agreement was inscribed in a tough language, the testing as well as compilation is completed via Remix Integrated Development Environment (IDE). For implementing and debugging the smart agreement codes, Remix a web-based tool is used and it can also check the toughness of codes. The smart agreement will be submitted by the producer and that agreement includes all the facts of the produced drug lot containing clarification and announcing the event in the supply chain environment. Whenever new members are supplementary to the system, they will be able to use the actions as they are fully stowed in the distributed ledger so they could easily observe the past transactions of some produced drug lot. The producer has the choice of uploading a picture of the drug lot to the InterPlanetary File System (IPFS) so that contributing individuals can easily access and view the drug lot tree. For the sale of drug lots in previous times, it must be crowded first then the producer will pronounce to other contributors that the freshly acquired drug lot is accessible for trade by

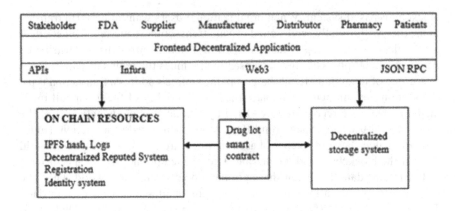

FIGURE 14.4   Ethereum-based blockchain architecture.

posting an event. Contributing producers who want to buy newly acquired drug lots will need to find a special job in marketing of drug lots, and when the work is completed, the event will inform the contributors to announce a new drug lot owner [45]. The producer will not be able to submit a smart agreement of drug lot until it is permitted through the FDA but then again due to ease, this authorization has not been submitted in the smart agreement (Figure 14.4 shows the Ethereum based blockchain architecture).

14.4.3.1   Flow of Drug Tracking with Ethereum Based Architecture

The smart agreement will be implemented by the features such as holder ID, with the location of Ethereum of the recent agreement holder [46]. The key point to be noted is that the holder ID is the main location as well as not mapping since the lot smart drug agreement can have only a single holder ID and whenever the holder ship has changed the transaction/action will be released and stowed in the blockchain, these actions are using to track the initials of drug lot [47]. A smart agreement denotes a certain lot of drugs, also having other characteristics like the name of the lot, the worth of the lot, the total count of boxes, the price of each box, and its real photo [48]. In addition, the three required mapping of certified attributes permitted the admittance of services inside a smart agreement such as producers, suppliers, and pharmacologists. A smart agreement has numerous roles that are required to perform the production procedure as well as the sale procedure of drug lots [49]. Furthermore, a generated drug lot's information is proficient with details of drug lot activity as input parameters, including name of the lot, worth of the lot, the total count of boxes, price of each box, and its real photo. Moreover, the producer has the choice to upload the photo on the IPFS, and the hash function of the IPFS photo is stored as well as retrieved by another attribute. The connection among smart agreements as well as IPFS is a ratio of 1:1 as each drug lot will have to upload a photo over IPFS at a time [50].

14.4.4 COMPARISON OF HYPERLEDGER FABRIC, HYPERLEDGER BESU, AND ETHEREUM ARCHITECTURES

This section elaborates a deep and practical evaluation of three discussed blockchain-based platforms, emphasizing their pros and cons. While Ethereum may be set as a private system, this association will emphasize it as a societal web. Comparative features were aggregated, constructed on suggestions from previous research and expansion, and real literature, and a few continuing projects [51].

As paralleled to Ethereum-based architecture, in cooperation with Hyperledger fabric-based architecture and Hyperledger besu-based architecture are intended to be used as independent, valid commercial-to-commercial systems. Ethereum is a slightly commercial-to-consumer concerned approach, without the natural maintenance of confidentiality or personal records/transactions deals. Hyperledger fabric and Hyperledger besu sustenance rapid understanding and provide a high rate of transaction toward speed. The smart agreements in Hyperledger fabric can be easily upgraded because they use standard software designing languages, unlike Hyperledger besu blockchain-based architecture along with Ethereum blockchain-based architectures, which use exact territory phonology. Hyperledger fabric blockchain-based architecture does not have the appropriate agreement of improved structure that is accessible for both besu and Ethereum. System arrangement, format, and distribution are very high on Hyperledger fabric, but they are easy to accomplish and upgrade because all modules are dockerized. Utilizing Hyperledger fabric blockchain-based architecture likewise arises through improved customer request function; however, it increases the number of controllers over the consumer end. Hyperledger fabric blockchain-based architecture is better as compared to Hyperledger besu blockchain-based architecture and Ethereum blockchain-based architectures for proprietary administration and admittance that regulate by containing both physical and logical, to manage. In the treatment schedule, both Hyperledger fabric blockchain-based and Hyperledger besu blockchain-based offer some of the best replacements and structures of an active tracking solution [52]. Table 14.3 aims to provide in-depth details on the comparison effect of the above-discussed architectures.

14.5 DISCUSSION AND OPEN CHALLENGES

This section describes the significant discussion and open challenges in implementing blockchain-based origin and track resolutions in the pharmaceutical business (Figure 14.5 highlights the open challenges in the drug tracking system).

14.5.1 STAKEHOLDER AGREEMENT

Blockchain setup is a dispersed platform, wherever all the pharmaceutical service providers stock their essential commercial records, as well as everybody takes admittance to given secretive records over the blockchain platform. Participants may be unwilling to contribute to these systems as it may result in the loss of their economic benefit, particularly while numerous commercial participants are on the identical supply list [54].

TABLE 14.3

Comparison of Above Discussed Three Architectures

Category	Hyperledger Fabric [53]	Hyperledger Besu [53]	Ethereum [53]
Network configuration complexity	High	Low	Always ready to use, very easy
Deployment of network	Used docker and docker-compose	Can be used docker and docker-compose	Publically available, setup is optional
Storage option	LevelDB, CouchDB	File storage	File storage
Multiple ledgers	Yes	No	No
Running cost	Depend on the size of the dynamic ledger	Depend on the size of the dynamic ledger	Depend on the dynamic ledger size
Size	1–4 GB	1–8 GB	4TB, 350 GB full node, 10 GB light node
Transaction	Unique execute order authenticate approach	Order execute approach	Order execute approach
Consensus protocols	Kafka, Raft	IBFT PoA and clique	Ethash PoW
Cost	Running cost only	The extra cost required along with the running cost	The extra cost required along with the running cost
Support of TLS	Yes	Yes	Yes
Privacy of data	Yes	Yes	No
User and node	Organized	Organized	Not organized
Identification of management and generation	Based on PKI	Based on public key	Based on public key
Smart contract execution platform	Isolate inside docker	EVM	EVM
Language	Java, Go, NodejS	Domain-specific	Domain-specific
Lifecycle of smart contract	Require installation again and again	Immutable	Immutable
Tokenization	No native support	Native support	Native support
Cryptography	Pluggable	Secp256kl	Secp256kl
Contributors	~220	~70	~475
Manner	Private, permissioned	Semi-private	Public
Maturity	High level	Middle	High level

14.5.2 Interoperability

It is well-defined as the widespread acceptance of commercial software and platforms through numerous governments to offer effective incorporation of policies. It works as a way for users of dissimilar software and platforms to interrelate and create sensible business activities freely. The remaining drug tracking resolutions like series, bar codes, RFID tags, solutions based on blockchain technology, and

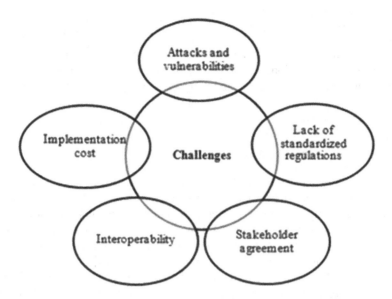

FIGURE 14.5 Discussion and open challenges in the drug tracking system.

platforms fail to work fully as there are no proven solutions to make combination, flexibility, and simplicity. In addition, dissimilar blockchain-based platforms further down the Hyperledger umbrella, deal with the challenges of providing collaboration, ensuring high scope and flexibility to allow interior and exterior communiqué among commercial administrations [55].

14.5.3 IMPLEMENTATION COST

Scheming a good blockchain system is not an easy job, as many of the surviving resolutions are still being established. Confidentiality, failure, and collaboration challenge similarly pay significantly to this problem. The cost of execution and energy efficiency is one of the important challenges facing most businesses, as well as the provision of the medicinal industry based on the supply chain. Surviving platforms and inherited software programs are incompetent and central to transaction processing, which creates significant costs for start-up and preservation overheads. For instance, Hyperledger fabric-based architecture that can be able to make further 4000 trades for each second along with its command depletion is meaningfully condensed as related to Ethereum, because of various consensus protocols [56].

14.5.4 ATTACK AND VULNERABILITIES

The main benefit and drawbacks of blockchain-based networks or technology are its ability to combat numerous categories of attacks, counting cyber-attacks. A current cybersecurity record enlightens a number of security threats, like malicious attacks on a centralized network, involvement in a blockchain network, and revealing network vulnerabilities. The recent use of blockchain is leaving the environment and bugs because of the growth of undeveloped procedures and organizations. Fraudulent theft of sensitive information, technological susceptibility, execution, and malware, because of the absence of ethics and processes, are currently major concerning challenges in order to move forward [57].

14.5.5 Lack of Standardized

The part of drug supervisory experts contains quality inspection, quality monitoring, security, and efficiency as well as monitoring the post-sales of pharmaceutical goods. It also supervises the production, circulation, and stowage of pharmacological goods hence unlawful acquisition, as well as trafficking in fake drugs, could be achieved rapidly and sufficiently. The key role of supervisory frameworks becomes more relevant and compound as it becomes too difficult for these organizations to describe the authorized and ecological limitations of blockchain technology. For example, whenever any new actions or transmissions are performed over a network, it is quite tough for these experts to undoubtedly explain the authority and to make right the legitimate compulsions of the attached shareholders. An additional challenge is to address future regulatory needs like FDA, QRC, DSCSA, and interest in blockchain-based systems. Hence, blockchain-based technology does not comply with the latest rules and guidelines about the provision of medicines [58].

14.6 CONCLUSION

Healthcare supply chains are intricate infrastructures that cross many administrative and territorial restrictions, offering essential support to essential facilities in daily life. The natural difficulty of these systems can lead to contaminations that contain imprecise data, ambiguity, and the provenance of limited data. Counterfeit drugs are a key sign of such restrictions contained by the surviving supply chains that not only have a devastating influence on human health but also lead to significant monetary losses in the healthcare industry. As a result, current research has highlighted the need for a vigorous, end-to-end tracing program and tracking of drug supply chains. The end-to-end tracking of goods through the pharmaceutical industry is critical to guaranteeing the security of goods and the removal of fake requests or unauthorized access. Furthermore, the surviving tracking systems are intermediate that lead to data confidentiality, visibility, and legitimacy in healthcare chains. The paper discovers the overview of blockchain with its different nature. Moreover, the paper discussed how blockchain technology can be applied in drug tracking and drug delivery. Additionally, the paper deliberated the most important and concerning the topic of today's research that is an overview of drug tracking in the healthcare domain. Furthermore, the paper enlightened the essential architectures for drug tracking systems based on blockchain. Hyperledger fabric, Hyperledger besu, and Ethereum based architectures are discussed with their drug tracking flow. These architectures offer a shared, reliable, authoritative, and community-based platform for maintenance as well as communication between the various drug supply shareholders in a way that can meet important needs or features counting safety, confidentiality, availability, limpidity, and scalability. In addition, evaluation of these three discussed platforms has been shown via table. Finally, this paper observes some open challenges and discussions that describe the many employment challenges that hamper the widespread acceptance of blockchain-based technology for real drug tracking. As a future reference, we plan to build smart contracts, by installing all parts of the system and creating a DApps user interface for the proposed properties.

REFERENCES

1. Malik, A., Gautam, S., Abidin, S. and Bhushan, B. (2019). Blockchain technology-future of IoT: including structure, limitations and various possible attacks. *2nd International Conference on Intelligent Computing, Instrumentation and Control Technologies (ICICICT)*, Kannur, India, 2019, pp. 1100–1104. doi: 10.1109/ICICIC T46008.2019.8993144.

2. Buettner, R., Blattner, M. and Reinhardt, W. (2020). Internet gaming more than 3 hours a day is indicative and more than 5 hours is diagnostic: proposal of playing time cutoffs for WHO-11 and DSM-5 internet gaming disorder based on a large steam platform dataset. *IEEE Sixth International Conference on Big Data Computing Service and Applications (BigDataService)*. pp. 189–192. doi: 10.1109/ BigDataService49289.2020.00037.

3. Saxena, S., Bhushan, B. and Yadav, D. (2020). Blockchain-powered social media analytics in supply chain management. *SSRN Electronic Journal*. doi: 10.2139/ssrn.3598906.

4. Salehi, S., Moayedian, N. S., Javanmard, S. H. and Alarcón, E. (2018, July). Lifetime improvement of a multiple transmitter local drug delivery system based on diffusive molecular communication. *IEEE Transactions on NanoBioscience*, *17*(3), 352–360. doi: 10.1109/TNB.2018.2850054.

5. Soni, S. and Bhushan, B. (2019). A comprehensive survey on blockchain: working, security analysis, privacy threats and potential applications. *2019 2nd International Conference on Intelligent Computing, Instrumentation and Control Technologies (ICICICT)*. doi: 10.1109/icicict46008.2019.8993210.

6. Mackey, T. K. and Liang, B. A. (2011). The global counterfeit drug trade: patient safety and public health risks. *Journal of Pharmaceutical Sciences*, *100*(11), 4571–4579. doi: 10.1002/jps.22679.

7. Gupta, S., Sinha, S. and Bhushan, B. (2020). Emergence of blockchain technology: fundamentals, working and its various implementations. *SSRN Electronic Journal*. doi: 10.2139/ssrn.3569577.

8. Gjini, E. and Wertheimer, A. I. (2016). Review of drug quality and security act of 2013: the drug supply chain security act (DSCSA). *Innovations in Pharmacy*, *7*(3). doi: 10.24926/iip.v7i3.462.

9. Dhiman, T., Gulyani, V. and Bhushan, B. (2020). Application, classification and system requirements of blockchain technology. *SSRN Electronic Journal*. doi: 10.2139/ssrn.3600745.

10. Hermansen, E., Moen, G., Barstad, J., Birketvedt, R. and Indrekvam, K. (2013). Laminarthrectomy as a surgical approach for decompressing the spinal CANAL:

assessment of preoperative Versus postoperative dural SAC cross-sectional areal (DSCSA). *European Spine Journal*, *22*(8), 1913–1919. doi: 10.1007/s00586-013-2737-1.

11. Saini, H., Bhushan, B., Arora, A. and Kaur, A. (2019). Security vulnerabilities in Information communication technology: blockchain to the rescue (A survey on Blockchain Technology). *2019 2nd International Conference on Intelligent Computing, Instrumentation and Control Technologies (ICICICT)*. doi: 10.1109/icic ict46008.2019.8993229.

12. Ray, P. P., Dash, D., Salah, K. and Kumar, N. (2021, March). Blockchain for IoT-based healthcare: background, consensus, platforms, and use cases. *IEEE Systems Journal*, *15*(1), 85–94. doi: 10.1109/JSYST.2020.2963840.

13. Kumar, A., Krishnamurthi, R., Nayyar, A., Sharma, K., Grover, V. and Hossain, E. (2020). A novel smart healthcare design, simulation, and implementation using healthcare 4.0 processes. *IEEE Access*, *8*, 118433–118471. doi: 10.1109/ACCESS.2020.3004790.

14. Li, P. et al. (2020, June). ChainSDI: a software-defined infrastructure for regulation-compliant home-based healthcare services secured by blockchains. *IEEE Systems Journal*, *14*(2), 2042–2053. doi: 10.1109/JSYST.2019.2937930.

15. Gamalo-Siebers, M. (2020). Journal of biopharmaceutical statistics editorial. *Journal of Biopharmaceutical Statistics*, *30*(1), 1–2. doi: 10.1080/10543406.2019.1709697.

16. Varshney, T., Sharma, N., Kaushik, I. and Bhushan, B. (2019). Authentication & encryption based security services in blockchain technology. *2019 International Conference on Computing, Communication, and Intelligent Systems (ICCCIS)*. doi: 10.1109/icccis48478.2019.8974500.

17. Pitts, P. (2020). The spreading cancer of counterfeit drugs. *Journal of Commercial Biotechnology*, *25*(3). doi: 10.5912/jcb940.

18. Goyal, S., Sharma, N., Bhushan, B., Shankar, A. and Sagayam, M. (2020). IoT enabled technology in secured healthcare: applications, challenges and future directions. *Cognitive Internet of Medical Things for Smart Healthcare*, 25–48. doi: 10.1007/978-3-030-55833-8_2.

19. Konkin, A. and Zapechnikov, S. (2021). Techniques for private transactions in corporate blockchain networks. *2021 IEEE Conference of Russian Young Researchers in Electrical and Electronic Engineering (ElConRus)*, 2021, pp. 2356–2360. doi: 10. 1109/ElConRus51938.2021.9396228.

20. Xu, B. et al. (2019, July). Incorporating user generated content for drug interaction extraction based on full attention mechanism. *IEEE Transactions on NanoBioscience*, *18*(3), 360–367. doi: 10.1109/TNB.2019.2919188.

21. Liu, N., Chen, C. B. and Kumara, S. (2020, January). Semi-supervised learning algorithm for identifying high-priority drug–drug interactions through adverse event reports. *IEEE Journal of Biomedical and Health Informatics*, *24*(1), 57–68. doi: 10.1109/JBHI.2019.2932740.

22. Ru, B., Li, D., Hu, Y. and Yao, L. (2019, July). Serendipity—a machine-learning application for mining serendipitous drug usage from social media. *IEEE Transactions on NanoBioscience*, *18*(3), 324–334. doi: 10.1109/TNB.2019.2909094.

23. Islam, T., Shitiri, E. and Cho, H. (2020). A simultaneous drug release scheme for targeted drug delivery using molecular communications. *IEEE Access*, *8*, 91770–91778. doi: 10.1109/ACCESS.2020.2994493.

24. Liu, Y., Zuo, Z. and Wu, G. (2020, July). Link prediction only with interaction data and its application on drug repositioning. *IEEE Transactions on NanoBioscience*, *19*(3), 547–555. doi: 10.1109/TNB.2020.2990291.

25. (2013). Tracking drug levels in blood in real time. *Nature Reviews Drug Discovery*, *13*(1), 9-9. doi: 10.1038/nrd4225.

26. Friedrich, M. J. (2011). Tracking drug quality. *JAMA*, *305*(19). doi: 10.1001/jama.2011.637.

27. Krstić, M. and Krstić, L. (2020). Hyperledger frameworks with a special focus on hyperledger fabric. *Vojnotehnicki Glasnik, 68*(3), 639–663. doi: 10.5937/vojtehg68-26206.

28. Wessling, F., Ehmke, C., Hesenius, M. and Gruhn, V. (2018). How much blockchain do you need? Towards a concept for building hybrid DApp architectures. *2018 IEEE/ ACM 1st International Workshop on Emerging Trends in Software Engineering for Blockchain (WETSEB)*, 2018, pp. 44–47.

29. Firdayati, D., Ranggadara, I., Afrianto, I. and Kurnianda, N. R. (2021). Designing architecture blockchain of hyperledger fabric for purchasing strategy. *International Journal of Advanced Trends in Computer Science and Engineering, 10*(2), 464–468. doi: 10.30534/ijatcse/2021/041022021.

30. Blockchain based warehouse supply chain management using hyperledger fabric and hyperledger composer. (2020). *International Journal of Innovative Technology and Exploring Engineering, 9*(3S), 147–151. doi: 10.35940/ijitee.c1033.0193s20.

31. Baliga, A., Solanki, N., Verekar, S., Pednekar, A., Kamat, P. and Chatterjee, S. (2018). Performance characterization of hyperledger fabric. *2018 Crypto Valley Conference on Blockchain Technology (CVCBT)*. doi: 10.1109/cvcbt.2018.00013.

32. Seo, J. and Cho, Y. (2020). Medical image sharing system using hyperledger fabric blockchain. *2020 22nd International Conference on Advanced Communication Technology (ICACT)*. doi: 10.23919/icact48636.2020.9061384.

33. Kumar S. N., and Dakshayini, M. (2020). Secure sharing of health data using hyperledger fabric based on blockchain technology. *2020 International Conference on Mainstreaming Block Chain Implementation (ICOMBI)*. doi: 10.23919/icombi4 8604.2020.9203442.

34. Park, W., Hwang, D. and Kim, K. (2018). A TOTP-based two factor authentication scheme for hyperledger fabric blockchain. *2018 Tenth International Conference on Ubiquitous and Future Networks (ICUFN)*, 2018, pp. 817–819. doi: 10.1109/ICUFN.2018.8436784.

35. Hua, S., Zhang, S., Pi, B., Sun, J., Yamashita, K. and Nomura, Y. (2020) Reasonableness discussion and analysis for Hyperledger Fabric configuration. *2020 IEEE International Conference on Blockchain and Cryptocurrency (ICBC)*, 2020, pp. 1–3. doi: 10.1109/ICBC48266.2020.9169444.

36. Praitheeshan, P., Pan, L. and Doss, R. (2021). Private and trustworthy distributed lending model using hyperledger besu. *SN Computer Science, 2*(2). doi: 10.1007/s42979-021-00500-3.

37. Azhar, M. T., Khan, M. B. and Zafar, M. M. (2019). Architecture of an enterprise project life cycle using hyperledger platform. *2019 13th International Conference on Mathematics, Actuarial Science, Computer Science and Statistics (MACS)*. doi: 10.1109/macs48846.2019.9024764.

38. Attia, O., Khoufi, I., Laouiti, A. and Adjih, C. (2019). An IoT-blockchain architecture based on hyperledger framework for healthcare monitoring application. *2019 10th IFIP International Conference on New Technologies, Mobility and Security (NTMS)*. doi: 10.1109/ntms.2019.8763849.

39. Kushwaha, R. and Singh, D. (2021). Hyperledger architecture for Internet of things and supply chain management services. *Blockchain Technology for IoT Applications*, 39–63. doi: 10.1007/978-981-33-4122-7_3.

40. Kienzler, R. (2016). Hyperledger – Eine offene blockchain technologie. *Blockchain Technology*. doi: 10.1515/9783110488951-005.

41. Klaokliang, N., Teawtim, P., Aimtongkham, P., So-In, C. and Niruntasukrat, A. (2018). A novel IoT authorization architecture on hyperledger fabric with optimal consensus using genetic algorithm. *2018 Seventh ICT International Student Project Conference (ICT-ISPC)*. doi: 10.1109/ict-ispc.2018.8523942.

42. Xu, R., Nikouei, S. Y., Chen, Y., Blasch, E. and Aved, A. (2019). BlendMAS: a blockchain-enabled decentralized microservices architecture for smart public safety. *2019 IEEE International Conference on Blockchain (Blockchain)*, 2019, pp. 564–571. doi: 10.1109/Blockchain.2019.00082.

43. Wessling, F., Ehmke, C., Hesenius, M. and Gruhn, V. (2018). How much blockchain do you need? towards a concept for building hybrid DApp architectures. *2018 IEEE/ACM 1st International Workshop on Emerging Trends in Software Engineering for Blockchain (WETSEB)*, 2018, pp. 44–47.

44. Mohanty, D. (2018). Ethereum architecture. *Ethereum for Architects and Developers*, 37–54. doi: 10.1007/978-1-4842-4075-5_2.

45. Kadam, S. B. and John, S. K. (2020). Ethereum based IoT architecture. *Second International Conference on Computer Networks and Communication Technologies*, 179–184. doi: 10.1007/978-3-030-37051-0_20

46. Mohanty, D. (2018). Testing strategy for ethereum dapps. *Ethereum for Architects and Developers*, 197–201. doi: 10.1007/978-1-4842-4075-5_8.

47. Paavolainen, S. and Carr, C. (2020). Security properties of light clients on the ethereum blockchain. *IEEE Access*, 8, 124339–124358. doi: 10.1109/ACCESS.2020.3006113.

48. Toyoda, K., Machi, K., Ohtake, Y. and Zhang, A. M. (2020). Function-level bottle-neck analysis of private proof-of-authority ethereum blockchain. *IEEE Access*, 8, 141611–141621. doi: 10.1109/ACCESS.2020.3011876.

49. Huang, Y., Wang, B. and Wang, Y. (2020). MResearch on ethereum private block-chain multi-nodes platform. *2020 International Conference on Big Data, Artificial Intelligence and Internet of Things Engineering (ICBAIE)*, 2020, pp. 369–372. doi: 10.1109/ICBAIE49996.2020.00083.

50. Yavuz, E., Koç, A. K., Çabuk, U. K. and Dalkılıç, G. (2018). Towards secure e-voting using ethereum blockchain. *2018 6th International Symposium on Digital Forensic and Security (ISDFS)*, 2018, pp. 1–7. doi: 10.1109/ISDFS.2018.8355340.

51. Gautam, S., Malik, A., Singh, N. and Kumar, S. (2019). Recent advances and countermeasures against various attacks in IoT environment. *2019 2nd International Conference on Signal Processing and Communication (ICSPC)*. doi: 10.1109/icspc46172.2019.8976527.

52. Malik, A. (2020, December 12). Steganography: step towards security and privacy of confidential data in insecure medium by using LSB and cover media. *SSRN Electronic Journal*. doi: 10.2139/ssrn.3747579.

53. Kumar, A., Abhishek, K., Bhushan, B. and Chakraborty, C. (2021). Secure access control for manufacturing sector with application of ethereum blockchain. *Peer-to-Peer Networking and Applications*. doi: 10.1007/s12083-021-01108-3.

54. Bhushan, B., Sahoo, C., Sinha, P. and Khamparia, A. (2020). Unification of block-chain and Internet of Things (BIoT): requirements, working model, challenges and future directions. *Wireless Networks*. doi: 10.1007/s11276-020-02445.

55. Bhushan, B., Khamparia, A., Sagayam, K. M., Sharma, S. K., Ahad, M. A. and Debnath, N. C. (2020). Blockchain for smart cities: a review of architectures, inte-gration trends and future research directions. *Sustainable Cities and Society*, 61, 102360. doi: 10.1016/j.scs.2020.102360.

56. Wang, G., Shi, Z., Nixon, M. and Han, S. (2019). ChainSplitter: towards blockchain-based industrial IoT architecture for supporting hierarchical storage. *2019 IEEE International Conference on Blockchain (Blockchain)*, 2019, pp. 166–175. doi: 10.1109/Blockchain.2019.00030.

57. Guo, H., Li, W., Nejad, M. and Shen, C. (2019). Access control for electronic health records with hybrid blockchain-edge architecture. *2019 IEEE International Conference on Blockchain (Blockchain),* 2019, pp. 44–51, doi: 10.1109/Blockchain.2019.00015.
58. Desai, H., Kantarcioglu, M. and Kagal, L. (2019). A hybrid blockchain architecture for privacy-enabled and accountable auctions. *2019 IEEE International Conference on Blockchain (Blockchain),* 2019, pp. 34–43, doi: 10.1109/Blockchain.2019.00014.

15 Securing Privacy and Integrity of Patient's Data in Healthcare 4.0 by Countering Attack using Blockchain

Avinash Kumar and Snigdha Kashyap
Sharda University

Tanmayee Prakash Tilekar
ISAC India

Tabassum Jahan
Sharda University

Azedine Boulmakoul
Hassan II University of Casablanca

CONTENTS

DOI: 10.1201/9781003224075-15

15.1　INTRODUCTION

Industry 4.0 has revolutionised human society by providing services offered using technologies with low latency, higher throughput and real-time monitoring. healthcare 4.0 branched from Industry 4.0 and made the healthcare system more successful as it constitutes Internet of Things (IoT), Artificial Intelligence (AI), Embedded Systems (ES) and various other recent technologies. These technologies have helped healthcare 4.0 to be more efficient, precise and provide preventive measures to various diseases and ailments. The heterogeneous nature of healthcare 4.0 attracts adversaries to perform malicious activities for financial gain and other disruptive intent [1]. Thus, it is vital to protect and secure healthcare 4.0 to restrict adversaries. In addition, when the availability of information is to be guaranteed to end users in a healthcare 4.0 network, security implementation becomes a major concern [2]. The below subsections explain various elements that are discussed to analyse healthcare 4.0 components, vital information, vulnerabilities and their resolution.

Healthcare is transforming the healthcare domain into a more inter-related information-driven one. Moreover, it is exceptionally directed, capital intensive and fulfils educational necessities for the individuals who are a part of the healthcare system. Accordingly, changes in healthcare are slow, although the changes are significant enough. From the last century, techniques such as sedation, anaesthesia and antiseptic surgery have been introduced in healthcare. With time, antimicrobials as well as antiseptics were having a tremendous effect on wellbeing and life span. Presently in the 21st century, the progress is driven by innovation [3]. In the future, by 2030, we are probably going to witness sensational changes in how medical services or healthcare is delivered due to the expanded admittance to information, added substance assembling, AI as well as wearable and embedded gadgets to monitor humans' wellbeing to fight diseases [4].

Currently, almost every healthcare services' framework possesses electronic records, and even reception at small country healthcare frameworks is huge in number. There is an enormous amount of information, which can assist with diagnosing infection, assess the adequacy of treatment, and even give an endorsement for care. When electronic records and information are combined with the features of AI, one can optimally imagine the future of healthcare. Soon, AI can turn into an advanced assistant for doctors or physicians, effectively gathering the data for medicine requirements, treatments as well as diagnostics. It can provide relevant data on request to a doctor or healthcare personnel [5]. Finally, numerous decisions made by doctors and individuals at present can be taken over by intelligent machines. As of now, AI can determine cellular breakdown in the lungs with far higher accuracy than humans. AI can assist with tracking and monitoring of patients' health through information examination and data analytics. AI has been a breakthrough in enabling safe, convenient, connected living and healthcare for human society [6].

Data plays a crucial role in healthcare. Thus, collection, maintenance and analysis of data are emphasised, when healthcare 4.0 is introduced. Patients' health status, illness and diseases can be instantly monitored by making use of specialised IoT sensors. Moreover, sensors are able to alert the healthcare personnel in emergency situations, such as patients' critical health or detection of some anonymous symptoms [7]. Raw data collected from sensors is processed and then analysed for respective purposes in healthcare as well as other domains. Along with IoT, industrial IoT (IIoT) also affects healthcare 4.0 positively within a decentralised network, by making use of cognitive computing, fog computing and edge computing [8]. IoT is also an important aspect for storage of the personal data of patients and keeping the records conveniently.

Since healthcare 4.0 deals with newer technologies and collection and management of sensitive data, security has to be preserved. Moreover, an increasing number of users pose a threat to healthcare systems when data is to be managed over the cloud servers [9]. Advancements in medical sciences such as nanotechnology and synthetic biology require the use of embedded devices in computing the health data from biological cells [10]. Thus, ensuring security while implementing healthcare 4.0 is a high-priority task. The risk of exposure of sensitive data outside a network is a possibility while implementing IoT, AI and other technologies in the healthcare domain. Sensors and devices in a decentralised network require patch updates for their consistent functioning, but few devices do not have the functionality to update themselves. Moreover, while receiving the updates, there is a need to monitor intrusions and malicious activities within the network. Any compromise with the patients' data or personal data of healthcare personnel and hospitals ought to be prevented and protected from being intercepted or modified.

This paper tries to analyse and present the most important features of blockchain that could make healthcare 4.0 more secure and resistant to cyber-attacks. The paper tries its best to investigate vulnerabilities in healthcare 4.0 and provides blockchain as one of the important solutions for the same. In summary, the major contributions of this paper are as follows.

- This work presents the heterogeneous nature of healthcare 4.0 and its components.
- This work presents blockchain features that are vital to achieve privacy and security in heterogeneous systems.
- This work presents the role of cyber security in healthcare 4.0.
- This work presents blockchain as one of the concrete solutions for protecting and securing healthcare 4.0.

The remainder of this paper is organised as follows: Section 15.2 presents healthcare 4.0 and its components. Section 15.3 describes the features of blockchain. Section 15.4 presents cyber security and its relevance in healthcare 4.0. Section 15.5 presents blockchain as a solution for privacy and security issues in healthcare 4.0. Finally, Section 15.6 concludes itself followed by future research directions.

15.2 HEALTHCARE 4.0

Healthcare 4.0 is a major transition in the healthcare sector. With the advent of Industry 4.0, features of current technologies in healthcare have transformed the complete view of the medical industry. Enhancement in medical care convenience is at its initial stage, and is accompanied by new technologies including AI, IoT, cloud computing, big data and advanced data analytics. Tissue implants by making the use of 3D printing technology can be considered an instance of healthcare 4.0 [11]. Newer technologies are enabling transmission and storage of data efficiently, and automate most of the functions in the healthcare domain, thereby reducing manual efforts. Constant monitoring of medical data is helped with the advent of healthcare 4.0 [12]. Real-time data analysis in the healthcare domain is yet another plus point of healthcare 4.0. Healthcare 4.0 can be considered a useful application of Industry 4.0, which has helped develop the methods of monitoring patients' health, maintaining and analysing personal data [13].

15.2.1 EVOLUTION OF HEALTHCARE

The emergence of the new concepts in healthcare led to revolutionisation of the healthcare industry with the introduction of silo Information Technology (IT). This emergence was termed healthcare 1.0 [14]. Healthcare evolved further with the introduction of networking as well as the Electronic Health Records (EHRs) integrated with medical imaging. This period was referred to as healthcare 2.0 [15]. Post healthcare 2.0, the year 2000 witnessed the development of genomic data along with the rise of wearables and implantables as well as networked EHRs of patients. However, because of data incompatibility and resistance to healthcare providers in a large healthcare network, acceptance of IT projects in healthcare 3.0 rarely led to serious advancements in society. At present, a new era of healthcare and science called healthcare 4.0 is being observed in the healthcare and scientific domain. The purpose of healthcare 4.0 is to implement the principles of Industry 4.0 by merging IoT and emerging technologies for information collection and processing. To mention a few applications, healthcare 4.0 supported augmenting the utilisation of AI and using blockchain for securing medical records of the patients. Focus on integration of advanced methods has made healthcare more speculative and customisable [16,17]. The improved amount of information available from doctors is a benefit provided by healthcare 4.0. Moreover, the benefit can be extended to extraction, computation and storage of data using blockchain. Data handling can permit patients as well as doctors to receive information anytime, anywhere. A better insight can allow various sorts of analyses for clinical response estimation as well as constructing and upgrading methods for detecting new diseases [18]. Healthcare 4.0 enables information to be utilised productively, and possibly identify domains for development and empower humanity to witness further advancements. It is driving the entire healthcare industry through an efficient and focused service billing system to a system that is based on value, which determines results in addition to promoting efficiency. Table 15.1 demonstrates the progress of methods and technologies from healthcare 1.0 to healthcare 4.0.

TABLE 15.1
Significant Changes in Healthcare from Healthcare 1.0 to Healthcare 4.0

	Healthcare 1.0	Healthcare 2.0	Healthcare 3.0	Healthcare 4.0
Principle aim	• Further develop productivity and lessen paperwork	• Further develop information sharing with productivity	• Provide patient-centred arrangements	• Provide capability to track real-time and reaction arrangements
Specialty	• Straightforward robotisation	• Availability to different organisations	• Collaboration with patients	• Coordinated ongoing testing of health with AI support
Data sharing	• Within an organisation	• Within a bunch of medical services	• Within a country	• Worldwide medical services store network
Key innovations utilised	• Regulatory frameworks and laboratory information management system (LIMS)	• Cloud computing and electronic data interchange	• Wearable gadgets, electronic medical records, big data	• Data analytics, AI, Blockchain

15.2.2 Drivers for Healthcare 4.0

Several features contribute to the development of better healthcare. First, many evolved countries including Singapore, the USA and the UK have raised the domestic "backbone" of IT that can encourage the integration of electronic medical records, making them more manageable. The government organises programs that are crucial in meeting community goals such as improving access to healthcare along with the provision of better patient results [19]. Secondly, healthcare consists of pathologists, doctors, specialists and emergency units and hence, healthcare 4.0 gives more precise results for all of them and is a key to implementing efficient treatment methods [20]. The third feature is openness of coordinated consideration [21]. Considering the features of healthcare 4.0, the patients can monitor their vital concentration and note guidelines to be followed during treatment. Family history in databases can help with identifying the patients' health data. Looking at the mentioned aspects, present healthcare systems seem to emphasise contributing quality care by empowering and organising the medical domain. They are efficient in taking care of people with sympathy as well as respect. Healthcare 4.0 drives a major change in healthcare that deals with data conversion occurring in several countries. The designed approaches in healthcare 4.0 result in less expensive, faster data communication due to private sector involvement and allow doctors as well as patients from small townships to get benefitted by the advantages of healthcare 4.0. To summarise, the centre of attention shifts to the combination of resources and integrated care.

15.2.3 Healthcare 4.0 and Its Main Technology

The advancement of healthcare using Information and Communication Technologies (ICT) began with the internet when forums about general wellbeing and diseases were first introduced. The advent of organisation-empowered and IoT-EHR frameworks incorporated with information logic followed ICT. ICT has now reduced the openness of EHRs alongside portable-based and cloud-based synergistic projects. These days, we witness the openness of healthcare 4.0 that gathers the entirety of mechanisation, in accordance with continuous information coordination. The primary objective of healthcare 4.0 is to associate patients, clinical suppliers with clinical gadgets, centres and emergency clinics. Medical service providers are providing services using networks for real-time coordination. The points below explain ICT progression by healthcare 4.0.

- **IoT**: IoT connects clinical gadgets to the web and includes testing clinical projects associated with X-beam machines and different clinical gear [22]. This IoT is known as the web of wellbeing offices, and more specifically Internet of Healthcare Things (IoHT).
- **Internet Providers**: They ensure the wellbeing of people through specialised gadgets, frameworks and associations. They are offered as programming administration with an exact interface between people or end users and the web and are known as the Internet of Services [23].

- **Clinical Cyber-Physical Systems (CPS)**: Medical CPS is known to make successful correspondence in the real and the digital world through consistent monitoring of health with administrative support [24].
- **Wellbeing Cloud**: Large cloud framework uses programming instruments for wellbeing applications [25]. This can enhance the healthcare 4.0 efficiency via interaction between users and applications over the cloud.
- **Wellbeing Fog**: Health Fog (or Edge) regions are useful for frequent speed-up cooperation of clinical gadgets and frameworks with medical care [26].
- **Huge Data Analytics**: A lot of data increments in medical care frameworks on an everyday basis. Thus, it becomes hard to manage by the administration in an efficient manner [27]. ICT helps to provide effective data analytics, especially for big data.
- **Versatile Networks (5G)**: 5G organisation mechanisation tries its best to supply more developed characteristics of healthcare management; for example, quick and low defer associations and information power [28]. This increases the real-time processing in healthcare 4.0.
- **Square Chain**: Healthcare benefits consistently by incorporating the assortment, stockpiling and using delicate and sectioned information. Healthcare requires dependable activity and arrangements with adequate information on examining and guaranteeing consistency in the system [29]. Square chain methods help to maintain consistency of medical information in healthcare 4.0.

15.2.4 HEALTHCARE 4.0 APPLICATIONS

There are a variety of healthcare systems that have made good use of high-quality ICT to achieve healthcare development goals. Designing and submitting applications to enable core functionalities of healthcare 4.0 need a clear vision of the skills and assets which they provide. Additionally, it requires technical skills along with design essentials to efficiently develop and use them. Healthcare 4.0 considers every single coordinated innovation, instruments, hardware, individuals, and programming to convey top-notch medical care benefits such as the application of custom-fitted assets. Applications in healthcare 4.0 can be classified into four main types based on their specific functionalities: patient services, healthcare services, healthcare management system and resource management applications. The available healthcare applications can assist with different identified uses. However, the discussion of the following sections provides a summary of the types of applications in healthcare 4.0.

- **Application for Patients**: Effective healthcare systems should be able to ensure copyright, better quality as well as experience. Healthcare 4.0 applications that provide patients' medical information vary depending on the purpose of the specific healthcare applications [30].

- **Application for Healthcare Professionals**: People, except patients, who participate in healthcare programs and contribute their services, can benefit tremendously from the healthcare 4.0 application. These programs can help to upgrade their working skills, perform repetitive tasks and incorporate high-quality and quick services in their future work.
- **Application for Resource Management**: Healthcare systems are generally large and include hundreds, perhaps thousands of assets. This includes the construction of infrastructure and related services such as water, energy, fire alarm systems as well as Heating Ventilation and Air Conditioning (HVAC) and other amenities [31].
- **Applications for Healthcare Management System**: There exist different methodologies in the healthcare domain that help quality administration, control, arrangement and proficiency in the system including healthcare 4.0. The approaches help in further developing the vitality of the healthcare framework [32].

15.3   BLOCKCHAIN

As the term suggests, blockchain refers to blocks chained together in a manner that they can store transactions using a public ledger and verifies each transaction individually using cryptographic methods. All the mining nodes sign a transaction. Each block is composed of a body and a header. They store the transaction information using a reference hash. The block to which reference hash belongs is called hash block, and the root block is called the genesis block.

15.3.1   TYPES OF BLOCKCHAIN

A blockchain system is classified into three broad types, based on authentication schemes and control methods; private, public and consortium blockchain. These are discussed in the below subsection.

15.3.1.1   Private Blockchain

Blockchain, which allows sharing of data privately among individuals or a group of people using a decentralised network, is known as a private blockchain. Puthal et al. [33] stated that private blockchain requires a dedicated team or individual to control the mining process in order to restrict the access of unauthorised users.

15.3.1.2   Public Blockchain

Blockchain, which allows an individual to carry out mining without requiring specific permissions, using a decentralised platform, is known as a public or permissionless blockchain. A crucial role is played by consensus mechanisms in allowing a node to consist of contradicting multiple blocks [34]. As participants are unknown before mining and nodes are free to operate, public blockchain is prone to Sybil attack [35]. However, it can be overcome using Proof-of-Work

(Pow), an efficient consensus mechanism according to which an adversary must hold 51% of the mining strength for controlling a transaction [35].

15.3.1.3 Consortium Blockchain

Consortium blockchain refers to a blend of private and public blockchain wherein some specialised people are responsible for consensus and block validation. Miner blocks are validated when the controlling node signs and approves them and the mining takes place using multi-signature schemes. However, a tampering attack makes consortium blockchain vulnerable when a group of nodes may act maliciously, thereby compromising its immutable and irreversible nature [36,37].

15.3.2 ARCHITECTURE OF BLOCKCHAIN

The architecture defines the working nature of the blockchain. Blockchain is constituted by six layers which are detailed in the below subsections.

15.3.2.1 Data Layer

Wang et al. [38,39] stated that the data layer is responsible for the manipulation of data of various types, collected from social, physical spaces as well as cyberspace. Data blocks are time-stamped and encapsulated with the help of this layer, which helps to trace blockchain data. Merkle tree is another component of the blockchain ledger, which stores transactions in the form of a hash binary tree and maintains data integrity.

15.3.2.2 Network Layer

It verifies, forwards and distributes transactions in a blockchain. A blockchain network topology is constructed in a manner similar to a Peer-to-Peer (P2P) network, where participants possess equal privileges. As soon as a transaction is created, it is broadcasted to all neighbouring nodes to be verified. The transaction is discarded in case it is found invalid. A digital signature mechanism based on asymmetric key cryptographic methods is used for validating transactions' authenticity [40].

15.3.2.3 Consensus Layer

Due to blockchain being decentralised, a protocol to ensure consensus among the nodes is required to overcome the absence of a central authority. One of the prominent consensus algorithms is PoW, wherein nodes make use of hash functions to ease the validation process by other nodes. Other consensus algorithms include Proof-of-Stake (PoS) [41] and Practical Byzantine Fault Tolerance (PBFT) [42].

15.3.2.4 Incentive Layer

This layer integrates allocation methods and the issuance of economic incentives into a network. Based on the contributions of individual nodes in the network, economic incentives, namely digital currencies are issued and distributed to the corresponding nodes. However, the layer is optional and serves as a driving force for nodes to participate in data verification.

15.3.2.5 Contract Layer

This layer utilises specific algorithms, scripts and smart contracts to allow complex blockchain transactions. A smart contract refers to a cryptographically signed group of rules, used for expressing logic as well as formulating and controlling participants' rights. It is self-executing in nature and is verified by every node in the network. In order to implement transaction logic, each blockchain system has its own programming language; for instance, Bitcoin uses non-Turing complete languages, whereas Ethereum uses Turing complete languages [43].

15.3.2.6 Application Layer

This layer is present at the client end and acts as soon as a transaction is initiated by the client application. It is composed of business applications including the IoT, digital identity, etc. The client application uses Software Development Kit (SDK) or Command Line Interface (CLI) to enable communication among the nodes in a blockchain network. The application layer facilitates interaction between end-users and the blockchain network with the help of some specific frameworks, Application Programming Interfaces (APIs), and scripts. The execution layer is its sub-layer, which contains the actual code to be executed.

15.3.3 Consensus Protocols

Consensus protocols are responsible for ensuring consensus among the nodes' respective blockchain ledgers in a distributed blockchain network. Some of the important consensus protocols are described in the below subsections.

15.3.3.1 Proof of Work

PoW is an algorithm based on proofs to identify nodes and is allowed to add the newly-mined blocks at the end of an existing chain, provided there is a necessary proof [44]. This algorithm resolves the issue of ambiguity on deciding nodes that can put transactions into blocks.

15.3.3.2 Proof of Stake

PoS is an algorithm according to which miners emphasise on having a sufficient stake in the blockchain, which also helps mitigate possible suspicious activities in the blockchain network [45]. It highly emphasises energy efficiency.

15.3.3.3 Delegated PoS

Unlike the direct approach of PoS, Delegated PoS (DPoS) follows a democratic approach in which delegates are elected by stakeholders to validate a block [46]. In contrast to PoS, it facilitates faster block generation and quick confirmation of transactions. However, the delegates may vote themselves and manipulate other participants to vote.

15.3.3.4 Proof of Burn

The Proof of Burn (PoB) scheme is used for the destruction of cryptocurrencies with verification. Two important functions constitute PoB; a function to generate an address for cryptocurrency and a verification function to check if the address is actually not spendable. PoB follows a coin-burning strategy as a result of which fewer coins are used in blockchain, thereby increasing the coin's value. PoB possesses three prominent properties; uncensorability, binding and unspendability.

15.3.3.5 Proof of Elapsed Time

According to Proof of Elapsed Time (PoET), a random number is generated by each node for estimating the waiting time before it generates blocks. It does not involve all users' invalidation; instead, it elects a leader within the chain for creating new blocks. Every node has a random timer associated with it. PoET is efficient in tracing a malicious user if the same node is chosen to be the leader again and again.

15.3.3.6 Proof of Capacity

The Proof of Capacity (PoC) scheme prefers the utilisation of nodes' hard drive spaces over the random generation of nonce values. Therefore, it is computationally less intensive compared to PoW protocols. The node possessing more disk space is eligible to own more stake as per PoC.

15.3.3.7 Practical Byzantine Fault Tolerance

When two communicating nodes in a network safely reach a consensus, even when few misbehaving nodes are present, such a condition is called Byzantine Fault Tolerance (BFT). Thus, PBFT is a replication algorithm in which nodes are ordered sequentially with a leader node, and other nodes act as backups. The integrity and origin of data are verified through voting. Three phases exist in PBFT: pre-prepared, prepared and commit.

15.3.3.8 Proof of Authority

This protocol solves certain energy consumption as well as dependency problems that occur in PoW and is used in a private blockchain. Li et al. [47] stated that trusted nodes are given the authority to exploit the majority criteria of forming the consensus and create new blocks. "N" trusted nodes in the chain are called authorities, assuming at least (N/2)+1 out of N to be honest.

15.4 CYBER SECURITY IN HEALTHCARE 4.0

Cyber security issues are burgeoning in any technology if it consists of sensitive and private data, heterogeneous structure and complex compliance. Healthcare 4.0 is a combination of the latest technologies that include IoT and AI, which drive the working of healthcare in the most efficient manner. The heterogeneous nature of healthcare makes the database, network, frontend more vulnerable to cyber-attacks. There are various devices used in healthcare such as Closed Circuit

Television (CCTV) and sensors, which do not have the capability to update themselves [48]. This makes them vulnerable to the attacks which are introduced in the cyber world after their manufacturing. The below subsection deeply focuses on various vital parameters that make healthcare more vulnerable to cyber-attacks.

15.4.1 NETWORK VULNERABILITY AND ATTACKS

A network is the backbone of healthcare 4.0. All the devices work together in an interconnected pattern. These devices in healthcare fetch first input from the field sensors or devices which further receive input from the surrounding environment. The network of healthcare is vulnerable because of the lack of patch update features in various devices. This results in making the network vulnerable to various network-based attacks such as Denial-of-Service (DoS), Jamming, Node Tampering (NT), Denial of Sleep, Spoofing and Flooding. It can affect either foremost devices such as routers, switches, CCTV cameras, sensors, or internal computation devices of healthcare such as web servers and database servers. The below-enumerated points furthermore explain network-based attacks.

- The DoS attacks can shut down the network of healthcare 4.0 and make it inaccessible to the employees, admins and patients in a healthcare system. This attack crashes the traffic or makes it unavailable for the intended users. The DoS attack either floods the network or crashes it. Buffer overflow attacks, Internet Control Message Protocol floods and SYN floods are the three main attacks the DoS uses to flood the healthcare network. Moreover, the crash is a result of DoS due to the existing vulnerability in the network or networking devices [49]. This attack becomes more devastating when it is executed in a distributed manner that is many devices attacking a single network.
- A jamming attack is another network-based attack that mainly targets wireless network systems [50]. Since healthcare 4.0 consists of various wireless communications and mostly for sensors, this attack has become prominent in the healthcare 4.0 system. There are various types of jamming attacks such as Deceptive jammer [51] and Random jammer that can affect wireless communication in the network of healthcare 4.0.
- NT is highly probable in healthcare 4.0 as it is performed by physical means. Many networking devices and field sensors of healthcare 4.0 are left unattended and can be easily accessed by the adversary. The adversary can replace the real node with its infected node (router, hub, switch, etc.).
- Denial of Sleep targets those devices, which have batteries as a source of power for their working [52]. These batteries have limited time; after which they require charging. When the battery charges, the device goes into sleep mode. The attack restricts the device from switching to sleep mode and hence, the device permanently gets shut down.

15.4.2 Policy Check Based Vulnerability and Attack

The policy plays an important role in minimising the attacks that are triggered via weak passwords, weak authentication mechanisms, weak Internet Protocol (IP) scanning, and filtration mechanisms. The below points explain these parameters in a detailed manner.

- User authentication is a highly crucial part of healthcare 4.0 as it consists of data that are personal in nature. The user can ensure that his identity is authenticated safely, especially in healthcare. Medical data is accessed by healthcare personnel, patients and other staff. It demands that emergency access to the data is guaranteed to the users in case of criticality. The method to ensure user authentication is using biometric security, being one of the most efficient mechanisms to verify user identity. It can be effectively used in healthcare 4.0. Also, biometric data can be fetched from the devices used in the medical domain or healthcare sector [53]. The password management system should be very intelligently covered in the policy so that authentication bypass using brute force and other social engineering attacks could be restricted.
- Another crucial parameter is device authentication, in which a personal device or server needs to authenticate the identity before receiving the medical data from sensors [54]. It is crucial because wrong data or any miscommunication may result in critical issues while monitoring and diagnosing patients' health. Thus, in healthcare 4.0, authentication methods should be implemented in a highly secured manner and be able to ensure the integrity and confidentiality of personal medical data. In healthcare 4.0, there should remain zero scopes for alteration of data to prevent compromising the personal information of healthcare personnel, patients and staff in the healthcare sector.

15.4.3 Sensor, Physical Vulnerability and Attacks

In healthcare 4.0, protecting medical data is a task of the highest priority. Thus, the source of data from where the data is fetched needs to be secure. Sensors are responsible for data collection. Hence, implementing security at the level of sensors is crucial. The possible security measures emphasise carrying maximum computation on personal devices and reducing overheads during data exchange. Below are the solutions for establishing sensor-level security.

- Sensors, being physical in nature, possess the risk of being stolen and tampered with by an adversary. It poses a threat to the healthcare sector while implementing healthcare 4.0. Thus, designing a tamper-proof system that should not allow any third party to access the medical data is important.

- Localisation is yet another factor in sensor security [55], in which the position of sensors is identified on the human body. However, identifying sensor position on the human body is of importance to healthcare personnel and hence cannot be eliminated. In such a scenario, there are possibilities that devices may shift from the network range frequently. A solution to resolve localisation issues is to design a real-time system to detect intrusion in a healthcare 4.0 network, which can be able to efficiently report malicious activities and alert users for the same.
- Security can also be ensured by self-healing methods. A self-healing method can detect an attack within a healthcare 4.0 network, and apply security measures on its own. However, each attack can be diagnosed in a different manner; thus, self-healing methods should be designed accordingly [56].
- Healthcare 4.0 includes Over-The-Air (OTA) programming techniques for updating nodes in a healthcare 4.0 network with a high number of IoT nodes [57]. However, they may lead to a possibility that an attacker node senses updates and impersonates legitimate nodes. So, it requires stringent security mechanisms to be designed such that any malicious node within the healthcare 4.0 network is not able to exploit other legitimate nodes and affect the healthcare 4.0 system.
- Since sensors are physical devices, they may have faults introduced and misbehave within the network, thereby affecting the data and communication in healthcare 4.0. Thus, ensuring security before and after the transmission of data is highly important. That is, backward and forward compatibility issues need to be properly addressed [58]. For the same, OTA programming for the delivery of updates about the same can be used.

15.5 ACHIEVING PRIVACY AND SECURITY USING BLOCKCHAIN FOR HEALTHCARE 4.0

In the current scenario, patients' records and related healthcare data are digitised, and the data are expanding each day. Moreover, the data are distributed on multiple devices, facilitated by cloud servers, and are not confined to a single device. Specialised IoT devices and sensors are responsible for collecting and processing data [59]. Also, there are multiple sources of information such as EHRs to deliver healthcare information to required users [60]. A number of datasets of patients contain sensitive and personal information. Thus, ensuring privacy and security in healthcare is highly important and approaches for the same are required to be implemented effectively. One of the suitable approaches to guarantee security of healthcare data is using blockchain. Blockchain supports changelessness and information discernibility. However, if integrated with cryptographic methods, blockchain can provide stronger security and consistency of healthcare data in a network [61]. The difficulties related to the protection of data in blockchain are explained below.

- **Identity Security**: Safeguarding patients' or users' identity and sensitive information.

- **Transaction Security**: Guaranteeing secure exchange of information and ensuring authorised and authenticated transactions (viewing or modifying data).

Identity of any user can be sensitive and must not be exposed to an unauthorised or illegitimate system or individual. Specifically, in healthcare 4.0, patients' personal data may contain information such as individual enlistment number and quantity of the charge card that the patient uses to make an installment in a private organisation. Thus, protecting the identity of a user in healthcare is a prime concern and cannot be overlooked. One of the strategies that assist with implementing and ensuring identity security is zero-information evidence [62]. Other robust security procedures include homomorphic cryptography, zk-snarks (as interpreted from the zero-information evidence), Trusted Execution Environment (TEE) and differential protection [63–66]. TEE can be used as one of the selective techniques to guarantee protection in the medical services and strengthen healthcare 4.0 framework. In addition to security procedures, stringent laws of data privacy can guarantee a noteworthy protection of healthcare 4.0 data. The Healthcare Insurance Portability and Accountability Act (HIPAA) rule aids to improve security in a healthcare 4.0 network with blockchain, with certain characteristics; enabling secure data sharing, providing improved medical services, enhancing public norms and securing individual healthcare information. The HIPAA security rules cover the attributes of Business Associates (BA), healthcare 4.0, Clearing Houses (CH) as well as prominent medical services. With the help of similar protection laws and rules, blockchain innovation can ensure quality and security of patients' individual data in healthcare 4.0 [67].

Along with the identity, transactions of data in healthcare also need to be secured and safeguarded. A secure communication environment needs to be set up so that information exchange within a healthcare 4.0 network is not compromised or affected by malicious activities. Blockchain is beneficial in transaction security as well. Decentralised Sharing of Healthcare Records is a design that investigates the idea of implementing security procedures for data as well as users in a healthcare 4.0 network [68]. In addition, alerts and warnings can facilitate security in the network. That is, whenever an unauthorised entry or intrusion into the network is detected, the network must be ready to resist the same. Another approach to guarantee security in a healthcare 4.0 network is generating information access logs in blockchain-based storage. Hence, information can be accessed directly from the respective blockchain organisation. Additionally, blockchain can also provide consistent quality assurance and security of big data [69]. Furthermore, information protection can be achieved suitably with the help of a strong legal base. Adhering to the data protection laws such as the General Data Protection Regulation (GDPR) is also a contribution to ensuring transaction security in healthcare 4.0 [70]. Implanting a watermark to strengthen copyrights is also a plus to these laws, and implies that the information in the blockchain is changeless [71,72]. Apart from laws, security and privacy issues in healthcare can be moderated by methods of zero-information confirmation and trait-based encryption.

Some updated security measures include using a blockchain-dependent differential security to further enhance and upgrade resistance to cyber-attacks in healthcare 4.0 frameworks [73,74]. It is required to emphasise that information protection is fundamental in a wellbeing setting, and blockchain innovation can help with strengthening security in healthcare 4.0.

15.6   CONCLUSION AND FUTURE RESEARCH DIRECTION

Healthcare 4.0 has become an essential part of human society where it cures and prevents diseases to serve humankind. Healthcare 4.0 is a heterogeneous system that consists of the most advanced technologies that include AI, IoT and other relevant recent technologies used for processing of data. The paper deeply discusses healthcare 4.0, explains its evolutionary phases and tries to explain the heterogeneity nature of healthcare 4.0 because of adopting recent technologies such as IoT and AI. The paper also dives deep into the dominant features of blockchain and its vitality. Moreover, the root cause of vulnerability in the various components of healthcare 4.0 has been analysed and the attacks that become prominent because of these vulnerabilities have been covered. The paper provides blockchain as one of the best solutions to counter and prevent cyber-attacks on healthcare 4.0 to preserve privacy and security.

The paper presents various vital components of healthcare 4.0 that could be used as a reference to carry out future research work. The paper also emphasises two distinct areas, that is, personal data and inefficient security patch management present in healthcare 4.0. The security aspect of networks in healthcare 4.0 can be used precisely to enhance research work on network-based vulnerabilities in healthcare 4.0. The inclusion of AI and IoT makes healthcare 4.0 a more heterogeneous system and hence can provide various elements for research. Hence, this paper provides a platform for various future research directions.

REFERENCES

1. Surati, S., Patel, S., & Surati, K. (2020). Background and research challenges for FC for healthcare 4.0. *Fog Computing for Healthcare 4.0 Environments*, 37–53. Doi: 10.1007/978-3-030-46197-3_2.
2. Hathaliya, J. J., Tanwar, S., Tyagi, S., & Kumar, N. (2019). Securing electronics healthcare records in healthcare 4.0: a biometric-based approach. *Computers & Electrical Engineering*, 76, 398–410. Doi: 10.1016/j.compeleceng.2019.04.017.
3. Azad, C., Bhushan, B., Sharma, R., Shankar, A., Singh, K. K., & Khamparia, A. (2021). Prediction model using SMOTE, genetic algorithm and decision tree (PMSGD) for classification of diabetes mellitus. *Multimedia Systems*. Doi: 10.1007/s00530-021-00817-2.
4. Khamparia, A., Singh, P. K., Rani, P., Samanta, D., Khanna, A., & Bhushan, B. (2020). An internet of health things-driven deep learning framework for detection and classification of skin cancer using transfer learning. *Transactions on Emerging Telecommunications Technologies*. Doi: 10.1002/ett.3963.

5. Parfett, A., Townley, S., & Allerfeldt, K. (2020). Ai-based healthcare: a new dawn or apartheid revisited? *AI & Society*. Doi: 10.1007/s00146-020-01120-w.

6. Alshehri, F., & Muhammad, G. (2021). A comprehensive survey of the Internet of Things (IoT) and ai-based smart healthcare. *IEEE Access*, 9, 3660–3678. Doi: 10.1109/access.2020.3047960.

7. Goyal, S., Sharma, N., Bhushan, B., Shankar, A., & Sagayam, M. (2020). IoT enabled technology in secured healthcare: applications, challenges and future directions. *Cognitive Internet of Medical Things for Smart Healthcare*, 25–48. Doi: 10.1007/978-3-030-55833-8_2.

8. Kumar, A., Krishnamurthi, R., Nayyar, A., Sharma, K., Grover, V., & Hossain, E. (2020). A novel smart healthcare design, simulation, and implementation using healthcare 4.0 processes. *IEEE Access*, 8, 118433–118471. Doi: 10.1109/access.2020.3004790.

9. Wang, S., Wang, H., Li, J., Wang, H., Chaudhry, J., Alazab, M., & Song, H. (2020). A fast CP-ABE system for cyber-physical security and privacy in mobile healthcare network. *IEEE Transactions on Industry Applications*, 1–1. Doi: 10.1109/tia.2020.2969868.

10. Zafar, S., Nazir, M., Bakhshi, T., Khattak, H. A., Khan, S., Bilal, M., Choo, K.-K. R., Kwak, K.-S., & Sabah, A. (2021). A systematic review of bio-cyber interface technologies and security issues for internet of bio-nano things. *IEEE Access*, 9, 93529–93566. Doi: 10.1109/access.2021.3093442.

11. Wehde, M. (2019). Healthcare 4.0. *IEEE Engineering Management Review*, 47(3), 24–28. Doi: 10.1109/emr.2019.2930702.

12. Narasima, A., & Venkatesh, D. (2019). Reimagining the future of healthcare industry through Internet of Medical Things (IoMT), Artificial Intelligence (AI), Machine Learning (ML), big data, mobile apps and advanced sensors. *SSRN Electronic Journal*. Doi: 10.2139/ssrn.3522960.

13. Sharma, N., Kaushik, I., Bhushan, B., Gautam, S., & Khamparia, A. (2020). Applicability of WSN and biometric models in the field of healthcare. *Deep Learning Strategies for Security Enhancement in Wireless Sensor Networks Advances in Information Security, Privacy, and Ethics*, 304–329. Doi: 10.4018/978-1-7998-5068-7.ch016.

14. Ranchal, R., Bastide, P., Wang, X., Gkoulalas-Divanis, A., Mehra, M., Bakthavachalam, S., Lei, H., & Mohindra, A. (2020). Disrupting healthcare silos: addressing data volume, velocity, and variety with a cloud-native healthcare data ingestion service. *IEEE Journal of Biomedical and Health Informatics*, 24(11), 3182–3188. Doi: 10.1109/jbhi.2020.3001518.

15. Katehakis, D. G. (2018). Electronic medical record implementation challenges for the national health system in Greece. *International Journal of Reliable and Quality E-Healthcare*, 7(1), 16–30. Doi: 10.4018/ijrqeh.2018010102.

16. Chanchaichujit, J., Tan, A., Meng, F., & Eaimkhong, S. (2019). An introduction to healthcare 4.0. *Healthcare 4.0*, 1–15. Doi: 10.1007/978-981-13-8114-0_1.

17. Yuan, X.-M. (2020). Impact of industry 4.0 on inventory systems and optimization. *Industry 4.0- Impact on Intelligent Logistics and Manufacturing*. Doi: 10.5772/intechopen.90077.

18. Wang, L., & Alexander, C. (2021). Big data in personalized healthcare. *Big Data in Psychiatry and; Neurology*, 35–49. Doi: 10.1016/b978-0-12-822884-5.00017-9.

19. Sligo, J., Gauld, R., Roberts, V., & Villa, L. (2017). A literature review for large-scale health information system project planning, implementation and evaluation. *International Journal of Medical Informatics*, 97, 86–97. Doi: 10.1016/j.ijmedinf.2016.09.007.

20. Bender, J. L., Feldman-Stewart, D., Tong, C., Lee, K., Brundage, M., Pai, H., Robinson, J., & Panzarella, T. (2019). Health-related internet use among men with prostate cancer in Canada: cancer registry survey study. *Journal of Medical Internet Research*, 21(11). Doi: 10.2196/14241.
21. Yang, L. (2020). Construction of integrated health care and elderly care Talent training system for health care and elderly care major in higher vocational education under combination of medical treatment and endowment. *2020 International Symposium on Advances in Informatics, Electronics, and Education (ISAIEE)*. Doi: 10.1109/isaiee51769.2020.00059,
22. Chander, B. (2020). Wireless body sensor networks for patient health monitoring. *Advances in Healthcare Information Systems and Administration*, 132–154. Doi: 10.4018/978-1-7998-0261-7.ch006.
23. Cardoso, J., Voigt, K., & Winkler, M. Service engineering for the Internet of services. *Proceedings of the 18th International Conference on Enterprise Information Systems*. Berlin, Germany: Springer, 2008, pp. 15–27.
24. Rana, M. M., & Bo, R. (2019). IoT-based cyber-physical communication architecture: challenges and research directions. *IET Cyber-Physical Systems: Theory & Applications*, 5(1), 25–30. Doi: 10.1049/iet-cps.2019.0028.
25. Kumar, S., Srivastava, R., Pathak, S., & Kumar, B. (2020). Cloud-based computer-assisted diagnostic solutions for e-health. *Intelligent Data Security Solutions for e-Health Applications*, 219–235. Doi: 10.1016/b978-0-12-819511-6.00012-1.
26. Ahmad, M., Amin, M. B., Hussain, S., Kang, B. H., Cheong, T., & Lee, S. (2016). Health fog: a novel framework for health and wellness applications. *The Journal of Supercomputing*, 72(10), 3677–3695. Doi: 10.1007/s11227-016-1634-x.
27. Bora, D. J. (2019). Big data analytics in healthcare: a critical analysis. *Big Data Analytics for Intelligent Healthcare Management*, 43–57. Doi: 10.1016/b978-0-12-818146-1.00003-9.
28. Yu, T., Wang, X., & Zhu, Y. (2019). Blockchain technology for the 5G-enabled Internet of Things systems: principle, applications and challenges. *5G-Enabled Internet of Things*, 301–321. Doi: 10.1201/9780429199820-14.
29. Al-Jaroodi, J., & Mohamed, N. (2019). Blockchain in industries: a survey. *IEEE Access*, 7, 36500–36515. Doi: 10.1109/access.2019.2903554.
30. Xu, J., & Xu, L. (2017). Sensor system and health monitoring. *Integrated System Health Management*, 55–99. Doi: 10.1016/b978-0-12-812207-5.00002-x.
31. Gong, H., Jones, E. S., Alden, R. E., Frye, A. G., Colliver, D., & Ionel, D. M. (2020). Demand response of HVACS in large residential communities based on experimental developments. *2020 IEEE Energy Conversion Congress and Exposition (ECCE)*. Doi: 10.1109/ecce44975.2020.9235465.
32. Betcheva, L., Erhun, F., & Jiang, H. (2020). Healthcare supply chains. *The Oxford Handbook of Supply Chain Management*. Doi: 10.1093/oxfordhb/9780190066727.013.13.
33. Puthal, D., Malik, N., Mohanty, S. P., Kougianos, E., & Das, G. (2018). Everything you wanted to know about the blockchain: its promise, components, processes, and problems. *IEEE Consumer Electronics Magazine*, 7(4), 6–14. Doi: 10.1109/mce.2018.2816299.
34. Haque, A. K., Bhushan, B., & Dhiman, G. (2021). Conceptualizing smart city applications: requirements, architecture, security issues, and emerging trends. *Expert Systems*. Doi: 10.1111/exsy.12753.
35. Bhushan, B., Sahoo, C., Sinha, P., & Khamparia, A. (2020). Unification of blockchain and Internet of Things (BIoT): requirements, working model, challenges and future directions. *Wireless Networks*. Doi: 10.1007/s11276-020-02445-6.

36. Saxena, S., Bhushan, B., & Ahad, M. A. (2021). Blockchain based solutions to secure IoT: background, integration trends and a way forward. *Journal of Network and Computer Applications*, 103050. Doi: 10.1016/j.jnca.2021.103050.

37. Bhushan, B., Sinha, P., Sagayam, K. M., & J, A. (2021). Untangling blockchain technology: a survey on state of the art, security threats, privacy services, applications and future research directions. *Computers & Electrical Engineering*, 90, 106897. Doi: 10.1016/j.compeleceng.2020.106897

38. Wang, X., Li, L., Yuan, Y., Ye, P., & Wang, F.-Y. (2016). ACP-based social computing and parallel intelligence: societies 5.0 and beyond. *CAAI Transactions on Intelligence Technology*, 1(4), 377–393. Doi: 10.1016/j.trit.2016.11.005.

39. Wang, X., Zheng, X., Zhang, X., Zeng, K., & Wang, F.-Y. (2017). Analysis of cyber interactive behaviors using artificial community and computational experiments. *IEEE Transactions on Systems, Man, and Cybernetics: Systems*, 47(6), 995–1006. Doi: 10.1109/tsmc.2016.2615130.

40. Zhang, S., & Lee, J.-H. (2020). A group signature and authentication scheme for blockchain-based mobile-edge computing. *IEEE Internet of Things Journal*, 7(5), 4557–4565. Doi: 10.1109/jiot.2019.2960027.

41. Saleh, F. (2018). Blockchain without waste: proof-of-stake. *SSRN Electronic Journal*. Doi: 10.2139/ssrn.3183935.

42. Chen, L., Xu, L., Shah, N., Gao, Z., Lu, Y., & Shi, W. (2017). On security analysis of proof-of-elapsed-time (poet). *Lecture Notes in Computer Science*, 282–297. Doi: 10.1007/978-3-319-69084-1_19.

43. Hildenbrandt, E., Saxena, M., Rodrigues, N., Zhu, X., Daian, P., Guth, D., Moore, B., Park, D., Zhang, Y., Stefanescu, A., & Rosu, G. (2018). KEVM: a complete formal semantics of the Ethereum virtual machine. *2018 IEEE 31st Computer Security Foundations Symposium (CSF)*. Doi: 10.1109/csf.2018.00022.

44. Wang, W., Hoang, D. T., Hu, P., Xiong, Z., Niyato, D., Wang, P., Wen, Y., & Kim, D. I. (2019). A survey on consensus mechanisms and mining strategy management in blockchain networks. *IEEE Access*, 7, 22328–22370. Doi: 10.1109/access.2019.2896108.

45. Kiayias, A., Russell, A., David, B., & Oliynykov, R. (2017). Ouroboros: a provably secure proof-of-stake blockchain protocol. *Advances in Cryptology – Crypto* 2017, 357–388. Doi: 10.1007/978-3-319-63688-7_12.

46. Skh Saad, S. M., & Raja Mohd Radzi, R. Z. (2020). Comparative review of the blockchain consensus algorithm between proof of stake (POS) and delegated proof of Stake (DPOS). *International Journal of Innovative Computing*, 10(2). Doi: 10.11113/ijic.v10n2.272.

47. Li, K., Li, H., Wang, H., An, H., Lu, P., Yi, P., & Zhu, F. (2020). PoV: an efficient voting-based consensus algorithm for consortium blockchains. *Frontiers in Blockchain*, 3. Doi: 10.3389/fbloc.2020.00011.

48. Al-Turjman, F., Zahmatkesh, H., & Shahroze, R. (2019). An overview of security and privacy in smart cities' IoT communications. *Transactions on Emerging Telecommunications Technologies*. Doi: 10.1002/ett.3677.

49. Bhushan, B., & Sahoo, G. (2017). Recent advances in attacks, technical challenges, vulnerabilities and their countermeasures in wireless sensor networks. *Wireless Personal Communications*, 98(2), 2037–2077. Doi: 10.1007/s11277-017-4962-0.

50. Bhushan, B., & Sahoo, G. (2019). A hybrid secure and energy efficient cluster based intrusion detection system for wireless sensing environment. *2019 2nd International Conference on Signal Processing and Communication (ICSPC)*. Doi: 10.1109/icspc46172.2019.8976509.

51. Sharma, M., Bhushan, B., & Khamparia, A. (2021). Securing Internet of Things: attacks, countermeasures and open challenges. *Advances in Intelligent Systems and Computing*, 873–885. Doi: 10.1007/978-981-15-9927-9_84.

52. Chang, S.-Y., Kumar, S. L., Hu, Y.-C., & Park, Y. (2019). Power-positive networking. *ACM Transactions on Sensor Networks*, 15(3), 1–25. Doi: 10.1145/3317686.

53. Pandey, P., Pandey, S. C., & Kumar, U. (2019). Security issues of Internet of Things in healthcare sector: an analytical approach. *Algorithms for Intelligent Systems*, 307–329. Doi: 10.1007/978-981-15-1100-4_15.

54. Chen, F., Tang, Y., Cheng, X., Xie, D., Wang, T., & Zhao, C. (2021). Blockchain-based efficient device authentication protocol for medical cyber-physical systems. *Security and Communication Networks*, 2021, 1–13. Doi: 10.1155/2021/5580939.

55. Tondwalkar, A., & Vinayakray-Jani, P. (2016). Secure localisation of wireless devices with application to sensor networks using steganography. *Procedia Computer Science*, 78, 610–616. Doi: 10.1016/j.procs.2016.02.107.

56. Lin, H., Chen, C., Wang, J., Qi, J., Jin, D., Kalbarczyk, Z. T., & Iyer, R. K. (2018). Self-healing attack-resilient PMU network for power system operation. *IEEE Transactions on Smart Grid*, 9(3), 1551–1565. Doi: 10.1109/tsg.2016.2593021.

57. Nugroho, A. P., Okayasu, T., Horimoto, M., Arita, D., Hoshi, T., Kurosaki, H., Yasuba, K.- ichiro, Inoue, E., Hirai, Y., Mitsuoka, M., & Sutiarso, L. (2016). Development of a field environmental monitoring node with over the air update function. *Agricultural Information Research*, 25(3), 86–95. Doi: 10.3173/air.25.86.

58. Breiter, M., & Nowak, R. M. (2019). The new C++ serialization library supporting backward and forward compatibility. *Photonics Applications in Astronomy, Communications, Industry, and High-Energy Physics Experiments*. Doi: 10.1117/12.2536387.

59. Moussa, M., & Demurjian, S. A. (2017). Differential privacy approach for big data privacy in healthcare. *Privacy and Security Policies in Big Data*, 191–213. Doi: 10.4018/978-1-5225-2486-1.ch009.

60. Correa-de-Araujo, R. (2017). Enhancing data access and utilization: federal big data initiative and relevance to health disparities research. *Big Data-Enabled Nursing*, 227–251. Doi: 10.1007/978-3-319-53300-1_12.

61. De Hert, P., & Kumar, A. (2021). Blockchain, privacy, and data protection. *Blockchain and Public Law*, 141–156. Doi: 10.4337/9781839100796.00014.

62. Carlo, E. D., Shin, H., & Lu, H. (2018). Using location k-anonymity models for protecting location privacy. *The Routledge Companion to Risk, Crisis and Security in Business*, 296–306. Doi: 10.4324/9781315629520-19.

63. Tsaloli, G., Banegas, G., & Mitrokotsa, A. (2020). Practical and provably secure distributed aggregation: verifiable additive homomorphic secret sharing. *Cryptography*, 4(3), 25. Doi: 10.3390/cryptography4030025.

64. Ziegeldorf, J. H., Matzutt, R., Henze, M., Grossmann, F., & Wehrle, K. (2018). Secure and anonymous decentralized bitcoin mixing. *Future Generation Computer Systems*, 80, 448–466. Doi: 10.1016/j.future.2016.05.018.

65. Philip, J., & Raju, M. (2020). Security impact of trusted execution environment in rich execution environment based systems. *Indian Journal of Computer Science*, 5(4&5), 26. Doi: 10.17010/ijcs/2020/v5/i4-5/154785.

66. Joseph, M., Mao, J., Neel, S., & Roth, A. (2019). The role of interactivity in local differential privacy. *2019 IEEE 60th Annual Symposium on Foundations of Computer Science (FOCS)*. Doi: 10.1109/focs.2019.00015.

67. Oyeleye, O. A. (2021). The HIPAA privacy rule, COVID-19, and nurses' privacy rights. *Nursing*, 51(2), 11–14. Doi: 10.1097/01.nurse.0000731892.59941.a9.

68. Kshetri, N. (2018). Blockchain and electronic healthcare records [cybertrust]. *Computer*, 51(12), 59–63. Doi: 10.1109/mc.2018.2880021.
69. Jarka, S. (2020). Blockchain and big data. *Management in the Era of Big Data*, 165–175. Doi: 10.1201/9781003057291-1.
70. Manoj, M. K., & Krishnan, S. S. (2020). Decentralizing privacy using blockchain to protect private data and challenges with IPFS. *Transforming Businesses with Bitcoin Mining and Blockchain Applications*, 207–220. Doi: 10.4018/978-1-7998-0186-3.ch012.
71. Bhushan, B., Khamparia, A., Sagayam, K. M., Sharma, S. K., Ahad, M. A., & Debnath, N. C. (2020). Blockchain for smart cities: a review of architectures, integration trends and future research directions. *Sustainable Cities and Society*, 61, 102360. Doi: 10.1016/j.scs.2020.102360.
72. Madaan, G., Bhushan, B., & Kumar, R. (2020). Blockchain-based cyberthreat mitigation systems for smart vehicles and industrial automation. *Studies in Big Data Multimedia Technologies in the Internet of Things Environment*, 13–32. Doi: 10.1007/978-981-15-7965-3_2.
73. Mironov, I. (2017). Rényi differential privacy. *2017 IEEE 30th Computer Security Foundations Symposium (CSF)*. Doi: 10.1109/csf.2017.11.
74. Khedekar, V. B., Hiremath, S. S., Sonawane, P. M., & Rajput, D. S. (2020). Protection to personal data using decentralizing privacy of blockchain. *Transforming Businesses with Bitcoin Mining and Blockchain Applications*, 173–194. Doi: 10.4018/978-1-7998-0186-3.ch010.

Index

Printed in the United States
by Baker & Taylor Publisher Services